DYSLEXIA

Theory & Practice
of
Remedial Instruction

Second Edition

DYSLEXIA
Theory & Practice
of
Remedial Instruction
Second Edition

DIANA BREWSTER CLARK
JOANNA KELLOGG UHRY

YORK
PRESS *BALTIMORE*

This book was manufactured in the United States of America. Typography by The Type Shoppe, Inc., Chestertown, Maryland. Printing and binding by BookCrafters, Fredericksburg, Virginia. Cover design by Joseph Dieter, Jr.

Clark, Diana Brewster.
    Dyslexia : theory & practice of remedial instruction / Diana
  Brewster Clark, Joanna Kellogg Uhry. -- 2nd ed.
       p.   cm.
    Includes bibliographical references and index.
    ISBN 0-912752-43-2 (pbk.)
    1. Reading disability. 2. Dyslexia. 3. Reading--Remedial
  teaching. 4. Dyslexic children--Education.   I. Uhry, Joanna
  Kellogg. II. Title.
  LB1050.5.C548 1995
  371.91'44--dc20   95-33423
                                                        CIP

Table of Contents

Preface to the First Edition

This book is written primarily for teachers engaged in language arts instruction for dyslexic students: remedial reading specialists, special education teachers, and reading and language arts teachers who are required to adapt instruction for disabled readers in their classrooms. These practitioners undoubtedly have the greatest influence over the educational outcome of dyslexic children. The book is also intended for undergraduate and graduate students of education who plan to work with dyslexic children, for they are the practitioners of the future. Additionally, it is my hope that professionals who make educational planning decisions for dyslexic children will be among its readers: school administrators, psychologists, and counselors.

The book's primary purpose is to provide practical information on methods of instruction in reading, writing, and spelling for dyslexic students. It presents this information against a backdrop of current research findings related to dyslexia and its treatment in order that its readers will understand the theoretical rationale behind these methods and thereby be able to judge their relative value.

The need for such a book became apparent in light of an extensive review I undertook of the research on dyslexia, or developmental reading disorder, and methods of instruction designed to treat this disorder. Added to my experience as a reading disabilities specialist engaged in both practice and research, the review led to several important realizations. The first is that a cure for dyslexia does not lie "just around the corner." Despite the considerable knowledge we have acquired over the last fifty years about the nature of this disorder, a multitude of unanswered questions remain, many of which may not be satisfactorily answered in the near future. It is encouraging to know that rapidly advancing techniques of neuropsychological investigation are helping us to identify the biological underpinnings of dyslexia; however, it may be a long time before we learn how to utilize this knowledge effectively in treating the disorder.

A second realization is that most of us involved in reading disabilities research have tended to overlook the fact that understanding developmental reading disorder is dependent upon understanding the process of normal reading development. Our disregard may be due in part to the fact that the psychology of normal reading development has been a field of inquiry hardly more enlightened than our own. In the last decade, however, significant progress has been made in reading research, and many of the findings, as well as newer theories, have enormous relevance for the study of dyslexia.

Another realization is that the separation of reading education, special education, and remedial reading education into three ostensibly autonomous domains of instruction—the first two residing in schools, the third for the most part in the private sectors—has been extremely detrimental to dyslexic students, causing unnecessary confusion over their identification and treatment. Sharing and integrating ideas between these three, now separate, disciplines is essential if dyslexic students are ever to be served effectively.

A fourth realization is that over the last twenty years considerable effort has been directed toward developing remedial methods and programs for teaching reading, writing, and spelling to dyslexic students. Some of these instructional approaches have been in practice for a notable length of time, yet information about them has been poorly disseminated. The major impetus for writing this book was my growing awareness that teachers and other professionals who work with dyslexic students need to be better informed about existing instructional methods for these students.

The development of remedial practice can not afford to wait for definitive pronouncements from the field of research. However, as the research reviewed indicates, we have available a significant amount of potentially useful data on the nature of the reading process, the acquisition of reading skills, the characteristics of disabled readers, and the instructional conditions that enhance their learning. This information needs now to be recognized, synthesized, and brought to bear on the problem of dyslexia. Knowledge thus derived can then be imparted to teachers and educational planners so that they will be able to evaluate not only existing instructional methods and programs for dyslexic students but also those that might be developed in the future. That is what this book is meant to accomplish.

Diana Brewster Clark
1988

Preface to the Second Edition

Diana Brewster Clark died early in 1991. She had begun working on the revisions for a second edition of this book. I am pleased to be carrying out this work for two reasons. First, Diana was a good friend and I wanted to see her work brought to completion. Second, I thought that the book was a valuable addition to the field and I wanted to see it stay in print as an up-to-date resource.

I have retained the three-part structure of the book. Part I continues to outline the psychological processes involved in both skilled and beginning reading, as well as historical and contemporary theories on what goes wrong in the reading acquisition process in children with dyslexia. There is greater clarity in the field than there was in 1988; there now exists a compelling body of evidence pointing to a very specific linguistic disorder in the realm of phonology that is associated with dyslexia. I have added a third chapter to Part I with information about assessment for the symptoms of dyslexia. This chapter includes a case history as an example of an educational evaluation.

Part II continues to focus on general principles derived from research on effective techniques for working with children with dyslexia (e.g., direct instruction, mastery learning, and multisensory instruction). There is a chapter on the application of these techniques in specific areas of the language arts: phonological awareness, phonics knowledge, automaticity and fluency in word reading, reading comprehension, spelling, handwriting, and composition. Part II ends with a chapter on the relationship between reading, writing, and spelling instruction.

Part III begins with a series of chapters, each devoted to a particular program designed to promote the acquisition of reading. Most, but not all, of these programs were designed for children or young adults with dyslexia. I have added two new programs to this section of the book: Reading Recovery is an early intervention program for first grade children and the Wilson System is a traditional multisensory program for adolescents and young adults with dyslexia. The final chapter has been revised as a continuation of the case history in Chapter 3. It describes the process of transforming test results into an educational plan which draws on a number of the programs outlined in Part III.

In addition to the four new chapters, there are a number of other changes throughout the book, intended to update findings from recent research studies. A number of large-scale federally funded projects have clarified the symptoms of dyslexia since 1988, and have begun to clarify appropriate treatments.

There are two changes involving style. In 1988 the pronoun he was justified, as most children considered to be dyslexic were boys. This is no longer the case (see Chapter 2); up-to-date research indicates almost equal numbers of boys and girls. Rather than the awkward term he or she, I have alternated pronouns throughout the book, sometimes referring to a girl and sometimes to a boy in descriptions of symptoms and in examples of treatment procedures.

The second stylistic change involves using the term *child with dyslexia* rather than *dyslexic child*. The former is suggested now in a number of style manuals because it does not suggest, as does the latter term, that the child is defined by the disability. This is common usage now for all handicapping conditions because it expresses a view of the child as an individual, first and foremost. It is particularly appropriate for children with dyslexia because these children have so many areas of strength. Provided with appropriate early remediation, they should be able to lead lives which are not defined by their dyslexia.

Joanna Kellogg Uhry
1995

ACKNOWLEDGMENTS

I am grateful to Linnea Ehri, Nancy Ellsworth, Kay Gorenson, Kathryn Hathaway, and Katherine Maria for reading and commenting on earlier drafts of chapters, and to Elinor Hartwig for her thoughtful readings and good advice.

I appreciate the information and help in updating information on their programs provided by Nanci Bell, Judith Birsh, Jeffrey Black, Phyllis Bertin, Connie Burkhalter, Robert Calfee, Aylett Cox, Nancy Eberhardt, Marcia Henry, Patricia Lindamood, Clara McCulloch, Connie Russo, and Phyllis Shavi. Special thanks to Trika Smith-Burke and Barbara Wilson for being generous with their materials, advice, and time, all of which were invaluable in preparing the two new program chapters. A number of practitioners participated in what we called *the dyslexia project* at the Teachers College, Columbia University Child Study Center during the early 1990s. These colleagues contributed to an ongoing dialogue that has helped to shape my thinking and the book: Judith Birsh, Kay Brigham, Ann Dooney, Betsy Horowitz, and Susan Nachamie. Margaret Jo Shepherd's contributions have been especially important ones. All of us are grateful to KM and other children like her who have allowed us to study their struggle to read.

JKU

To Elise, Ashley, and Brewster - DBC

To my family, and especially to Alene Uhry
who has been reading for more than eighty years, and
to Alene Rhea who is learning - JKU

I

Reading and Dyslexia

1

Perspectives on Reading and Learning to Read

It is the intent of this book to provide an overview of the nature of dyslexia and of how children with this reading disorder can be helped to be better readers. In order to understand what goes wrong with reading in children with dyslexia, the acquisition of skilled reading in normally achieving children needs to be examined. What processes are involved in mature skilled reading? And how do these processes develop? These two questions are crucial to the understanding of dyslexia.

The psychology of reading has been under investigation since the beginning of this century. Combined efforts of reading educators and researchers from related disciplines (e.g., psychology, neurology, linguistics) have led to new theoretical perspectives on the acts of reading and of learning to read, several of which have contributed substantially to the understanding of reading disability. One such perspective views reading as an *information processing system*. It attempts to identify the psychological processes involved in the act of skilled reading and to determine how they are coordinated. A second perspective focuses on reading as a *developing process*. Understanding how normal reading is acquired is crucial to the understanding of what goes wrong during the development of reading in children with dyslexia.

INFORMATION PROCESSING THEORIES OF SKILLED READING

The main purpose of reading is to become informed, or to gain meaning from text, whether for educational or recreational purposes.

3

How does comprehension happen? How do skilled readers look at a page filled with letters and understand a message written by someone else in another time and place, a process involving movement from sensory input to higher level thought?

One model for analyzing such interactions is called *information processing*. The mind is viewed as a system for taking in information at the sensory level, organizing and interpreting it, keeping it temporarily in short-term memory or storing it in categories for later retrieval. Executive control processes or monitoring mechanisms, which are affected by prior experiences both with life and with print, help in guiding this process. For example, expectations about what will come next in a story affect the way incoming information is perceived and organized.

Viewing reading as information processing provokes questions about what subprocesses are involved, the order in which they occur, and the relative contribution of the various available information sources. One extremely important query, for example, concerns the extent to which reading might be guided by print, the small pieces of information that enter the system at the sensory level, or by meaning and context, which are influenced by prior experiences and which guide the self-monitoring process. Reading theorists have developed *models*, or theoretical representations of the reading process, to explain their points of view on these issues. Three distinctly different positions on the reading process are discussed below.

Top-Down Theory

Proponents of the *top-down* theory of reading, led by Kenneth Goodman and Frank Smith, take a strong meaning-based position. They maintain that reading is primarily dependent upon the reader's intention, or purpose, for reading a text and is driven by their understanding of the text. According to these theorists, rather than processing every word, good readers sample, or select out, only the essential textual information for meeting this purpose (Goodman 1967; Smith 1978, 1979). Such readers rely heavily on their acquired knowledge of the world and of conventional graphemic, syntactic, and semantic structures to hypothesize or predict the words to come and to confirm the sense of what they have read. Only when they find that the text does not make sense do they go back and focus on individual words or examine letters in words. Sensory input in this model is guided by metacognitive monitoring.

Goodman calls reading a *psycholinguistic guessing game* (Goodman 1967). This phrase refers to a process conceptualized as the use of multiple knowledge sources (e.g., syntactic context, background knowledge, purpose for reading) to read text. The reader makes an informed guess that is consistent with what is known so far from the text in regard to both part of speech and meaning. Both Goodman and Smith describe reading as a *top-down* procedure, moving from higher order (cognitive) to lower order (sensory and perceptual) mental processes, that is to say, from the attachment of meaning or purpose for reading to the perception of visual cues in the text. One argument used to support this model is that skilled reading is so rapid and automatic that it could not possibly involve a close look at every letter in every word.

The implication for instruction from this model involves reading instruction aimed from the beginning at the meaning level and limiting instruction at the letter and word level to situations within the context of a meaningful passage of text. Classrooms adhering to this model are commonly referred to as *whole language* classrooms. Teachers adhering to a *whole language* philosophy consider beginning reading to be an extension of oral language development. In these classrooms, a teacher reads aloud to emerging readers who then build print knowledge from an oral language meaning base. Beginning reading is practiced by matching oral language, memorized from several readings, with written language. For this, young readers use a strategy called *fingerpoint-reading* (Ehri and Sweet 1991; Morris 1981). A child says a line of text from memory while pointing at each word, making use of, and expanding upon, letter-sound knowledge and the alphabetic principle to guide in fingerpoint-reading. Another common activity in *whole language* classrooms is called *writing workshop*; classrooms are organized so that children simulate the steps used by professional adult writers (e.g., brainstorming, writing, sharing for feedback, revising, publishing). Even very young children write on a daily basis, with the emphasis on expression of thought rather than mechanical correctness. This text is another source for beginning reading instruction. During the mid-1990s, *whole language* classrooms are common but not the rule.

Goodman and Smith's *top-down* model, in fact, has been called into question by studies that demonstrate that proficient readers do not skip over words and phrases, nor do they rely on context alone to gain information. Instead, they read as many as five words each second (Raynor and Pollatsek 1987) and fixate on almost all words in text (e.g., Just and Carpenter 1980). Fluent readers are less reliant on context in processing textual information than poor readers because they are more adept at recognizing individual words within the text (Stanovich 1986b). Thus accurate word recognition indeed appears to be an essential component of proficient reading.

Speed of word identification has also been shown to be a major determinant of reading ability (Perfetti 1984; Stanovich 1980). Correlations as high as .80 have been demonstrated between the rate of context-free word recognition and reading comprehension (Stanovich, Cunningham, and Feeman 1984). The strength of this relationship seems to bear out the *limited capacity mechanism* thesis of LaBerge and Samuels (see below). Charles Perfetti (1984, 1985b), another leading reading theorist, offers a similar explanation for this relationship which he calls *verbal efficiency* theory. In his view, the more automatic the ability to recognize individual words in reading text, the greater the resources available for comprehending it.

BOTTOM-UP THEORY

Diametrically opposed to the Goodman-Smith perspective on reading is the *bottom-up* perspective. This model describes reading as a hierarchical procedure that moves from processing the smallest bits of graphemic information, individual letters, to ever larger chunks of information and only attaches semantic meaning after words have been identified (LaBerge and Samuels 1974). In this model a series of associations must be built between low level pieces of information, such as sounds and letters, before they can be interpreted and associated with specific meanings.

An important contribution of the *bottom-up* model is its emphasis on the subprocesses of the reading act and its contention that many of these subprocesses, such as letter and word identification, must become automatic in order for readers to be fluent. David LaBerge and S. Jay Samuels (1974), who were among the first investigators to focus on the attentional demands of reading, hypothesize a *limited capacity mechanism* in human information processing that controls the distribution of attentional resources. As they explain it, during execution of a complex skill such as reading, many component processes must be coordinated within a very short time; if none of these processes is carried out automatically, there will not be enough attention available to execute the reading act successfully.

The implication for instruction here involves teaching letter sounds before words, words before sentences, and sentences before passages. Only then can passages be read and understood. Carrying the theory into practice would imply teaching decoding in isolation and mastering decoding before teaching reading comprehension. There are few classroom examples of this theory in pure form, but several Orton-Gillingham remedial reading programs follow this model (e.g., see Chapter 13, Alphabetic Phonics). However, there are numerous examples of classrooms using basal reading series that outline a program of activities including workbook exercises for teaching letter-sounds in isolation and for pre-teaching sight words in isolation before they are encountered in a reading passage. While comprehension instruction is not absent in such programs it is not a major focus in the early grades.

INTERACTIVE THEORY

Top-down and *bottom-up* models represent extreme theoretical perspectives on the act of reading. Both describe reading as a series of sequentially ordered processes and are therefore referred to as *serial processing models*. In both models, control over the reading process operates in one direction; each processing event triggers another processing event, either one step up or one step down in a hierarchy. In contrast, another view of reading holds that many of the component processes occur at the same time or in *parallel.* David Rumelhart (1977), who originally proposed this theory, contends that readers simultaneously initiate word identification and predict meaning, and he maintains that these are reciprocal events. He cites several sources of knowledge that the good reader has available to help extract the message in the text: knowledge of the grapheme–phoneme system, knowledge of particular sight words in the lexicon, knowledge of the syntactic and semantic aspects of language, background knowledge, and metacognitive knowledge of how to self-monitor during reading. Note that the first knowledge source involves print and its relationship with the phonological aspects of spoken language, whereas the remaining sources refer to oral language alone. Rumelhart believes that these knowledge sources can be activated concurrently and that they operate reciprocally; he refers to his theory as an *interactive* model of the reading process.

Rumelhart's colleague Mark Seidenberg, in collaboration with James McClelland, developed what they call a *connectionist* model which is similar to the interactive model. Their reasoning is that reading involves a series of associations or connections resulting in accumulated lexical knowledge. The model involves connections in both directions between context and meaning, and then additional two-way connections between meaning, orthography, and phonology (i.e., meaning-orthography, orthography-phonology, and phonology-meaning). The term phonology refers to the sounds in spoken language and the term *orthography* refers to the letter patterns in written words. In other words, connections or associations between any two processors can trigger other associations in any direction and contribute to the overall reading process. Seidenberg and McClelland have used computational simulations of word learning to provide evidence of the interactive nature of the relationship between phonology and orthography. Theoretical *hidden units*, to which Seidenberg and McClelland assign statistical weights, mediate these connections (1989).

Skilled reading involves rapid decoding; an often cited study by Raynor and Pollatsek (1987) puts the rate at more than five words every second. As described by Seidenberg and McClelland, rapid word reading triggers associations with several other processors. Pronunciations and word meanings are generated by visual word recognition, as are hypotheses about possible syntactic patterns. All of this contributes to comprehension, so that "text and discourse are interpreted essentially as the signal is perceived" (Seidenberg and McClelland 1989, p. 523). The point here is that these connections are made all at once rather than in a linear, hierarchical fashion (i.e., either *top-down* or *bottom-up*). As Marilyn Adams puts it:

> In order for the connections, and even the connected parts, themselves, to develop properly, they must be linked together in the very course of acquisition. And, importantly, this dependency works in both directions. One cannot properly develop the higher-order processes without due attention to the lower. Nor can one focus on the lower-order processes without constantly clarifying and exercising their connections to the higher-order ones (Adams 1990, p. 6).

Instruction following from applications of this theory involves not merely introducing all the processors or cue systems at the same time rather than in a hierarchical sequence, but actively helping children connect each cue system with the others. Questions such as, "What does a cow say? What letter would you expect to see if the word is *moo*?" encourage the child to interconnect the system of processors.

Sylvia Farnham-Diggory describes an idealized model for reading instruction that she attributes to ancient Greece and Rome and that is consistent with the *interactive* model. First-order skills (enciphering and deciphering) and second-order skills (comprehension and composition) are taught together. She describes a teaching/learning model that resembles *whole language* instruction in combination with systematic, direct instruction designed to highlight the rule-based nature of what she calls the *orthographic cipher* or letter-sound system of English. Both first- and second-order skills are taught in a way that emphasizes the reciprocal relationship between reading and writing and both are taught within the context of meaningful projects (Farnham-Diggory 1990). Her teaching model is consistent with one proposed by Adams (1990) in which meaning-based and code-based strategies are taught together.

The *interactive* model has gained acceptance among some of the more prominent researchers in the field of reading who claim that serial (one-way) processing models fail to hold up under scrutiny through research. According to Keith Stanovich (1980), bottom-up models are unable to explain the effects of context on reading speed that have been observed under experimental conditions; top-down models must be rejected for the reasons cited above. *Interactive* models, on the other hand, can account for concurrent influences at all levels of processing because, as he expresses it, "... higher-level processes constrain the alternative of lower-level processes but are themselves constrained by lower-level analyses" (Stanovich 1980). By *lower-level* Stanovich is referring to graphemic (letters) and orthographic (letter clusters) features in words.

WHAT HAPPENS WHEN ONE OF THE SYSTEMS DOES NOT WORK EFFICIENTLY?

Stanovich's Compensatory Model

Stanovich emphasizes the potentially compensatory nature of these interacting processes and calls his own view of reading an *interactive-compensatory* model. The finding that readers with poor word recognition are more reliant on context than good readers is one example of such compensation. Stanovich's interactive-compensatory model, because it illustrates so well the trade-offs that can occur among the component subskills of reading, helps to explain individual differences in reading ability, and therefore has considerable appeal for those of us concerned with disabled readers. There is much similarity between this theory and Perfetti's verbal efficiency theory.

Gough's Simple View of Reading

Philip Gough and William Tunmer present a model of skilled reading comprehension that is dependent on two components: 1) the ability to look at print and recode it into spoken language, and 2) the ability to understand spoken language (Gough and Tunmer 1986). In order to function effectively in regard to reading comprehension, the reader must be good at both components. Gough and Tunmer concede that the model is an oversimplification and that reading, in reality, is a highly complex task, rather than a simple one. However, the model provides a very clear view of what might go wrong in skilled reading. To refer back to the connectionist model, if the processors that are involved in turning print to speech, or if the processors that are involved in prior knowledge, understanding of words, or comprehension of complex oral syntax are not working efficiently, then the connections between them will break down. Without all systems working well, text cannot be understood. According to Gough and Tunmer, in skilled reading both word reading and listening comprehension must work well to facilitate proficient reading comprehension.

DEVELOPMENTAL PERSPECTIVES ON READING

CHALL'S DEVELOPMENTAL MODEL

Reading at proficient levels and reading as a developing skill are quite different behaviors. Reading is learned over many years, and for most people important changes in reading behavior occur over this span of time.

Jeanne Chall (1983b), a leading researcher in reading education in this country, has developed a stage theory of reading development, which she prefers to call a scheme or model. She hypothesizes six qualitatively different stages from readiness to maturity. She maintains that most people progress through these stages in the same order, though not necessarily at the same rate and despite the fact that many people do not reach the higher stages, or expert levels, of reading ability. She believes that rate and success in learning to read are determined by the interaction between learner and environment. Borrowing from Jean Piaget's stage theory of cognitive development (Inhelder and Piaget 1958; Piaget 1970), Chall describes reading as "a form of problem solving in which readers adapt to their environment through the processes of assimilation and accommodation" (1983b). *Assimilation* refers to the learner's application of previously acquired skills to a particular task or problem. *Accommodation* refers to the learner's ability to adopt new skills or new ways of thinking in performing an unfamiliar task or solving a new problem. Chall provides ages and grade levels at which the average student may be expected to reach each of the six stages, but urges that they be considered only approximations.

Stage 0: The Prereading Stage

The longest stage in Chall's model is Stage 0, the prereading stage. It lasts from birth to age six and goes from the very beginnings of an individual's language awareness to the ability (in the case of many pre-school children) to recognize and name letters of the alphabet and even to read some popular names on signs and packages or some words in familiar books. Readiness concepts such as understanding the purpose of reading, understanding the relationship between pictures and print, understanding the relationship between written and spoken words, being able to rhyme, to alliterate (match initial sounds), and to segment units of speech (words in sentences and syllables in words, if not phonemes in words) are some of the readiness concepts acquired by most children during this stage. The time frame and developing competencies in Chall's readiness stage are commonly referred to as *emergent literacy* in much of the literature today. At this point, as Chall puts it, children bring more to the printed page than they take out.

Stage 1: Decoding

Stage 1, the initial or decoding stage, is attained by most children between the ages of six and seven while in first and second grades. The major accomplishment of this period is grasping the alphabetic principle and learning the letter-sound correspondences, or the alphabetic code. Children increasingly attend to graphic elements in words rather than treating words as wholes. Chall explains the successful transition from Stage 0 to Stage 1 as a process of accommodation. Children apply their newly acquired readiness concepts and skills, which include the ability to analyze parts within wholes, to the challenge of reading unfamiliar words. However, if these readiness skills are lacking, children approach new challenges through assimilation, continuing to use the strategies learned in the previous stage, viewing all words holistically and relying on contextual cues such as pictures and memory for stories.

Stage 2: Confirmation

Stage 2 involves confirming what has been learned in the previous stage and gaining fluency. While phonics knowledge continues to develop during this period and even later, it is confirmation of old knowledge that is the focus here. Children gain confidence in "their decoding knowledge, the redundancies of the language, and the redundancies of the stories" (Chall 1983b, p. 19). They begin to develop speed as well as accuracy in word recognition. At this point, the learner should be attending to both meaning and print and using cues from these information sources interactively. Stage 2 is a particularly critical period for the developing reader; if progress breaks down, the individual can remain "glued to print," as Chall expresses it.

Stages 3–5: Reading to Learn

Stage 3, which commences in fourth grade at roughly nine years of age, is primarily distinguished from the previous stage by a change in motivation for reading. At this point, the individual begins to read in order to learn new information. Where Stages 1 and 2 are referred to by Chall as *learning to read*, Stages 3 through 5 are called *reading to learn.* Reading in content area subjects (science and social studies) is introduced in school. Vocabulary enlargement and expansion of world knowledge become increasingly important. For the most part, the material encountered during this stage presents only one point of view. The ability to deal with multiple viewpoints is more fully developed in Stage 4 (ages fourteen through eighteen), which covers the high school years. This ability is acquired mainly through formal education.

Readers who attain the highest level of reading development, Stage 5, have learned to read selectively and are able to develop their own opinions and make their own judgments about what they read. As Chall expresses it, the reading process at this stage is "essentially constructive"; readers construct their own knowledge from that of others. Stage 5 is not usually reached until college age or later and may, in fact, be reserved for individuals who have an intellectual bent.

Each stage builds on the skills acquired in previous stages, and success in meeting the challenges confronted at each stage is to a large extent dependent upon mastery of those skills normally acquired in earlier stages, according to Chall.

STAGES WITHIN CHALL'S EARLY STAGES

Even within Chall's stages, growth in reading acquisition represents qualitative changes. For example, in a year-long study of first graders,

Andrew Biemiller observed reading errors that suggested three distinct and hierarchical word-reading strategies (Biemiller 1970). A number of reading researchers have used observations and research findings to construct stage models for reading acquisition. These models usually involve four phases in which four strategies develop, each dependent on those that come before.

PHASE 1: THE LOGOGRAPHIC PHASE

British reading theorist Uta Frith calls the earliest reading phase *logographic* (Frith 1985, 1986) and Linnea Ehri calls it the *visual-cue* phase (e.g., Ehri 1989). When using this strategy, young children are highly dependent on the look of a word within a particular context. Some researchers claim that a few words are recognized instantly at this stage through memorization of the exact shape of the word. Others say that the word needs to be linked to context-dependent cues. For instance, the word *McDonald's* might be recognized under the golden arches but not on its own. *Xepsi* on a soda-can logo might be read as "Pepsi" (Masonheimer, Drum, and Ehri 1984). Letters can be used in a limited way at this stage but attending to letter order is not a characteristic of the logographic strategy (Frith 1985, 1986; Marsh et al. 1981). For many years it was a widely held belief, both by researchers and by teachers, that children needed to acquire a sight vocabulary of roughly 40 memorized words before they could take advantage of letter cues. The lexicon of sight words was believed to provide insight into the letter-sound relationship and to provide a base for the next strategy.

Ehri has questioned the size of this pre-phonics lexicon through an experiment showing that even readers who knew only a few words could use letter cues to learn new words (e.g., GRF for *giraffe* and LFT for *elephant*), and that the use of letter-sound cues was a more efficient strategy for them than the use of visually distinctive letter patterns (Ehri and Wilce 1985). Letter-sound associations are built on letter-name knowledge. For instance, the name of the letter *g* provides a clue to its sound and helps children remember how to read a particular word. That is, this initial visual-cue or logographic phase may last only a very short time. Some researchers doubt that the stage exists at all.

PHASE 2: THE PHONETIC-CUE PHASE

Linnea Ehri has called the next phase the *phonetic-cue* phase (Ehri and Wilce 1987a, 1987b) or *rudimentary alphabetic* phase (Ehri 1995). Here letters play a more important role, but children still do not use every letter in a word. Associations are made between salient letters, such as the initial *j* and final *l* in the printed word *jail* and a stored memory of the word *jail* (Ehri and Wilce 1987b). When phonetic-cue readers see the *j* and *l* together in a word they scan their lexicon for a match that sometimes involves the correct word and sometimes a look-alike word. The phonetic-cue strategy helps children remember particular words but it does not help them sound out new words.

PHASE 3: THE CIPHER OR ALPHABETIC PHASE

The *cipher* phase (Gough and Hillinger 1980) is also called the *alphabetic* phase (Frith 1985, 1986). This strategy takes full advantage of the alphabetic system upon which our writing system is based. Letters are sounded out, one at a time, from left to right, and then the sounds are blended together into words. To do this, a child needs to have knowledge of letter-sound associations, some of which are learned intuitively through knowing letter names (e.g., *j* and *m*), and some of which need to be taught more explicitly (e.g., *y* and *w*). The beginning cipher reader also needs metacognitive knowledge about units of sound in speech, a knowledge that is called *phonological awareness, and of how these speech-sound units, once segmented, can be mapped onto letters in print, which is called the *alphabetic principle*. Only at this phase of strategy development can the beginning reader actually read a word that has not been memorized. A reader at this phase should be able to read accurately using letter-sound associations.

PHASE 4: THE ORTHOGRAPHIC PHASE

The term *orthography* comes from Greek roots that can be translated as *perfect writing*. In the context of reading stage theory the term refers to spelling patterns, or units of letters commonly occurring together. The *orthographic* (Frith 1985, 1986) or *analogy* strategy (Goswami 1986, 1988) involves recognizing a unit of letters that forms a spelling pattern that represents a sound. Both Goswami and Rebecca Treiman (1985) provide evidence that the natural break-point in a word for young readers is after the initial consonant or consonants (e.g., *c-* or *cl-*), which is called an *onset*, and before the vowel-consonant or vowel-consonants units (e.g., *-at* or *-ink*), which is called a *rime*. Being able to read *cat* allows a child to recognize the *at* portion of *sat*. Capitalizing on this phenomenon is a method of instruction called *word families* in which same-spelling-pattern words are taught together. According to a version of the four-phase model proposed by Marsh and his colleagues (Marsh et al. 1981) analogies can be made at the *morphological* level as well. This involves groups of letters that are units of meaning, or *morphs*, such as the unit *know* in *knowledge*. Note that here the unit of letters actually differs in sound from word to word while the meaning remains constant.

While the analogy strategy is considered the most sophisticated form of decoding according to the four-phase model, British researcher Usha Goswami has carried out experiments demonstrating that even very young children can read unknown words through analogy to a known word (e.g., Goswami 1986, 1988). Goswami chose analogous words with similar endings using the argument that end-analogies or *rimes* (e.g., *beak, peak*) are easier to learn than beginning-analogies (e.g., *beak, bean*) because the break between *onset* (i.e., initial letter or letter cluster) and *rime* (i.e., vowel unit and final consonant unit) is an easier form of segmentation for young children. In Goswami's training studies, a target word was taught and then embedded in a word list of unknown words which included a few rimes of the target word. More of the rime words were read successfully than were other unfamiliar words (Goswami 1986, 1988). These experiments have been used by practitioners as evidence that children should be taught using a word-families approach right from the start.

Linnea Ehri carried out an experiment that confirmed Goswami's finding that very young readers can read by analogy, but she found that those subjects who knew how to use a cipher strategy were better at using the analogy strategy than were the children who were still using a phonetic-cue strategy. The phonetic-cue readers, who read using associations between partial letter cues and a stored lexicon could not figure out new words from old words, whereas the cipher readers could (Ehri and Robbins 1992). Goswami, too, has found evidence that skill in phonological awareness, a crucial factor in cipher reading, contributes to *analogy* reading (Goswami and Mead 1992).

EHRI'S CONTRIBUTIONS TO STAGE THEORY

Through her research, Linnea Ehri has done much to clarify the role of reading strategies at each of these four phases, as noted above. She has produced much of the evidence that demonstrates just what processing demands are associated with each phase. Her subjects are carefully screened so that she is able to document differences between children she considers nonreaders, novices, and beginning readers.

Another important contribution made by Ehri (1992) is in regard to the relationship between word attack skills, used to decode or decipher unfamiliar words based on letter-sound relationships, and the acquisition of *sight words*, which have been memorized and can be recognized instantly. It is part of both historical theory and school lore that instruction involves either one approach or the other. For example, teachers talk of using either a *sight approach* or a *phonics approach* to teaching reading. Often they try to fit a particular approach to a particular child depending on whether they view the child as a *visual learner* or an *auditory learner*. The term *dual route* is used to express these alternate routes to meaning. According to the dual route theory, there are two avenues to meaning. The first of these hypothesized routes involves sounding out a word, or turning print into speech, in order to trigger a connection with its meaning in a *lexicon* or stored bank of vocabulary words. The second depends on a rote-learned arbitrary connection between print and meaning without the intermediate step of recoding the letters to a phonological system.

Ehri's model of the relationship between what she calls *recoding* (or moving from print to speech through the use of letter-sound associations) and sight word acquisition casts doubt on this dichotomy. Ehri is critical of the connectionist notion that arbitrary associations can be made between a printed word and its meaning. She notes that the research literature does not support either a *phonological route* or a *visual-semantic route*. Ehri suggests a third route, which she calls the *visual-phonological route*. According to her theory a series of complex connections are made on several levels. Letters are connected with phonemes. In Ehri's example, the letter *l* in *belt* is connected with the sound /l/. Units of letters are connected with parts of spoken words (e.g., the letter unit *elt* is connected with the sound /elt/). The whole printed word is connected with the whole spoken word (e.g., *belt*). In addition, the printed word *belt* is connected with its meaning. Ehri uses the term *cipher sight word reading* when words are recognized quickly as a result of connections made through the cipher strategy. In other words, the cipher strategy facilitates decoding until a word has been read enough times to be recognized rapidly through what Ehri calls "a complete network of visual-phonological connections in lexical memory" (Ehri 1992, p. 138).

The implication of Ehri's theory in terms of word-reading stage theory is that at each phase in strategy acquisition (e.g., logographic, phonetic-cue, cipher, orthographic) the connections between print and oral language become more elaborated and the lexicon of sight words is more easily built and more automatically retrieved. She suggests that instruction can facilitate sight word learning most effectively if phonics instruction is linked to acquisition of a few highly practiced, phonetically regular words at any one time. That is, when short *a* is taught in phonics instruction, sight word instruction should involve short *a* words (Ehri 1992).

FRITH'S CONTRIBUTIONS TO READING STAGE THEORY

British researcher Uta Frith presents a model of decoding acquisition, cited in descriptions of the phases outlined above (1985, 1986). Note that her model skips the phonetic-cue phase and moves directly from logographic to alphabetic reading. Frith's model is insightful in two regards. Her first contribution to stage model theory is her notion that there are two steps at each of her three phases, one involving the acquisition of the strategy for reading and the other for spelling. At each of her three phases, these skills develop, one behind the other, but not always in the same order. Reading develops first, before spelling, at the *logographic phase*. That is, children become aware of letters and written words through exposure to environmental print, on cereal boxes and traffic signs for example, before they learn to write letters or words.

At the alphabetic phase, the order is reversed. Children can spell using an alphabetic, left-to-right, letter-by-letter strategy before they can read alphabetically. That is, they continue to use a logographic strategy to recognize a few memorized words while spelling alphabetically. Often they can spell phonetically regular words that they cannot read.

The notion of using alphabetic spelling instruction as a way of leading young children into using the alphabetic strategy for reading appears to be quite sound. Linnea Ehri and Lee Wilce (1987b) found that kindergarten children trained in listening carefully to the sounds in words and then representing these sounds with letters were able to read words composed of these letters more accurately than children trained in letter-sound associations alone. Ehri presents evidence, however, that these kindergarten children were using a phonetic-cue strategy (the strategy omitted by Frith's theory) rather than the full cipher or alphabetic strategy.

Spelling-to-read instruction appears to work in school settings as well. Uhry and Shepherd (1993a), working with small groups of children over the course of their first-grade school year, taught them phoneme segmentation (e.g., "What sound do you hear at the beginning of *pig*?") in combination with spelling (e.g., "What letter spells the /p/ sound?"). Children trained in segmentation/spelling showed an advantage in nonsense word reading (e.g., *ift, bim*) in comparison with children trained in letter-sound associations and whole word reading but not trained in phonemic analysis. This advantage in nonsense word reading suggests an advantage in alphabetic decoding. Instruction here was carefully sequenced in terms of introducing words composed of relatively transparent letter sounds (e.g., *map,*) early in the training and limiting instruction to words that are phonetically regular.

A somewhat less formal, less carefully sequenced approach appears to work as well. The term *invented spelling* indicates spellings that children construct themselves, using letter-name knowledge to deduce letter-sound relationships. Invented spelling is used as an instructional approach in many whole language classrooms. Clarke (1988) reports a study of four Canadian classrooms using two different spelling approaches for weekly writing activities. In one, children were encouraged to spell correctly with the teacher supplying model spellings. In the other, children were encouraged to invent their own spellings. By March of the first-grade year the invented spellers had become stronger decoders. Results were particularly striking when the initially lowest achievers from each classroom were compared across groups. Thus, there is support in these three studies for using spelling involving analysis of phoneme segments as a method of teaching beginning reading. This seems to support Frith's model of alphabetic spelling preceding and leading the way into alphabetic reading.

At the *orthographic phase*, again, the order of spelling and reading acquisition is reversed according to Frith. Exposure to print in books helps children recognize units of letters in order to read by analogy while they are still producing phonetic rather than orthographically conventional spellings. Using memorized units to spell appears to be the last strategy to develop.

Frith's second contribution to stage theory is the notion that it is at the *alphabetic phase* that children with dyslexia begin to fail in reading. In other words they are able to memorize a few words using *logographic* strategies, but are unable to use the alphabetic principle to invent spellings or to decode new words they have not seen before (1985, 1986). This is consistent with detailed descriptions of individuals with dyslexia from the research literature presented in Chapter 2 of this book. Support for acquisition of the alphabetic principle is the basis for most of the programs currently in use for the remediation of dyslexia, as outlined in Part III of this book.

EDUCATIONAL IMPLICATIONS OF DIFFERING PERSPECTIVES ON READING

Not all reading authorities agree that knowing the graphophonetic code is essential for learning to read, nor do they acknowledge to the same extent the inherent challenges of the alphabetic system. Perspectives on these issues have important implications for reading instruction. Theorists who espouse a strong meaning-based or *top-down* view of reading tend to minimize the importance of learning the code. Kenneth Goodman, for instance, is critical of the use of phonics instruction in the early stages of reading (1993). He argues that English phonics rules are arbitrary and unreliable, and are not helpful out of context. What Jeanne Chall calls the *great debate* in reading instruction goes back long before the advent of whole-language philosophy (Chall 1983a). In the 1930s, for instance, advocates of John Dewey's philosophy recommended teaching whole words, rather than letter sounds, because, they assumed, whole words put children directly in touch with meaning right from the start. During the late 1960s and early 1970s advocates of open classrooms suggested teaching reading using meaningful materials, such as the children's own writing, as well as *language-experience* text generated by groups of children and written down by teachers. Historically, periods in which naturalistic, child-centered approaches to reading instruction dominate have alternated with periods characterized by a swing toward an emphasis on word-level skills.

The terms *basal readers* and *basal series* refer to packaged programs that include student readers and workbooks, complete teacher instruction guides and even scripts for teachers to follow in using the materials. They tend to be structured in a way that is consistent with the currently popular approach to teaching reading (e.g., sight word learning, phonics, literature-based, etc.). The majority of basal reading programs include some form of phonics instruction while still emphasizing a meaning-based, whole-word approach to reading. That is, they tend to be both eclectic and conservative, rather than expressing an extreme in point of view. Jeanne Chall (1983b) observes in her analysis of existing beginning reading programs that phonics instruction in most basal series is provided nonsystematically in follow-up activities and often not coordinated with the stories to be read. For these reasons, some teachers may opt to omit phonics instruction altogether from basal-reader lessons.

In 1967 Jeanne Chall published a massive review of the literature on reading instruction, which she later updated (Chall 1983a). After examining the relevant research studies, Chall concludes that early intensive phonics instruction produces greater gains in reading by third grade in comparison with other approaches. She makes the point that because English is an alphabetic language, all children who learn to read will learn some phonics, either by figuring it out themselves from exposure to words, or through *direct instruction*. Chall finds convincing evidence that direct, systematic phonics instruction is significantly more effective than the alternative, often called *indirect* or *intrinsic* learning.

Like Chall, Marilyn Adams has carried out an extensive review of the literature on learning to read (Adams 1990). However, Adams is much more explicit than Chall in outlining the importance of connections between meaning processors and letter-sound processors. She concludes that to be effective, phonics instruction must be linked with language-based reading instruction. She provides a detailed description of this in discussing Reading Recovery, an individual reading program for beginning readers who are behind their peers in whole language classrooms (see Chapter 23, Reading Recovery). In this reading model, children are explicitly instructed in how to coordinate the use of various cue systems.

Reading acquisition, then, involves a series of developmental stages in which more and more features of printed words are used to recode print as oral language. A crucial aspect of this developmental sequence involves linking print with meaning right from the start. Skilled reading involves rapid connections between processing systems for almost instantaneous print-to-meaning operations. What goes wrong in this process for children with dyslexia? Why are some children able to master skilled reading while others are not?

2

The Nature of Dyslexia

DEFINING DYSLEXIA

The term *dyslexia* is derived from the Greek *dys* (difficult) and *lexicos* (pertaining to words) and was first used by Berlin in 1887 to describe extreme difficulty reading and spelling words. The World Federation of Neurology defines dyslexia as follows.

> *Specific developmental dyslexia* is a disorder manifested by difficulty learning to read despite conventional instruction, adequate intelligence, and adequate sociocultural opportunity. It is dependent upon fundamental cognitive disabilities which are frequently of constitutional origin (1968; cited in Critchley 1970).

The qualifier *developmental* refers to a disorder of suspected congenital or hereditary origin, in contrast to acquired dyslexia, a disorder resulting from brain injury after the onset of reading (Frith 1986). It is important to state that the word *developmental* does not mean that the disorder will disappear with maturity. A distinguishing characteristic of dyslexia is, in fact, its persistence, although appropriate remedial treatment and the development of compensatory strategies may moderate its effects.

The qualifier *specific* is intended to connote a disorder limited specifically to reading rather than involving a general learning problem. As Keith Stanovich describes this notion,

> Simply put, it is the idea that a dyslexic child has a brain/cognitive deficit that is reasonably specific to the reading task. That is, the concept of a specific reading

19

disability requires that the deficit displayed by the disabled reader not extend too far into other domains of cognitive functioning (Stanovich 1988a, p. 155).

Stanovich refers to poor readers who are poor in cognitive ability as well as in all academic areas as *garden variety poor readers* (Stanovich 1988b). Reading is not discrepant from IQ in these children as it is in children with dyslexia.

There is even evidence that dyslexia is limited not just to reading, but to very specific aspects of reading. Philip Gough's theoretical *simple view of reading* (see chapter 1) holds that there are two contributors necessary to skilled reading comprehension: 1) decoding and 2) listening comprehension (Gough and Tunmer 1986). That is, children with reading problems could be having difficulty at either the word reading level or with understanding what they have read once they have decoded or deciphered written words into spoken words. Wesley Hoover has tested Gough's model using data from 900 children on the Iowa Test of Basic Skills. He analyzed subtest results for listening comprehension, decoding, and reading comprehension to confirm Gough's two independent contributors to reading comprehension and found that each is necessary but not sufficient for reading success (Hoover 1994). Dyslexia is conceptualized as difficulty at the word-reading level. Reading comprehension is affected, but it is decoding, and not listening comprehension, that causes the difficulty.

Dyslexia is considered a learning disability in the Federal Register under Public Law 94–142 (see Kavanagh and Truss 1988). As with other learning disabilities covered under this law, dyslexia involves what is called an *exclusionary* diagnosis. That is, instead of describing characteristics directly, the definition describes all the conditions that must be ruled out (e.g., low IQ, physical handicaps, environmental factors, etc.) before making a diagnosis.

The term *learning disabilities* is actually a political label coined by Samuel Kirk (see Farnham-Diggory 1992). The term was adapted to secure special services for students with mild learning handicaps. Some of these children had not previously qualified for placement in already-established special education categories — mentally handicapped, emotionally handicapped, physically handicapped. Others' parents did not want their children classified with those more-severely handicapped. Although the majority of students who are classified as *learning disabled* have reading difficulties, in many cases these difficulties can be attributed to mild handicapping factors or conditions other than dyslexia, such as low average intelligence. These children, in terms of Gough's *simple view of reading* are poor at both decoding and listening comprehension. They are considered *garden variety poor readers*. Much of the research on reading disorder has been muddied by failure to distinguish between children who are dyslexic and those who are classified for school instruction as learning disabled, with poor reading as part of a more extensive set of difficulties (e.g., borderline IQ, poor mathematics skills, poor listening, etc.).

Stanovich and Gough base their models on a very specific language deficit in the area of phonological processing, a deficit that will be discussed later on in this chapter in great detail. The idea of a specific deficit distinguishes dyslexia from other, less specific learning disorders.

HISTORICAL AND CURRENT VIEWS ON ETIOLOGY

While the term *dyslexia* has been used consistently since 1887 to indicate reading disorder at the word-reading level, theories about the exact etiology or causes of dyslexia have changed over time. Much of the very early thinking about possible causes grew out of work with brain injured adults who had lost the ability to read. James Hinshelwood, an ophthalmologist practicing in Scotland at the turn of the Century, was one of the first scientists to describe clinical studies of children who failed to read (e.g., 1896; 1917). He surmised that his patients with reading disorder, which he called *congenital word blindness*, must have had either birth injuries to the brain or brain defects. Hinshelwood believed that these defects were in the left hemisphere of the brain in areas related to the storage of visual memory because these children seemed to have difficulty remembering the names of letters and words.

Samuel Orton, an American neurologist, also published theoretical work in which visual processes were implicated. According to Orton, reading reversals (e.g., *b* for *d* and *saw* for *was*) were caused by problems with cerebral dominance in the early stages of reading. He theorized that both right and left visual fields received visual input and relayed this as mirror images to the visual cortices. While in most people one side of the brain becomes dominant over the other and suppresses the image from the non-dominant hemisphere, he believed that dominance was poorly established in people with dyslexia and that the backwards image was often perceived rather than inhibited or suppressed, resulting in what he called *strephosymbolia*, or twisted symbols (1928). Thus, children with dyslexia would see the word *saw* but perceive its mirror image, the word *was*. Orton's model is often misinterpreted, however, as a deficit at the sensory input level involving actually seeing mirror images. This was never his intention.

Orton was also one of the first to associate dyslexia with language disorders (Geschwind 1982), and this constituted the major thrust of his work. Orton's work on language formed a basis for many of the remedial programs that are currently in use. However, it is his visually based mirror-image explanation that caught on in the popular literature and that continues to be a widely held misconception.

VISUAL EXPLANATIONS OF DYSLEXIA
The Visual-Perceptual Deficit Hypothesis

Orton's mirror-image theory had been discredited by the 1970s on several grounds, one being that reversal and sequencing errors did not appear to account for a greater proportion of the total reading errors made by readers with dyslexia than by normal readers (Stanovich 1986a). In other words, while children with dyslexia may make more oral reading errors than do children who are good readers, the ratio of reversal errors to other errors is the same; most readers make occasional reversals.

Another reason to question the visual-perceptual deficit hypothesis is that readers with dyslexia were not found to differ from average readers in their performance on nonlinguistic tasks, such as the ability to distinguish visual designs or faces (Liberman and Shankweiler 1979). In studies performed by Frank Vellutino and his colleagues, poor readers had no more difficulty than good readers in copying or recognizing letters or words from a novel alphabet, which were essentially nonverbal stimuli (Vellutino et al. 1975; Vellutino, Steger, and Kandel 1972). Furthermore, Vellutino (1978, 1983) demonstrates that poor readers are almost as adept as good readers at copying visually confusable letters and words from memory, although they are significantly less good at naming or pronouncing these items on second exposure. He attributes the naming problems of poor readers to less well established verbal codes for letter or word forms rather than to visual-perception deficits. Vellutino (1987) suggests that the mirror writing exhibited by some dyslexics (as well as some normally developing readers) reflects their incomplete grasp of letter-sound relationships rather than a visual-perception deficit. That is, it is not the case that they confuse the look of the letters; rather, they cannot remember which name goes with which letter.

In a recent review of the literature, however, Dale Willows and Megan Terepocki suggest that there is some evidence for non-linguistic directional confusions in children with reading disorder. While the look-alike and sound-alike properties of b and d could indeed result in a naming-based reversal problem consistent with Vellutino's model, we ought to continue to refine research methods for examining directional confusions in children with reading disorder (Willows and Terepocki 1993).

Probably the most compelling arguments against attempting to correct dyslexia through correcting visual-perception come from two additional lines of research. First, there is little evidence of a significant correlation between early visuo-spatial or visuo-motor problems and later reading ability (e.g., Robinson and Schwartz 1973). Consistent with this, a second line of research from the 1970s indicates that visual-perception training is generally ineffective in improving reading skills in individuals with dyslexia (Bateman 1979; Bryant 1979). This training was once quite popular. For example, during the 1960s Marianne Frostig developed a test for visual perception and a remedial training program involving tracing, and copying shapes and patterns (Frostig 1967; Frostig, Lefever, and Whittlesey 1964). While Frostig apparently meant these materials to supplement rather than replace reading training, many training programs were misguidedly based on her materials alone. There simply were no studies from that period indicating that this training had any positive affect on reading ability.

Optometric training for visual-perception deficits is another historical trend. As Larry Silver points out, optometric training programs that proliferated in the 1960s and 70s have been both controversial and generally unsuccessful in promoting reading acquisition (Keogh and Pelland 1985; Metzger and Werner 1984). Optometric training alone is not sufficient to improve reading. This point of view grows out of a compelling body of research in the mid- to late-1970s suggesting that *diagnostic-prescriptive teaching* or *process training* (remediation of weak processes, usually visual-perception processes) did not produce gains in reading (e.g., Arter and Jenkins 1979). The most effective remedial therapy for children with reading problems involves direct instruction in reading (Silver 1987).

The Intersensory Deficit Hypothesis

Another hypothesized explanation for dyslexia involves difficulty integrating information that must be processed simultaneously in two or more modalities (Birch 1962). This seemed logical, for in reading, both auditory and visual systems are involved. Herbert Birch, who first proposed the intersensory deficit hypothesis, developed a test of auditory-visual integration that requires children to match rhythmic patterns with dot patterns, and found that some poor readers were markedly less proficient than good readers at this task (Birch and Belmont 1964). However, subsequent efforts by Birch and his associates to substantiate this theory have been criticized for failing to control for deficiencies within, rather than between, sensory channels (Bryant 1968). Other researchers, such as Naomi Zigmond (1966), find that disabled readers are inferior to readers of normal ability when processing in a single modality, as on auditory tasks; therefore, their inferior performance on intersensory tasks can be expected.

In a further challenge to the intersensory or cross-modal deficit hypothesis, Frank Vellutino and his colleagues (Vellutino, Steger, and Pruzek 1973) find no significant differences between poor and adequate readers on nonverbal paired-associate matching tasks that measure both within and between modality functioning (visual-visual; auditory-auditory; visual-auditory). By contrast, similar studies carried out with verbal stimuli, such as words and letters, reveal notable differences for poor and adequate readers. These investigators conclude that verbal, rather than intersensory, deficits distinguish dyslexics from normal readers.

Erratic Eye Movements

The above research has centered on misperception or failure to integrate stationary visual forms. Other work has focused on the temporal aspects of vision. One such line of research involves questions about eye movements. According to Alexander Pollatsek (1993) when the eyes view letters and words, or any other stationary visual stimuli, they fixate briefly (for roughly 200 to 300 ms) while constructing an image to be perceived by the brain before performing a *saccade* or eye movement (for roughly 10 to 40 ms) to the next fixation. Visual information from the saccade is suppressed. This *saccadic suppression* insures a series of discrete rather than overlapping images. In reading, most movements are from left-to-right but there are also right-to-left movements when we go back to confirm a letter or word.

Because erratic eye-movement patterns have been observed in children who are poor readers, it has been hypothesized that this is a cause of dyslexia (Pavlidis 1985; Punnet and Steinhauer 1984). However, it seems likely that erratic eye movement is the result rather than the cause of reading problems; in most cases it is not observed when poor readers are reading at their independent reading levels, but rather when they read text that is too hard for them. Consistent with this explanation, Richard Olson and his colleagues compared younger good readers with older poor readers in a reading-age-match study (Olson, Conners, and Rack 1991) and found similar eye movement for the two groups during the reading of similar text.

At the same time, some researchers continue to suggest that there may be a small percentage of children who are dyslexic and whose abnormal fixation patterns reflect a primary visual-spatial disorder (Benton 1985; Eden et al. 1995; Keogh and Pelland 1985; Raynor 1985). For example, there is recent research suggesting that both language and visual skills contribute to reading ability and that this is true for good as well as poor readers (Eden et al. 1995). Guinevere Eden administered visuospatial and oculomotor measures to subjects who were already participants in a longitudinal study of reading disability conducted by Frank Wood and his colleagues at Bowman Gray Medical School (see below). These children were discrepantly poor readers, with IQs significantly stronger than reading ability, and with deficits in phonological skills. In comparison with normal readers of comparable IQ they were poor at several visuospatial skills (i.e., vertical tracking and fixation stability with the left eye, which is ordinarily used as the lead eye during movement). Note that they were no poorer at these visual tasks than a third group of garden variety poor readers. Eden states that her results are consistent with the sort of temporal visual deficits in poor readers reported by Lovegrove and his colleagues (see below).

Deficits in Timing in the Visual Pathways

Another, more complex visual explanation for reading disorder in some children has emerged recently. In this model, there is a deficit in regard to *saccadic suppression* (see above) involving one of the two systems that transmit information from the eye to the brain. The sustained or *parvocellular* system operates during fixations and the transient or *magnocellular* system operates during saccades or movements to the next fixation. Keep in mind that it is information from the fixation rather than the saccade that is perceived. During the saccade, in normal readers the image from the first fixation is suppressed before the next fixation.

A number of researchers have demonstrated that the transient system operates somewhat sluggishly in some poor readers in comparison with normal readers (e.g., Livingstone 1993; Lovegrove 1992; Lovegrove and Williams 1993), and fails to suppress the initial fixation as efficiently as is the case for good readers. Note that this body of research is based on tasks designed to measure identification of images under both quickly and slowly changing conditions, but that the tasks are not reading tasks. However, it has been hypothesized that during reading, failure of the transient system to suppress one fixation before moving on to the next would result in perception of two overlapping sets of letters, which would gradually fade to a single set. Children with *saccadic-suppression deficits* should be able to read words in lists more easily than in connected text (Breitmeyer 1993; Lovegrove and Williams 1993). However, as Charles Hulme points out, this is not the case (Hulme 1988).

If Livingston and Lovegrove are correct, some forms of dyslexia involve a neural deficit that cannot be corrected and that causes a perceptual deficit (Breitmeyer 1993). The implications for instruction have not been addressed fully, but Breitmeyer and others suggest that reading may be improved by using colored lenses (i.e., Irlen lenses) or transparent colored overlays to cover text. This has been a highly controversial treatment for reading problems (e.g., Blaskey et al 1990; O'Connor et al 1990; Robinson and Conway 1990; Solan 1990). Up until this point there has been no theoretical model or research to explain why some individuals report increased ease in reading with these lenses. Breitmeyer suggests that while certain complex properties of red light would exacerbate the deficit, blue lenses could actually help to counteract the effects of the sluggish transient system. Note that there is insubstantial evidence to draw conclusions about either the model or the treatment.

Keith Raynor, an important figure in the development of research on eye movement, makes several important points in his concluding chapter to a recent book that reviews research on visual processes in reading (Raynor 1993). He points out that with the publication of Frank Vellutino's *Dyslexia* in 1979, the field began to shift away from a notion of dyslexia as a visual problem and toward the unitary view that dyslexia was caused by a language deficit involving phonological processing (Vellutino 1979). Raynor suggests that we need to be careful not to assume that dyslexia has a unitary cause. He advocates continuing examination of the most current models of skilled reading (e.g., Seidenberg and McClelland 1989) with attention to the various points at which reading might break down. At this time, though, there is no persuasive and comprehensive body of research pointing to a visual-deficit explanation for dyslexia.

DYSLEXIA AS A LANGUAGE-BASED DEFICIT

The more prevalent view for the past 15-20 years involves language problems (e.g., Catts 1986, 1989; Liberman 1973, 1984; Stanovich 1986a; Vellutino 1979). Language is a highly complex function, however, and not all aspects of language appear to be implicated as primary causes in developmental dyslexia.

Early Language Difficulties and Dyslexia

Research substantiates a significant relationship between early language processing and/or production problems and later reading problems. Follow-up studies of children diagnosed with early specific language impairment (SLI) have shown the incidence of later reading disability to be 90 percent or greater (e.g., Stark et al. 1984; Strominger and Bashir 1977). While the incidence of later reading difficulties for children with early language impairment is very high, the reverse is not always the case. Not all children with dyslexia have histories involving early language disorder. For example, in a prediction study, Natalie Badian used a screening tool that included a number of language measures with four-year-olds to predict sixth-grade reading (Badian 1988). Almost all of the four-year-olds with low screening scores developed later reading problems, but only a little more than half of the children with later reading problems had scored below the screening cut-off as four-year-olds. There are two groups of children here, those whose global language impairment causes later reading impairment, and those whose dyslexia affects only a specific area of language development (see Catts 1989).

Specific Linguistic Deficits in Phonological Processing

Speech Perception Deficits. One recurring question in the field is whether or not difficulty with the phonological aspects of reading is caused by difficulty with auditory perception. No differences have been found between children with and without dyslexia in perception of nonverbal environmental sounds (Brady, Shankweiler, and Mann 1983; Godfrey et al. 1981). Possible difficulties appear related to speech sounds alone. Susan Brady and her colleagues at Haskins Laboratories have carried out a series of experiments comparing good and poor readers in ability to listen to words and repeat them back. In an early study there were no differences except when stimuli were presented under conditions of background noise (Brady, Shankweiler, and Mann 1983). In this study the words were all a single syllable in length. In a later study differences were found in listening and repeating back nonsense words and multisyllable words even in the absence of background noise. Brady hypothesizes that the difficulty is not at the perceptual level but at the level of phonological representation. This results in poor ability to encode phonological information. That is, under less than optimal conditions (unfamiliar words, long words, and under noisy conditions), children with this reading-related deficit have difficulty remembering sounds and encoding them into spoken reproductions (Brady, Poggie, and Rapala 1989).

Paula Tallal, who works with children with language deficits, observed a group of reading impaired children, not diagnosed as language impaired, who were deficient in discriminating tone sequences presented at rapid rates (Tallal 1980). Tallal and her colleague Rachel Stark suggest that there may be a subgroup of individuals with dyslexia who have a subtle auditory perceptual deficit characterized by difficulty in perceiving and analyzing rapidly presented speech sounds. They believe that this problem interferes with the ability to detect fine discriminations between phonemes in words and, consequently, with the ability to make connections between graphemes and phonemes in attempting to read (Tallal and Stark 1982). Tallal has recently suggested that there may be links between this impairment in rapid auditory processing and difficulties in the rapid processing of visual information (see above). Consistent with Tallal's argument, Stein (1993) reports an association between unstable binocular control, indicative of a deficient transient visual system, and deficits in phonological processing. Like Tallal, he indicates that both may be affected by a deficit at the neural level involving ability to process rapidly changing information.

Verbal Short-term Memory. Measures of ability to listen, remember, and repeat auditory stimuli have also been used to assess verbal short-term memory, but the stimuli tend to be longer than the single words used above in the auditory perception tasks. Individuals with dyslexia have been found to perform less well than same-age normal readers on tasks requiring them to repeat information verbatim (e.g., Mann, Liberman, and Shankweiler 1980). A number of studies comparing children of equivalent IQ, but of both high and low reading ability report deficits on the Digit Span subtest of the Wechsler Scales for the poor readers (see Jorm 1983). The idea here is that verbal information is held in memory more efficiently when it is stored in a phonological code. Individuals with impaired phonological processing have difficulty doing this. Holding meaningless material in short-term memory involves heavier demands on phonological coding than does memory for materials that are meaningful. For example, in a group of 6- and 7-year-olds referred for reading disorder, there was a significant discrepancy between ability to repeat sentences, the easier task for this group, and unrelated word strings, which was more difficult (Shepherd and Uhry 1993).

As Peter Bryant and Lynette Bradley point out, verbal short-term memory is another area in which one can question the causal role in reading. (Bryant and Bradley 1985). Does the pre-reading level of facility in remembering oral linguistic material drive later reading ability? Or is verbal short-term memory exercised during reading through needing to remember strings of words until the end of a sentence is reached? Bryant and Bradley make a strong case for this practice effect, and thus for the effect of reading on verbal memory. To test their hypothesis, they measured memory in 368 children over a period of four years. They found that verbal short-term memory at age 4 was not a very good predictor of reading at age 6, but that reading at age 6 was a good predictor of verbal short-term memory at age 8. Contradictory results are reported by Virginia Mann and Isabelle Liberman who found that memory for word strings in kindergarten predicted some of the variance in first-grade reading (Mann and Liberman 1984).

Speech Articulation Rate. It can be argued that at least some of the variance in verbal short-term memory tasks may be accounted for by motoric elements affecting articulation rate. That is, as a child prepares to repeat lists or sentences, they are retained in an *articulatory loop* in which material is rehearsed subvocally in order to retain it in short-term memory. Slowness in vocalization can cause the phonological impression to deteriorate and can interfere with accuracy of reproduction. This could be caused by speech-motor deficits. Peter Wolff and his colleagues at the Children's Hospital in Boston report evidence that both children and adults with dyslexia are slow and dysrhythmic when asked to repeat the same sequence of syllables (e.g., *pa-ta-ka*) over and over to the rhythm of a metronome. Furthermore, these speech motor deficits are correlated with deficits in reading (Wolff, Michel, and Ovrut 1990b). Hugh Catts reports similar findings. He found children with reading disorder to be significantly slower in repeating multisyllabic words when compared to normal readers (Catts 1986).

Rapid Naming. The length of time it takes to look at a visual stimulus and say its name is a good predictor of reading ability. Inability to retrieve the names of objects previously known is symptomatic of adult acquired aphasia. Early studies of children with anomia or word-finding problems have grown out of the literature on adult aphasia. One of the two formats commonly used for testing retrieval rate involves what is called *discrete trial* or *confrontational* naming in which objects are presented for naming one at a time. Earlier studies found that this format did not appear to be linked with dyslexia. For example, Maryanne Wolf found that confrontational naming using the Boston Naming Test (Kaplan, Goodglass, and Weintraub 1983) in kindergarten was correlated with later comprehension but not with decoding ability (Wolf and Goodglass 1986). In other studies, poor readers named colors, digits, and pictures as quickly as did good readers. It was only when naming written words (i.e., reading but not name finding) that poor readers did less well (Perfetti, Finger, and Hogaboam 1978; Stanovich 1981). However, recent studies suggest that this is a highly complex issue worth reexamining (see Wolf 1991 for a fuller description of the tasks and their link with dyslexia).

The second format, *continuous* or *serial naming*, involves a number of stimuli presented in linear format, and named in a series, one after the other. This form of retrieval difficulty appears to be unequivocally linked with dyslexia. Seminal work with an instrument for measuring the dyslexia-related second form, continuous or rapid serial naming, has been carried out by Martha Denckla and Rita Rudel. Called the Rapid Automatized Naming Test (RAN; Denckla and Rudel 1974, 1976a, 1976b), the instrument uses matrixes of the same five colors (and then numerals, pictured objects, and letters) repeated over and over in random serial order. Denckla and Rudel found that the length of time it took to name these stimuli varied with age; older children were quicker than younger children. It also varied with reading ability; good readers were quicker than poor readers at any given age (Denckla and Rudel 1974). This has been confirmed through more recent studies (e.g., Wolf 1986; Wolff, Michel, and Ovrut 1990a).

This task is similar to the act of reading. In both cases a child looks at a visual stimulus and speaks a response. It could be argued that good readers, in effect, practice for the RAN test when they practice reading, whereas poor readers, who read far fewer words in a day or a week, practice less and thus are slower on the RAN. The Oxford psychologist Peter Bryant and his research colleague Lynette Bradley have criticized the methods used in the Denckla and Rudel studies. As in the case of verbal short-term memory, they make the point that only through reading-age–match studies can rapid automatized naming be linked specifically with dyslexia, rather than with the early stages of reading. That is, if older dyslexics and younger normal readers who read at the same level were compared, and the dyslexics were still poorer than the normal readers, then slow retrieval rate could be linked to dyslexia with more confidence (Bryant and Bradley 1985). On the other hand, there are a number of studies in which retrieval rate in prereaders has been found to be an accurate predictor of later decoding ability (e.g., Wolf 1986). That is, slow retrieval rate is a precursor to, rather than result of, poor reading.

Phonological awareness.   The term phonological awareness refers to the metacognitive understanding that spoken language is made up of a series of sounds and that these sounds occupy a particular sequential order . Keep in mind that this is quite different from skills in phonics knowledge, a low–level paired–associate form of learning that relates letters and sounds on an automatic or rote level. The seminal work on phonological awareness in the United States involves a tapping task used by Isabelle Liberman together with her students at the University of Connecticut and her colleagues at Haskins Laboratories (Liberman, 1973; Liberman et al. 1974; Liberman et al. 1977). Liberman asked children to use a wooden dowel to tap the number of sounds they could hear in spoken sentences and then in words. She found that there was a developmental hierarchy with words in sentences easier to segment than syllables in words, which in turn were easier to tap than phonemes in single syllables. Virtually none of the children could represent phonemes accurately at age four, a few at age five, and most by age six. Liberman's work suggests that these tasks develop in a sequence, and that they develop late in children with reading disorder.

Several British researchers have provided evidence of a link between deficits in phonological awareness and deficits in reading. In a series of often cited case histories, Maggie Snowling and her colleagues document the pervasive phonological deficits of children with dyslexia seen over a period of time in a clinical setting (e.g., Snowling and Hulme 1989). While it has been argued that phonological awareness may be an effect of mature reading rather than its cause (Morais et al. 1979), it has also been demonstrated that the degree to which phonological awareness is developed prior to reading instruction plays a powerful role in determining reading outcomes (e.g., Bradley and Bryant 1983). In a reading-age match study, Snowling (1980) found that older poor readers matched on reading level with normal younger readers were much poorer at phonological tasks. This suggests that the deficit has a cause beyond lack of exposure to reading. It is likely that the relationship is reciprocal; phonological awareness drives reading in the early stages and then exposure to print increases phonological awareness once reading catches on.

Keith Stanovich has suggested that the entire range of difficulties often attributed to dyslexia may stem from what he calls the *phonological core deficit.* He argues that failure to learn to decode words because of phonological processing problems causes subsequent deficits in reading comprehension, vocabulary development, and even IQ through lack of access to print experiences. Stanovich calls this the *Matthew effect* from Bible verses in which the rich get richer and the poor get poorer. There is evidence that this phonological core deficit is of organic origin. There is also evidence that its symptoms are responsive to remediation.

NEUROLOGICAL AND BIOLOGICAL CORRELATES

Historically, overt neurological problems have been difficult to identify among children with dyslexia (Rutter 1978). Therefore, investigative efforts to understand the neurological underpinnings of dyslexia were focused historically on individual behavioral differences, thought to indicate neurological differences, with much of the exploration in the area of divergences in hemispheric specialization. The basic assumption behind this research has been that language processing in dyslexics may not be controlled by the same areas of the brain as in individuals without dyslexia. For the majority of the population, these areas lie in the left cerebral hemisphere. Much of this research examined *laterality differences* which were presumed to reflect *lateralization differences*. *Laterality* refers to the choice of hand, eye, or foot in performing everyday activities. *Lateralization* refers to "the involuntary brain functioning of the left and/ or right cerebral hemispheres" (Obrzut and Boliek 1986), otherwise called *hemispheric specialization*.

The relationship between left-handedness and reading disability has received considerable attention. Within the general population, the incidence of left-handedness has been estimated to be 8 to 10 percent (Kinsbourne and Hiscock 1981); lateralization indices are not as easily determined. Drake Duane, a neurologist, reported in 1983 that 98 percent of right-handed people and 70 percent of left-handed people have language lateralized in the left hemisphere (Duane 1983b). An interesting finding from one study (Hardyck and Petrinovich 1977) is that left-handers with a family history of left-handedness appear to have less hemispheric specialization than right-handers, whereas left-handers with no family history of left-handedness seem to process language in the left hemisphere like most right-handers. Confounding the issue is the possibility that some cases of left-handedness may be the result of early brain injury (Satz, Saslow, and Henry 1985). Clinical investigations of reading disorder may involve such *pathological left-handers* and cognitive deficits in such cases would more likely be due to cerebral insult than to deviant cerebral lateralization (Hiscock and Kinsbourne 1982). Any data pertaining to the connection between left-handedness and dyslexia, therefore, would be falsely skewed.

Among educators, psychologists, and neuropsychologists, opinions on the theorized association between handedness patterns and reading disability vary considerably. Finding left-handedness to be more common in males than females, the late Norman Geschwind, a neurologist who pioneered neurological research on the etiology of dyslexia, proposed a theory, based on epidemiological research, that links male sex, left-handedness, and autoimmune diseases to dyslexia (Geschwind 1983; Geschwind and Behan 1982). Further exploration of this hypothesized association has been carried out by Geschwind's colleagues at Beth Israel Hospital in Boston, principally Albert Galaburda (Galaburda 1985). The majority opinion among respected professionals exploring the link between left-handedness and dyslexia, however, is that we lack enough substantial data to draw definitive conclusions (Hiscock and Kinsbourne 1982).

In contrast to the unresolved issues related to handedness and dyslexia, the research indicates quite firmly that there is no significant link between eye preference and reading disability (Hiscock and Kinsbourne 1982; Obrzut and Boliek 1986; Rutter 1978).

Lateralization

Several measures of central language processing have been devised that are now considered to be better indices of cerebral lateralization than handedness. One of these measures is dichotic listening, where paired stimuli are presented simultaneously to each ear and the subject's response pattern, favoring one or the other ear, is thought to indicate the dominant hemisphere for that particular stimulus type: a right-ear advantage (REA) reflecting left-hemispheric processing and vice versa. Another measure, visual half-field (VHF) technique, involves presenting verbal or nonverbal stimuli tachistoscopically to either the left or right visual fields, or to both fields simultaneously in bilateral presentations. Response performance comparisons are considered to reflect degree of lateralization to one or the other hemisphere.

Cerebral Anomalies

A few postmortem anatomical studies have been conducted on the brains of persons previously diagnosed as dyslexic (e.g., Galaburda 1983, 1985; Galaburda and Kemper 1979). Although biological anomalies were indicated, the number of cases has not been sufficient to draw any definitive conclusions about the occurrence of cerebral abnormalities in dyslexics (Geschwind 1986). However, in the opinion of the investigators, one finding is considered particularly significant. Whereas in most individuals the left hemisphere is larger than the right, the dyslexic brains examined by Galaburda "showed deviation from the standard asymmetry pattern of the language regions, i.e., instead of a larger size of the left temporal language region there was symmetry" (Galaburda 1985). The symmetry appears due to a larger-than-normal right hemisphere in the brains of individuals with dyslexia. This finding has led Albert Galaburda to postulate that the etiology of dyslexia lies in abnormal migration of neural cells during fetal development (Galaburda, Rosen, and Sherman 1989).

Early efforts to look for possible cerebral abnormalities in dyslexic individuals involved a number of noninvasive techniques, such as *electroencephalography* (EEG), an electrical scanning procedure, and *computerized tomography* (CT), a radiological scanning technique. Neither of these brain scanning methods has been effective in identifying dyslexia (Connors 1978; Denckla 1978; Denckla, LeMay, and Chapman 1985; Duane 1983b). In a literature review on a more recent technique, *magnetic resonance imaging* (MRI), the above-mentioned earlier devices are described as somewhat imprecise (Filipek and Kennedy 1991). Even the CT scan, which provided an image of the brain, failed to do this with much clarity.

Until recently, studies of blood flow in the brain involved the radioactive isotopes used in *positron emission tomography* (PET) scans, which limited experimental use with children. Experiments with *magnetic resonance imaging* (MRI) are far less invasive and provide the sort of detailed picture available prior to MRI only through postmortem studies. Work with MRI indicates that there are physiological differences between individuals who read normally and those who are dyslexic. For example, Lubs and his colleagues found differences in patterns of asymmetry in the two hemispheres; whereas normal readers tend to be asymmetrical in the angular gyrus area of the parietal lobe, with left side larger than right, the pattern is reversed with individuals who are dyslexic (Lubs et al. 1991). In another example of imaging techniques, Frank Wood and his colleagues at Bowman Gray Medical Center have carried out studies indicating that blood flow differences involving Wernicke's area of the left hemisphere are present in adults diagnosed with dyslexia as children, in comparison with those without a history of reading disorder. These studies were carried out during performance of an auditory-to-orthography task; subjects were asked to indicate whether a word they heard had four letters (Flowers 1993; Wood et al. 1991).

The value of this recent ability to form an image of the brain of a living person engaged in a specific linguistic task lies not so much in diagnostic benefit for individuals, as in its ability to confirm that dyslexia is an organic disorder.

Attention Deficit Disorder and Dyslexia

Up until fairly recently the distinction between children with dyslexia, and those classified as learning disabled who read poorly and also had behavior problems, was not made clear in much of the research literature. One important recent step has involved isolating *attention deficit disorder* with and without *hyperactivity disorder* (ADD/ADHD) as distinct from other learning disorders.

During the 1960s and 70s, the term *minimal brain dysfunction* (MBD) was used to describe children assumed to have subtle neurological problems causing both learning and behavior problems (e.g., Clements and Peters 1962). Neurological *soft signs* such as reflexes or borderline performance on the EEG were used diagnostically by the medical community. These children were often assumed to have suffered birth injuries resulting in erratic behavior and learning problems. They most likely shared symptoms with the brain injured children described earlier by Werner and Strauss (1940; or see Farnham-Diggory 1992). There was never clear agreement in the educational and medical communities on either diagnostic procedures or a clinical profile for MBD and the concept lost favor by the 1980s. It is now believed that many of these children may have suffered from ADHD among other conditions.

Recent work by Sally and Bennett Shaywitz of the Yale University School of Medicine, and others in the field, has helped to identify ADD more easily and to differentiate it from learning disabilities. The Shaywitzes have developed what they call the Yale Children's Inventory (YCI), which includes a parent questionnaire about behavior (Shaywitz et al. 1988). The YCI examines academic, language, and fine motor development as well as behaviors such as attention, activity, and negative affect. Portions of this questionnaire are reprinted in a book edited by the Shaywitzes that summarizes some of the recent work on ADD (Shaywitz and Shaywitz 1992). The YCI was used with 445 children who participated in the Connecticut Longitudinal Study. Data including the YCI as well as school-based testing were collected on all of the kindergarten children from 12 Connecticut towns at the beginning of the 1983-84 school year and again during the spring of their second- and fourth-grade years. Results from this study have helped clarify the relationship between ADD and reading and other academic problems. Based on findings from this unreferred population, as well as from other sources, the Shaywitzes report that somewhere between 10 and 20 percent of children have ADD (Shaywitz and Shaywitz 1991).

The relationship between reading disorder and ADD is complex. There is evidence that the two syndromes represent independent factors. That is, either syndrome can exist with or without the other. In a clinic-referred population of 192 children studied at the University of Arkansas Child Study Center, roughly 50 percent of those who met criteria for ADD from the Diagnostic and Statistical Manual of Mental Disorders (DSM III) also had specific reading problems using the criteria of reading scores that were significantly lower than Verbal scale IQ. That is, not all children with ADD have specific reading difficulty (Dykman and Ackerman 1991). The degree of overlap between these syndromes tends to depend on whether or not subjects are studied by researchers through a school system or through a referred clinic population. As many as 80 percent of clinic-referred children with academic disorders were found to have ADD in very early studies, whereas only about 30 percent of the children with reading disorder in the Connecticut Longitudinal Study had concomitant ADD (Shaywitz 1986).

In looking at the ADD-reading relationship Frank Wood and Rebecca Felton report three longitudinal studies carried out through the Bowman Gray Medical Center with both children and adults. These studies indicated that while ADD certainly predicts academic success in general, it does not predict specific success or failure at the word-reading level (Wood and Felton 1994). In one of these studies, 485 children were followed from first to fifth grade. Specific linguistic factors related to phonological processing were far better at predicting later word-level reading ability than were measures of ADD (Felton and Wood 1989). In other words, while ADD and dyslexia can be *comorbid*, or both present in the same child, they are separate factors and ADD does not appear to affect the acquisition of word-level decoding skills in a specific way.

The Shaywitzes have reported evidence that silent reading comprehension difficulties may be associated with ADD (Shaywitz 1993). This may be because ADD involves a generalized inability to attend during complex tasks that need a high degree of self-monitoring, rather than a difficulty specific to reading.

While ADD is a distinct neurological syndrome, it is not necessarily present as a condition of dyslexia. Failure in early research to describe the ADD status of subjects with reading disorder may have provided us with a picture of the child with dyslexia as having behavioral symptoms or reading comprehension difficulties more typical of ADD than of dyslexia. Researchers such as Wood and Felton and the Shaywitzes have helped to clarify these issues.

Heritability

Clinicians have long been convinced that dyslexia runs in families. They often find a parent or sibling with dyslexia when collecting data on family history in the initial phase of an evaluation or in preparation for tutoring a referred child.

Recent research carried out as part of the Colorado Twin Study has provided convincing evidence that relatives of dyslexics are more predisposed to dyslexia than individuals in families of good readers. With the genetic etiology of dyslexia in mind, the Twin Study was carried out by John DeFries and his colleagues. This involved collecting data on pairs of twins, both identical (*monozygotic* or MZ) and nonidentical or fraternal (*dizygotic* or DZ) twins, from 27 Colorado school districts. Initial data was used to screen for any set of twins in which there was at least one member with a history of school reading problems. Extensive testing of IQ, reading level, phonological awareness, and eye movements was carried out, as well as tests to confirm *zygosity* (the twin relationship). Ninety-nine identical pairs were identified, as well as 73 same-sex and 39 different-sex pairs of fraternal twins. If dyslexia were primarily of environmental influence one would expect roughly the same number of co-occurring instances of dyslexia in fraternal as in identical twins. That is, what the researchers call the *concordance* rate should be the same in the two sets of twins. However, this was not the case. In 70 percent of the identical pairs, when one twin had a reading disorder, the other did as well, while in the fraternal twins the concordance rate was only 48 percent (DeFries et al. 1991). These rates confirm findings from earlier, smaller studies from other researchers, in suggesting the heritability of dyslexia.

An interesting additional finding from the Twin Study involved analysis of phonological processing data. While there was a strong genetic influence on phonological skills, this was not the case with orthographic skills. That is, when subjects were poor at reading and weak phonological processing skills, there was a genetic link. This was not so when orthographic processing was considered. These findings are consistent with those of a British twin study in which the genetic component of spelling disorder appears to influence phonology but not orthography (Stevenson 1991).

Using a different model but asking a similar question, Herbert Lubs and his colleagues also find a familial predisposition to dyslexia. Eleven families with dyslexic members were traced for three generations in an attempt to locate a gene leading to dyslexia. The pattern of inheritance that emerges from this and other studies is called *autosomal dominant inheritance* (Lubs et al. 1993). Some unaffected members appear to carry the gene but remained asymptomatic, while others appear to have recovered or compensated. The latter are more apt to be women than men.

A number of recent studies have tried to identify a gene for dyslexia. For example, Shelley Smith and her colleagues have worked on gene localization using a technique called *sib pairs*, in which DNA samples are analyzed in pairs of siblings. The argument for this technique is that pairs of siblings who are both dyslexic will have similar DNA in regard to the dyslexia gene, while this will not be the case in disconcordant pairs. Smith found encouraging results for both chromosome 6 and chromosome 15 (Smith, Kimberling, and Pennington 1991). A more recent study favors chromosome 6 (Cardon et al. 1994). This work is in the very early stages and caution should be exercised in interpreting results.

While there is much still to be learned about the genetic characteristics of dyslexia, it does seem clear at this time that it can be inherited. Bruce Pennington, one of the principal researchers in the Colorado Reading Study, cites evidence that dyslexia is both "familial (about 35%-40% of first degree relatives are affected),", and "heritable (with a transmission rate of about 50%)" (Pennington 1991, p. 48).

GENDER

The stereotype of the male dyslexic grew out of statistical descriptions based on children referred to clinics and to special school placements.

Using these samples, it looked as though there were roughly four times as many boys as girls with dyslexia or severe reading disorder (Vogel 1990). Recent re-evaluation of these ratios has been carried out in projects involving, for example, the Connecticut Longitudinal Studies (Shaywitz et al. 1990), Bowman Gray Medical Center (Wood et al. 1991), and the Colorado Reading Project (DeFries et al. 1991). Instead of figuring ratios of boys to girls in samples of referred children, these studies tested large numbers of children within school districts. When tallies were kept of the number of children whose reading was lower than expectations based on IQ, there were close to as many girls as boys with reading deficits. One possible explanation of the discrepancy is that boys are referred more often than girls because they are more apt to have attentional and behavioral problems (Vogel 1990) and thus their reading problems are more visible than those of girls.

ACADEMIC MANIFESTATIONS OF DYSLEXIA

Dyslexia is generally perceived first and foremost as a word-reading disorder. At the time of the first edition of this book there was fairly general agreement in the field that along with this word-level reading disorder there might be a wide range of other disorders including persistent difficulty in spelling, phonological processing, reading rate, comprehension, expressive writing, and handwriting. The picture has shifted toward primary deficits in phonologically driven word-level reading as the area of deficit in dyslexia as several large-scale federally funded studies have provided better control in terms of careful description of the samples of children examined.

ORAL READING

Word Attack Skills

The most pronounced among the reading difficulties that individuals with dyslexia experience is the inability to decode unfamiliar words (e.g., Olson et al. 1985; Siegel 1985; Vellutino 1983). This problem appears to be the common denominator in all cases of dyslexia (Gough and Tunmer 1986).

The basis for the decoding deficiencies among dyslexic readers is believed to be a deficit in phonological processing that affects ability to make use of letter-sound associations (i.e., phonics knowledge) possibly as an effect of rapid retrieval problems. Deficits in understanding the sound structure of speech (phonological awareness) confound mastery of the relationship between sounds in speech and letters in words. In short, children with dyslexia have extraordinary difficulty in using word attack skills to read words they have not committed to memory. These children have trouble breaking down spoken words in order to identify their component parts when they spell, and in blending together these parts into words when they read. Sound sequencing errors (articulating letter sounds in the wrong order), as well as letter-sound confusions (producing the wrong sound for a given letter or letters), are often observed in their oral reading. Word attack skills have proven to be the most sensitive identifier of disabled readers (Read and Ruyter 1985; Richardson, DiBenedetto, and Adler 1982; Ryan, Miller, and Witt 1984; Siegel 1985).

Nonsense words are widely used to measure ability to use word attack skills to read unfamiliar words. This task seems artificial, especially to advocates of a meaning-based approach, but keep in mind that many syllables in long words are nonsense words until the full word has been decoded. For example, the syllable *lan* has no meaning until all of the word *Atlantic* has been decoded.

Studies documenting the nonsense-word-reading deficit are often carried out through matching dyslexic and normal readers by word recognition level. The question here is, do the older children with dyslexia, matched on real-word reading level with younger normal readers, have more difficulty in reading nonwords? Maggie Snowling provided early documentation of the nonword reading deficit in a *reading-age-match* (RAM) comparison in which children were asked to respond to words using pairs of modalities (visual-visual, auditory-auditory, visual-auditory) and say whether the words were the same or not. Children with dyslexia were as competent as normal readers in making same-different judgements in pairs such as *torp* and *trop* in the visual-visual and auditory-auditory modes. Only when they needed to see one word in print and listen to the other did they have substantially more difficulty than normal readers (Snowling 1980).

In another often-cited study, Richard Olson and his colleagues made a similar comparison of 15-year-olds with dyslexia and 10-year-old normal readers. They were asked which of a pair of written words (e.g., caik-dake) sounded like a real word. The older readers were poorer than the younger normal readers, despite the match in real word reading level (Olson et al. 1985). In a more recent study with much larger numbers of students, including twin pairs from the Colorado Twin Study, this phonological coding deficit was confirmed, as was its heritability (Olson et al. 1989).

Word Recognition

If individuals with dyslexia are not facile at decoding unfamiliar words, how do they read? One argument is that they compensate by using an area of strength to make up for their phonological weakness and that this strength involves visual memory for letter strings, which is considered an orthographic skill. Richard Olson tested this theory in an experiment using the same 15 year-old-dyslexic and 10-year-old-normal readers tested for phonological ability above. This time he asked them to choose between two phonologically similar written words, one real and the other its pseudohomophone (e.g., *street-streat*). The task here is essentially one of proof reading. Which word looks right? Here the two groups did not differ. Keep in mind, however, that the children with dyslexia were five years older than the normal readers. These children's strength in orthography is a relative one in comparison with their weakness in phonological skills. Compared to normal readers of their own age, they read far fewer words (Olson et al. 1989).

Dyslexia is most evident when words are presented in isolation (Perfetti 1984; Stanovich 1980). This is logical because children with dyslexia are relatively strong in comprehension. Understanding a paragraph can help in understanding an unknown word. Once enough words have been learned to enable at least some degree of comprehension, then comprehension enables decoding of unfamiliar words.

Reading Rate

Word recognition skills improve with remediation, and there is even evidence that word attack skills can be improved through intensive training in phonological awareness, but individuals with dyslexia continue to read more slowly than normal readers. That is, accuracy can be remediated more effectively than rate. Much of the recent research on reading rate has been carried out through the Colorado Reading Project in the laboratories of Richard Olson. He and his colleagues have found significant differences between readers with and without dyslexia in vocal response latencies — the time between presentation of a stimulus and a subject's response — when single words are presented on a computer screen.

Another way of looking at rate is to time entire passages of text. P. G. Aaron and Scott Phillips examined the academic skills of college students with dyslexia and found their reading comprehension scores to be well above these students' own scores for reading rate (Aaron and Phillips 1986).

SPELLING PROBLEMS

For individuals with dyslexia, spelling presents even greater challenges than reading. While reading is remediable to some degree, spelling deficits appear to persist through adulthood (Aaron and Phillips 1986; Cone et al. 1985; Ganschow 1984; Rutter 1978).

Roderick Barron (1980) observes that poor readers are more likely to use a visual-orthographic strategy in reading and to apply a phonological strategy to spelling. Lynette Bradley and Peter Bryant find this same strategy differential in young normal readers (Bradley 1985; Bradley and Bryant 1979). They believe that the independence of reading and spelling behaviors is a natural developmental phenomenon; young children who have not yet learned to read often spell words on the basis of sound. Are children with dyslexia simply behind on a developmental continuum, or do they spell differently from children without dyslexia?

In a recent analysis of the spelling errors of children who are dyslexic but have received intensive remediation, Mary Kibel and T. R. Miles found persistent difficulty with a type of errors not found in spelling-age matched controls. The errors involved both cluster reduction (e.g., spelling *blend* as "bend") and substitution of phonologically confusable pairs (e.g., *e/a, b/d, r/l*). These errors are consistent with Tallal's theory that individuals with dyslexia experience difficulty processing rapid acoustic information (Kibel and Miles 1994). These findings are consistent with several other studies. A similar analysis by Louisa Moats produced evidence of cluster reductions and unstressed syllable reductions in the spelling errors of third and fifth grade children with dyslexia, again in comparison with spelling-age matched controls (Moats 1993). Maggie Bruck and Rebecca Treiman have also found consonant clusters to be particularly troublesome for spellers with dyslexia (Bruck and Treiman 1990). These studies are more sophisticated than earlier ones that attempted to categorize errors as either phonological or orthographic, in that highly specific phonological processing deficits are the focus here, rather than a wider array of phonetic errors.

The unanswered question here is why individuals with dyslexia appear better able to compensate for phonological processing deficits in reading than in spelling. If orthographic spelling develops over time through exposure to print, this should fall into place eventually, after remediation of reading. It may be that orthographic processing in spelling is particularly dependent on successful phonological processing and subsequent representations of the sound structure of words.

READING COMPREHENSION

Children with dyslexia have been found to be poorer at reading comprehension than good readers, which is consistent with Philip Gough and William Tunmer's simple view of reading (1986). If decoding is poor, even in the presence of well developed listening comprehension, then reading comprehension will be poor. This is also consistent with Keith Stanovich's Matthew effect (1986b). Reading comprehension is a skill that needs development over time; it is difficult to practice comprehension if decoding is undeveloped.

Lack of reading accuracy and automatic recognition at the word level appear to place limitations on the comprehension of text, as well as on reading fluency (Stanovich, Cunningham, and Feeman 1984). David La Berge and S. Jay Samuels (1974) attempted to explain this apparent trade off in attentional resources by hypothesizing a limited capacity mechanism in working memory. In the same vein, Charles Perfetti (1984, 1985b) proposes a verbal efficiency mechanism to account for the strong relationship between speed and accuracy of word identification and reading comprehension shown in correlational studies.

Tests of the simple view of reading indicate that reading comprehension cannot surpass its two components, word decoding and listening comprehension (Hoover 1994). However, this data comes from very large numbers of readers drawn from the general population of school children. In examining the relationship between decoding and comprehension in readers with dyslexia in the Colorado Twin Study, Richard Olson and his colleagues provide a different story. When children with dyslexia were matched with controls in regard to timed word recognition ability, their comprehension levels were significantly higher on several measures. Keep several things in mind. The match was on *timed* word reading. Had accuracy been the matching criterion the match would have been with higher functioning controls. Also, the children with dyslexia were older and thus had an intellectual advantage.

Maggie Bruck reports similar data from a study of college-age students with dyslexia. Some of these subjects comprehended very well despite poor decoding skills. Bruck proposes the possibility of what she calls a *minimum threshold level* for word recognition, saying, "Once critical levels of word-recognition skill have been achieved, variation in comprehension levels may be best accounted for by higher level component processes" (Bruck 1990, p. 450). That is, bright individuals with dyslexia use their oral language strengths (e.g., vocabulary, general knowledge, interpretation of context) to compensate for weak decoding skills.

LISTENING COMPREHENSION

Counter to current definitions provided by research, historically, children described as dyslexic were found to have deficits in a range of oral language skills including listening comprehension (Smiley et al. 1977), understanding complex sentences in speech as well as reading (Byrne 1981; Vogel 1975), and in grammatical understanding and morphological knowledge (Byrne 1981; Menynuk and Flood 1981). Keep in mind that attention deficit disorder is associated with deficits in both listening and reading comprehension, but not with decoding deficits. Until recently, control for this factor has not been a systematic part of research studies on reading comprehension. It may account for some of the variation in listening comprehension in many individuals who are also dyslexic.

While the research is both clear and clearly articulated on this point, the term *dyslexia* continues to be used with many children who appear to have language deficits beyond the phonological domain. While The Orton Dyslexia Society has adapted a phonologically oriented definition of dyslexia for research purposes, it uses a second, broader definition in order to be able to procure special dyslexia-oriented services for children with a range of language-related problems. Their definition is not limited to phonological difficulties, but includes more global deficits in expressive and receptive language (The Orton Dyslexia Society 1994).

Keith Stanovich is an advocate of limiting the term *dyslexia* to individuals with a discrepancy between listening and reading comprehension (Stanovich 1988a, 1988b), which makes it strictly a reading problem. Hugh Catts calls it a language problem but limits it to those aspects of language that are phonological (Catts 1989). Catts' model is consistent with that of Isabelle Liberman and her colleagues, who have led this line of research. Liberman maintained that as we read or listen we must hold incoming linguistic information in working memory in phonological form while we process sentences (e.g., Liberman and Shankweiler 1985; Mann, Shankweiler, and Smith 1984). Thus, the deficit that affects reading also affects listening. Support for this view can be found in a recent study carried out in Australia by Gail Gillon and Barbara Dodd. They tested poor readers, ages 8-10 years, matched on reading level with younger good readers, using a number of measures of phonological processing as well as measures of syntax and semantics. While the poor readers were weaker than reading-age-match controls in all oral language areas, they were particularly poor in phonological processing (Gillon and Dodd 1994).

Another explanation of weak listening skills in older students with dyslexia is linked to Stanovich's Matthew effect. Because of their general lack of reading experience some dyslexic individuals may fail to develop a strong knowledge base, which further limits their ability to comprehend and remember text material (Stanovich 1986b; Torgesen 1985). Insufficient background knowledge can be considered a second-order comprehension problem. It is most likely that both phonological processing deficiencies and lack of reading experience contribute to lowered levels of listening comprehension when this occurs.

Maggie Bruck has not found diminished levels of either listening comprehension or verbal IQ in adults with dyslexia (1990). Her data suggest a hierarchy of skills in both high- and average-IQ adults with dyslexia, in which low-level, phonologically driven skills such as nonsense-word reading are less developed than high-level skills such as reading and listening comprehension. Whether or not listening has been diminished by phonological processing deficits, there is agreement that decoding is poorer than reading comprehension, which, in turn, is poorer than oral language skills.

EXPRESSIVE WRITING PROBLEMS

While poor spelling is a well documented characteristic of dyslexia, little research exists on the written expression problems associated with dyslexia. When we consider the three potential areas of writing difficulties for individuals with dyslexia — composition, spelling, and handwriting (Cicci 1983) — spelling stands out as by far the most prevalent area of deficit (Ganschow 1984; Poplin et al. 1980). Other types of deficiencies can also be found in the writing samples of dyslexic students — for example, poor punctuation, word omissions, lack of subject/ predicate number agreement, and lower percentages of compound and/ or complex sentences — but there is little consistent documentation of their prevalence. In a study in which students with learning disabilities were asked to dictate stories to an examiner and then to write stories by hand or on a word processor, the dictated stories were significantly longer, of better quality, and contained fewer grammatical errors. These findings suggest that "...mechanical and conventional demands of producing text appear to interfere with the fluency and quality of written expression" (MacArthur and Graham 1988). It can be argued that deficits in spelling absorb so much energy and attention that all other aspects of writing are diminished in quality (Uhry and Shepherd 1993b).

Perhaps the most serious writing problem among individuals who are dyslexic is a general resistance to writing. As Diana King (1985), who works with adolescents, affirms, without remedial intervention this resistance tends to build throughout the school years.

HANDWRITING PROBLEMS

Research on handwriting is minimal, and there is no reliable standardized measurement instrument to evaluate letter and word formations (Cicci 1983). Visual memory deficits, fine motor problems, or slow rate of execution may all interfere with handwriting, but these are not deficits specifically associated with dyslexia. It is not far-fetched to suggest that emotional factors may also contribute to poor handwriting, given the lack of confidence most individuals with dyslexia have in their spelling abilities. No systematic analysis of these difficulties or of their relationship to dyslexia has been made.

RECURRING QUESTIONS
SUBTYPES OR UNITARY DISORDER?

A question that has provoked specialists and researchers for some time is whether dyslexia is a unique syndrome or whether it comprises a number of identifiable subcategories. The question has led to studies aimed at classifying dyslexia into discrete subtypes based on patterns of symptoms.

Subtyping research began many years ago with M. Kinsbourne and E. K. Warrington (1963). They distinguish two groups of poor readers having more than a 20 point discrepancy between verbal and performance IQ on the Wechsler Intelligence Scale (Duane 1983a):

children with lower verbal IQ scores appear to have language related deficits whereas those with lower performance IQ scores demonstrate perceptual and visual–motor impairments. Note, however, that while low Verbal scale IQ is associated with language disorder, it is not a characteristic of dyslexia.

Some researchers have based subtypes on spelling errors. Elena Boder (1971), for example, claims to find three distinct spelling patterns among individuals with dyslexia. She terms these error patterns *dysphonetic* (reflecting deficits in sound-symbol association), *dyseidetic* (representing difficulty remembering visual aspects of words with nonphonetic spellings), and *dysphonetic-dyseidetic* (a combination of both problems). Attempts to validate Boder's subtypes, however, have not been successful (Carpenter , 1983; Moats 1983; Nockleby and Galbraith 1984). In a recent study, Dale Willows and Gillian Jackson found Boder's categorization measures to be unreliable in terms of consistency between examiners (Willows and Jackson 1992).

Rebecca Treiman and Jonathan Baron (1983) examine spelling behaviors in dyslexia from the perspective of rule application. They find evidence of individuals with dyslexia who are overly reliant on spelling-sound rules, whom they have labeled *Phoenecians,* and a group who depend on word-specific associations, whom they call *Chinese*. These investigators allege that the Phoenician is able to spell nonsense words but tends to over-generalize phonics rules to exception words.

Another approach to the subtyping of dyslexia involves a dichotomy between what is called *surface dyslexia*, or failure on an orthographic level to move directly from print to meaning, and *deep dyslexia*, or failure in using phonological processes to decode unfamiliar words. This dichotomy is consistent with the dual route theory of processing in which either the direct lexical route or the phonological route is used. The terminology comes from studies of adults who were once normal readers and who lost either one ability or the other following brain damage (Patterson, Marshall, and Coltheart 1985). When used with children these terms are altered to *developmental surface dyslexia* and *developmental deep dyslexia*.

In a review of the literature on nonsense word reading John Rack, Maggie Snowling, and Richard Olson make the point that while studies using large numbers of subjects generally fail to distribute all subjects into distinct subtypes, not all individuals with dyslexia have the same profiles (Rack, Snowling, and Olson 1992). Snowling and her colleagues have documented a number of case histories of children with average or higher IQ scores and extraordinary difficulty with word reading and these profiles fall into two types, children with phonological deficits and those with visual memory deficits (Goulandris and Snowling 1991; Snowling, Goulandris, and Stackhouse 1994; Snowling and Hulme 1989).

At this point there is no single subtype classification system that is supported by a comprehensive body of research or that is useful in choosing remedial programs for children with dyslexia. While 25 years ago practitioners tried to match children with instruction depending on whether they were considered to be *auditory learners* or *visual learners*, there is no research base to support this dichotomy as a construct. The best practice involves teaching children to coordinate these two systems because both are crucial to skilled reading.

How Distinct is Dyslexia from "Normal" Reading?

Another argument in the field involves the conceptualization of dyslexia as an *either-or* condition. Is it, like pregnancy, a condition that one either has or does not have? Or, like blood pressure, is it on a scale ranging from normal to abnormal by degrees? In an often cited study, Rutter and Yule (1975) tested a large number of children in reading and demonstrated a statistical hump toward the low end of the bell curve, creating a bimodal distribution. That is, in addition to the distribution of readers, ranging from poor, to average, to strong along a normal curve, clustered around the mean, there was a second, smaller cluster of poor readers at the low end of the curve. These readers, they argue, represent a group of disabled readers distinct from the normal distribution.

In a recent study that challenges this finding, Sally Shaywitz and her colleagues tested children participating in the Connecticut Longitudinal Study on a number of measures over several years. Twenty-four intact kindergarten classes in twelve schools were randomly chosen from the state of Connecticut to participate in the study. The sample is reported by the study to be 84 percent non-Hispanic white, 11 percent Black, 2 percent Hispanic, and .9 percent Asian. Data on the 445 children were collected over a number of years. Children with dyslexia were identified through discrepancies between IQ and reading scores in first grade and then tested again in grades three and five. The Rutter and Yule model of dyslexia as a discrete condition would predict that once children were classified as dyslexic they would remain in this category, but this did not turn out to be the case. There were substantial shifts, both into and out of the dyslexia category, with each new testing period (Shaywitz et al. 1992).

Is There Recovery from Dyslexia?

There was some initial criticism of the Shaywitz study, centered on the claim that the results were misleadingly optimistic in terms of the prognosis for individuals with dyslexia (e.g., Duane 1992). Other research leads us to believe that children do not spontaneously recover from dyslexia. Furthermore, symptoms such as slow reading rate and difficulty with nonsense-word reading often persist into adulthood, even in individuals with dyslexia who have become successful academically (e.g., Bruck 1990).

Symptoms persist on an organic level as well. Frank Wood and his colleague Lynn Flowers have examined adults first diagnosed by Samuel Orton. Many of these individuals with dyslexia were tutored as children by Orton's wife, June Lyday Orton. Brain differences in regard to blood flow were found in these individuals as adults even in cases where reading had been successfully remediated during childhood (Flowers 1993; Wood 1993). When these same adults were examined for neuropsychological residue of dyslexia, they were found to have deficits in nonword reading, phonological awareness and rapid automatized naming (Felton, Naylor, and Wood 1990). Of the three symptoms, rapid automatized naming seems to be the most pervasive and to determine the degree to which recovery from dyslexia is possible (Wood and Felton 1994). There is evidence, by contrast, that phonological awareness and nonsense word reading are remediable to some degree (e.g., Alexander et al. 1991; Kibel and Miles 1994; Shepherd and Uhry 1993; Uhry 1994; Wise et al. 1989). Put in terms of word-reading, accuracy can be improved over time, but reading rate remains slow.

Recovery-rate research is hard to interpret because of inconsistent documentation of the characteristics of subjects and instruction across studies. Are there some symptoms of dyslexia that are easier to remediate than others? Is it important to begin early? What methods work best? At present, two large-scale longitudinal treatment studies are being carried out by research teams in Florida (Torgesen 1985) and Texas (Foorman, Francis, and Fletcher 1995). Results should clarify the extent to which recovery from dyslexia is possible.

SUMMARY

Dyslexia, then, is a reading disability at the word-reading level. It runs in families and is of fairly certain organic origin. Historically, dyslexia has been associated with both visual deficits and phonological processing deficits but not with global language deficits. At this time, the most compelling body of evidence points to phonological processing as the predominant cause. A number of reading-related treatments have been found to be effective in remediating phonological awareness deficits, but low-level cognitive skills such as spelling and timed oral reading never develop as fully as reading comprehension, which is a high-level cognitive skill.

The following chapter presents a conceptual plan and practical suggestions for the educational assessment of individuals with dyslexia based on the research discussed above.

3

Assessment for Dyslexia

The assessment of a child who is struggling to learn to read should help to answer two important questions. Is the child dyslexic? And how can we formulate a plan to facilitate reading? In providing guidelines for assessing children with reading difficulty, this chapter draws on two sources of knowledge. The first involves the results of recent research. Since the first edition of this book (Clark 1988), substantial federal funding has culminated in clearer descriptions of dyslexia. Many of the references in this chapter are taken from the record of an April 1992 National Institutes of Health (NIH) conference on learning disabilities assessment (Lyon 1994). The second source involves practice at the Teachers College, Columbia University Child Study Center[1]. The following discussion of assessment for dyslexia is intended to answer the sorts of questions often asked by clinicians about putting theory into practice. The chapter ends with a description of the evaluation of a child with dyslexia.

---

[1] The Child Study Center is a site within the Department of Special Education at Teachers College, Columbia University designed for the practical training of graduate students in the diagnosis and remediation of children with special needs. Both authors worked there as clinicians, and the second author served as Director for five years. The pronoun *we*, used throughout this chapter, refers to the group of faculty, clinicians, and students who collaborated at the Child Study Center during the early 1990s on what we call *the dyslexia project*. This was an exploration of the clinical description of dyslexia and of effective strategies for its remediation (Shepherd and Uhry 1993; Uhry in press). Notes on the assessment of the student KM come from several formal evaluations conducted by Margaret Jo Shepherd and from ongoing, research-based assessment by Joanna Uhry.

BACKGROUND INFORMATION AND
PSYCHOLOGICAL PROFILE

The term *assessment*, means the general process of inquiry, both formal and informal, used to answer questions — in this case, questions about a child's learning problems. The term *educational evaluation*, refers to the formal process of gathering background information, formulating hypotheses, choosing and administering measures to test hypotheses, and writing up a report with a logical presentation of conclusions. In many ways the two terms refer to the same process, but assessment tends to be ongoing, whereas an educational evaluation takes place at a specific time.

An educational evaluation of a child suspected of having dyslexia should be carried out by an educational evaluator with special reading expertise, in consultation with a psychologist. The role of the psychologist is to provide IQ testing in order to explore cognitive functioning, as well as personality testing, which can provide insight into emotional issues that might be factors in school difficulty.

The purpose of the evaluation should be clarified at the onset. Is classification for special school services the goal? Is a new school or tutor the issue? Is the purpose to come up with a remedial plan including teaching materials and methods? Will an older student want to use the evaluation report to qualify for untimed school tests or college entry exams? Both family and student should have a voice concerning the purpose of the evaluation and should understand possible benefits. Both should be involved in feedback sessions.

An educational evaluation should begin with a thorough history. Have family members had reading difficulty? The Colorado Twin Study indicates that dyslexia is familial (DeFries et al. 1991; Olson et al. 1989; Olson et al. 1990). Have there been prolonged absences during critical periods in reading acquisition? What reading methods are used in school? Weakness in phonics can be exacerbated by lack of instruction. Virginia Berninger and Robert Abbott make the point that we ought to be looking at failure to respond to appropriate instruction over time as an indicator of disability (Berninger and Abbott 1994).

The actual testing process should be conceptualized as having three phases. Results from the first establish a diagnosis of dyslexia using a discrepancy model. The second phase looks for the phonological processing deficits often associated with dyslexia. The third provides an inventory of which reading and writing skills and strategies are solid and which ones remain to be taught. This third step serves as a guide in planning remediation. In reading the following, keep in mind that it is a framework for testing many possible hypotheses. All of the following would be too much for any one child. Tests and procedures should be selected to answer particular questions or to provide a baseline measure against which to measure future growth.

PHASE I: DISCREPANCIES

The first phase of evaluation for dyslexia includes the use of standardized test scores to establish average or higher IQ (i.e., an IQ above 85) and a discrepancy between word-reading and other verbal abilities. This discrepancy is the key element in the first phase; the diagnosis of dyslexia rests on evidence of specific reading-related weaknesses in the presence of statistically stronger oral comprehension.

DISCREPANCIES BETWEEN IQ AND READING ACHIEVEMENT

While there is controversy about the use of IQ testing in the diagnosis of dyslexia (e.g., Siegel 1989; Stanovich 1991), it is still standard practice to look for a discrepancy between Verbal Scale IQ[2] and reading comprehension achievement scores. The Reading Comprehension subtest from the Wechsler Individual Achievement Tests (WIAT; Wechsler 1992) provides an ideal way to do this because the WIAT is normed on the same population sample as the Wechsler Intelligence Scales for Children (WISC-III; Wechsler 1991). The WIAT manual provides tables of score differences that can be considered significantly discrepant. IQ-achievement discrepancies can also be established by using the Woodcock-Johnson (Woodcock and Mather 1989a; 1989b) and Kaufman (Kaufman and Kaufman 1983; 1985) batteries. However, the Wechsler is considered the IQ test of choice by most psychologists. Linda Siegel (1989) makes the point that the relationship between achievement and IQ is most likely bidirectional. In support of this point, in our clinical practice we have seen IQ scores fall over time when children are not reading. With older, reading-deprived and thus vocabulary- and knowledge-deprived children, an experienced clinician needs to weigh data from a number of tests to make a diagnosis.

DISCREPANCIES BETWEEN AND WITHIN ACADEMIC DOMAINS

Discrepancy evidence to support the hypothesis of dyslexia is routinely sought in other areas as well. Keith Stanovich (1991) suggests comparing listening comprehension and reading comprehension to avoid the use of IQ tests. It is important to choose two tests from the same battery; the two tests are thus normed on the same sample. It is

---

[2]A finding of low reading and high Verbal Scale IQ indicates a bright child with dyslexia. A finding of low reading, low Verbal Scale IQ, and High Performance Scale IQ indicates a bright child with a language disorder. A finding of low reading and low Full Scale IQ indicates low reading which is part of all-around low performance as in Stanovich's *garden variety poor reader.*

common practice in reading assessment to compare comprehension of a passage a child reads aloud with comprehension of a parallel passage read to the child by the examiner. Keep in mind that any conclusion needs to consider idiosyncratic background knowledge; does this child really understand better when he listens or does he just know a lot more about baseball than about the topic of the parallel passage he read himself? In contrast, scores on standardized tests tend to reflect performance over a number of passages. Use of the WIAT, for example, provides a standardized comparison between multiple reading passages and multiple listening passages. The listening versus reading comprehension comparison, interpreted in the light of Philip Gough's *simple view of reading* (Gough and Tunmer 1986), implies a deficit in word reading in the child who understands spoken text better than text he must read himself.

Richard Olson and his colleagues suggest a more direct focus on word reading (Olson et al. 1994). As evidence to support the hypothesis of dyslexia, we would expect to find either inaccurate or slow word reading. Olson suggests using computer-administered word lists to collect data on word-reading time as well as accuracy. If a commercial test is used, he suggests choosing one with enough words to keep results from being influenced by idiosyncratic knowledge. Note that the number of words provided to measure word reading in grades K–12 varies a great deal from test to test. There are 44 words listed on the Woodcock-Johnson Tests of Achievement, 55 on the WIAT, 66 on the Peabody Individual Achievement Test (PIAT-R; Markwardt 1989), and 106 on the Woodcock Reading Mastery Test (WRMT-R; Woodcock 1987).

A third way to look for specific word-reading problems involves looking at discrepancies between decoding and comprehension. In our clinical practice, we have worked with older, remediated children with dyslexia who can comprehend at reading levels close to those commensurate with age, IQ, listening ability, and school experiences, but who continue to decode somewhat inaccurately and extremely slowly. A discrepancy here makes a powerful argument for a specific decoding disorder.

A discrepancy between reading and math can also be used to support the hypothesis of a specific rather than general learning disorder. Some children with dyslexia are strong in math and weak in reading, and some are even strong in math concepts, but weak in computation. Lack of automaticity in retrieval can cause difficulties in both decoding and in computation. Batteries such as the WIAT, the PIAT-R, or the Kaufman Test of Educational Achievement (K-TEA) provide an opportunity for some or all of these comparisons. Keep in mind that a comparison must use tests normed on the same sample, and that each test or subtest needs to have high reliability, preferably close to .90 or higher (Hill 1981; Jensen 1980).

Another discrepancy often found in older children who have had good remediation involves accuracy versus rate in timed oral reading. We use the Gray Oral Reading Tests (GORT-3; Wiederbolt 1992) to make standard score comparisons between accuracy and rate in regard to passage reading. Note that even the timed GORT does not meet Olson's criteria (see above) for timing latencies on single word reading. We have found that accuracy is more responsive to remediation, in comparison to rate, in a group of third graders after two years of remediation in our clinic (Uhry 1994).

Children with dyslexia tend to be better at reading real words than at sounding out phonetically feasible nonsense words (see Rack, Snowling, and Olson 1992). Note that *nonsense words* are also called *nonwords* or *pseudowords* in the literature. It is crucial in making the nonsense word versus real word comparison to use tests normed on the same children, such as the Word Identification and Word Attack subtests from the WRMT-R. There is some evidence that this discrepancy may not be present after remediation (Alexander et al. 1991; Shepherd and Uhry 1993; Uhry 1994), and also, that the discrepancy may develop over time and not occur until the late elementary grades (Snowling 1994). Ellis Richardson and Barbara DiBenedetto provide a mechanism for looking at this discrepancy in their Decoding Skills Test (DST 1985). The DST uses both phonetically regular words (e.g., *shut*) and nonsense words that are their phonological analogs (e.g., *thut*), and then compares the two in what they call a *phonic transfer index*, which is the ratio of nonsense words to real words. A ratio close to or above 1 indicates strong phonetic strategies, while a ratio below 1 indicates poor phonetic strategies.

Spelling tends to be poor in young children with dyslexia, and to remain poor even after the decoding of real words improves. Louisa Moats (1994a) suggests choosing a spelling measure that has high reliability and that samples a broad domain of orthographic and morphological patterns. Note that to test reading, Richard Olson suggests an orthographic recognition task (e.g., *room* or *rume?*), a task that is similar to many group administered proofreading-type spelling tests (Olson et al. 1994). By contrast, Patricia Lindamood advocates looking at spelling without using letters at all, through the use her Lindamood Auditory Conceptualization Test, described below (Lindamood 1994). In our clinic, we use the WIAT Spelling test for three reasons. First, it has a balance of word types (phonetically regular words, high frequency words which are less regular, and words which are homonyms) . Second, it is reliable, and third, spelling can be compared with word reading, reading comprehension, and listening comprehension on the same measure.

Once standardized testing of some of the above discrepancies has been completed, it is helpful to arrange the scores into a pattern. We have developed the following model from our clinical work with children with dyslexia. It is consistent with findings from the Colorado Twin Study and with Maggie Bruck's work with adults previously diagnosed with childhood dyslexia (e.g., Bruck 1990). The pattern seems to hold for

> spelling / nonsense word reading
>   < decoding words in lists
>   < decoding words in text
>   < reading comprehension
>   < listening comprehension / IQ

most of the older children with dyslexia we see in our clinical work, particularly those who have had good remediation. While not every adjacent difference is statistically significant, the pattern of hierarchical nesting appears to hold.

PHASE II: PHONOLOGICAL PROCESSING

Three specific linguistic deficits are considered markers of dyslexia and are often grouped together as *phonological processing deficits*. Some researchers see 1) rapid automatized or serial naming, 2) verbal short-term memory, and 3) phonological awareness deficits as related symptoms of an underlying deficit while others see each as a separate construct. Rapid naming is also called *retrieval of phonological codes*, and verbal short-term memory is also called *phonological coding in working memory* (Wagner et al. 1993). There is evidence in the literature that all three are related to dyslexia, and that each can be present in the absence of the other two (e.g., Wood and Felton 1994).

RAPID SERIAL NAMING

Rapid serial naming is usually tested using a procedure developed by Martha Denckla and Rita Rudel (1976b). On the Rapid Automatized Naming Test (RAN) children are asked to name five colors (and then numbers, pictured objects, and letters) presented over and over in random order on a 50-item matrix. Scores are presented based on time rather than accuracy. Each subtest has age norms in seconds so that a clinician can see how quickly a child retrieves names in comparison with age peers. Evidence of slow retrieval by itself does not mean, necessarily, that a child is dyslexic. This information needs to be used as part of a collection of evidence. In our clinical practice we find that being at least one, and usually two, standard deviations slower than peers on more than one RAN subtest is common for children with severe and enduring difficulty acquiring speed in decoding.

VERBAL SHORT-TERM MEMORY

There is less agreement about the optimal way to measure verbal short-term memory. The Digit Span test from the WISC-III is a measure of recall of digits repeated by a child in both foreword and backward order. The advantage here is that this subtest can be viewed as part of an overall picture of language strengths and weaknesses on the Verbal Scale of the WISC-III. Another approach is to compare memory for rote material (e.g., lists of unrelated words) to memory for meaningful material (e.g., words in sentences). To do this, standard scores from the Word Sequences and Sentence Imitation subtests of the Detroit Tests of Learning Aptitude (DTLA-2; Hammill 1985) can be compared. Again, this information cannot be used alone to make a diagnosis of dyslexia, but should be presented as part of a pattern of evidence.

PHONOLOGICAL AWARENESS

There are a number of different ways to measure phonological awareness and most are correlated with each other (Stanovich, Cunningham, and Cramer 1984). Joseph Torgesen and Brian Bryant have recently developed the Test of Phonological Awareness (TOPA; Torgeson and Bryant 1994), a screening test that measures the ability of children in grades K-2 to match pictures of words by initial or final sound. Also designed to test readiness to read, Sawyer's Test of Awareness of Language Segments (TALS; Sawyer 1987) uses colored blocks to segment oral language. It builds on Isabelle Liberman's work on a developmental sequence moving from segmenting words in sentences, to syllables in words, to phonemes in single syllables (Liberman 1973; Liberman et al. 1974). Phoneme segmentation can also be measured using young children's invented spellings (Mann, Tobin, and Wilson 1987; Morris and Perney 1984). Morris's 12-word spelling list with its developmental scoring system is not normed but provides a source of good descriptive information for kindergarten or first-grade children (Morris 1992). We have found that by combining several of these tasks and looking at them together with early word recognition skills, in an instrument called the Early Reading Screening (Uhry 1993a), we can identify quite accurately in kindergarten those children who at risk for dyslexia.

Children without reading problems usually become adept at blending and segmenting phonemes during first grade. The Roswell-Chall Auditory Blending Test (Chall, Roswell, and Blumenthal 1963; Roswell and Chall 1963) is still widely used in reading diagnostic work. Here an examiner says parts of words aloud and then the child says the whole word. The most commonly used task for measuring the reverse procedure — full phoneme segmentation — is the Elkonin (1963, 1973) task using blocks or tiles, with or without letters, to represent sounds. Sawyer's TALS and the Lindamood Auditory Conceptualization Test

(LAC; Lindamood and Lindamood 1979) are two commercially available measures for this. The LAC uses colored blocks to distinguish, count, and sequence phonemes. The final items involve short nonsense words such as *ap*, with a different colored block for each phoneme. The Lindamoods' task differs from Sawyer's in that this representation is manipulated. The child is asked, "If that says *ap*, show me *pa* (e.g., change yellow-blue to blue-yellow).

Many of the above mentioned tasks can be used beyond the primary grades. The Roswell-Chall Auditory Blending Test includes norms through grade five. However, no more than three sounds are blended on the highest items (e.g., *map, pet*). The Sound Blending Test from the Illinois Test of Psycholinguistic Abilities (ITPA; Kirk, McCarthy, and Kirk 1968) includes longer words (e.g., *telephone*) and nonsense words (e.g., *opasto*). While the ITPA is not as reliable as the Roswell-Chall, its items are probably a more realistic match for blending demands at this age. *Deletion* or *elision* tasks (e.g., "Say *coat* without the sound /k/") are considered to be the most sophisticated of all phonological tasks (e.g., Adams 1990, Yopp 1988). On Rosner's Test of Auditory Analysis Skills (TAAS; Rosner 1975b; Rosner and Simon 1971), second graders are asked to delete the first consonant from a consonant cluster, and third graders are asked to delete an interior phoneme (e.g., "Say *smack*. Now say it again but don't say /m/"). Note that this complex manipulation task involves conceptualizing the location of the phonemes, deleting one, and then blending the others into a new word. The task assumes facility with consonant clusters, which are complex and difficult units for poor readers (Bruck and Treiman 1990). In our clinical practice we find that children who cannot manage these items inevitably have difficulty reading words with consonant clusters and usually benefit from training in consonant cluster *word changes* activities (Elkonin 1963, 1973), which are described in Chapter 5.

Keep in mind that none of these tasks should be used as the only measure in making instructional decisions and that phonological awareness deficits are not synonymous with dyslexia. Keith Stanovich (1986b) makes the point that it is poor decoding that is correlated with phonological awareness, not dyslexia. In other words, children with dyslexia most likely demonstrate deficits in phonological awareness, verbal short-term memory, or rapid automatized naming, but not all children with these characteristics are dyslexic. This information must be used together with discrepancy evidence from other academic and cognitive testing.

PHASE III: INVENTORY OF SKILLS AND STRATEGIES

Phase three of an evaluation involves an inventory of strengths and weaknesses in regard to skills and strategies. It involves generating lists of mastered material and lists of what needs to be taught next. Careful observation of oral decoding in connected text is crucial. We often videotape reading episodes for careful analysis of strategies. We always try to listen to a child read a familiar book from home or school. We also use a set of graded reading passages such as the Diagnostic Reading Scales (DRS; Spache 1981) or the Analytical Reading Inventory (ARI; Woods and Moe 1995) to establish both independent and instructional reading levels, and to note strategies and miscues. Observations can tell us whether the child is using a full range of cue systems (e.g., letters, pictures, contextual meaning, and prior information) and whether these systems are being used in isolation or in an integrated manner. Trial teaching using both phonetically controlled text and trade books can be useful in planning instruction.

Some practitioners use published tests to construct a record of which letter names, letter sounds, and sight words have been mastered by a child. Measures such as the Brigance Diagnostic Inventories (Brigance 1977, 1991) or Florence Roswell and Jeanne Chall's Diagnostic Assessment of Reading (DAR; Roswell and Chall 1992) provide procedures for collecting this data. The DAR has a particularly well constructed sequence of word types. However, the same information can be garnered by an experienced clinician through observations of miscues in text.

Analysis of spelling errors, both from test lists and from a writing sample, provides insight about phonological awareness and phonics knowledge that is useful in planning remediation. In our clinic we often follow an initial standardized spelling test such as the WIAT with the phonetically organized Spellmaster lists (Greenbaum 1987) in order to inventory basic letter-sound patterns.

In looking at writing in the absence of a comprehensive model for standardized assessment of written expression, Hooper suggests an informal measure such as a writing sample administered with think-alouds involving a dialogue with the child as she works at getting ideas down on paper, and trial teaching structured to focus on the presenting problem (Hooper et al. 1994). This is a sensible and workable suggestion.

An effective evaluation should clarify the nature of a child's reading difficulty but should also provide specific information for remediation. We like to end an evaluation with trial teaching, and we like to demonstrate possible methods and materials for parents and teacher/tutors as well. For example, we often administer a reading passage from an alternate form of an informal reading inventory at a student's instructional level, and ask the student to write a short essay under several conditions. We begin by asking the student to summarize the passage, and then we contrast this piece with a second one written with much more direct guidance. We ask the student whether any of the guided strategies we used were helpful, and if so, we include them in the educational plan.

At this point in an evaluation it should be possible to diagnose dyslexia. If there are discrepancies in test scores with IQ or oral language significantly stronger than reading ability in the absence of other causes, we can say that a student has dyslexia or reading disorder at the word reading level. Use of phonological processing tests should confirm characteristic linguistic deficits. In the third phase of the evaluation we have gathered information telling us where and how to begin treatment. The following case history is used to illustrate the above principles.

CASE HISTORY OF AN EDUCATIONAL EVALUATION: KM
BACKGROUND INFORMATION AND PSYCHOLOGICAL PROFILE

KM first came to the Child Study Center to be tested at the end of her first-grade year at the suggestion of her school because she could not read. Counter to our own advice, we did not begin, in KM's case, with an initial consultation with a psychologist because her school supplied results from the Wechsler Preschool and Primary Scales of Intelligence (WPPSI-R; Wechsler 1989). KM's IQ was reported to be in the superior range. Information provided in an initial family interview indicated that KM's father had experienced difficulty in reading as a child, and that her mother thought that she herself had had attention deficit disorder (ADD) as a child. Her parents were divorced, which ordinarily would have presented the possibility of emotional issues interfering with the development of reading, but all sources reported an amicable relationship between the parents with successfully shared custody.

KM had attended kindergarten and first grade in an independent school with small classes and assistant teachers which meant that she had received a great deal of personal attention in an enriched and supportive atmosphere. She was first identified as being at risk for reading difficulty when her school administered a kindergarten screening (Uhry 1993a). Results indicated mild difficulty with phonological awareness (e.g., segmenting, blending, invented spelling), and with recognition of environmental print (e.g., names of classmates and other words from the classroom). Results from the Rapid Automatized Naming Test (RAN; Denckla and Rudel 1976a) indicated extraordinarily slow response time in naming. KM was not immediately referred for assessment but her school did provide some small-group help during first grade. KM was not provided with systematic direct instruction in letter-sound associations; her school used a whole language approach to reading. A visit to observe KM's classroom convinced us that while lack of direct instruction may have exacerbated her difficulties, it was not the cause; many other children read quite well. KM's restless behavior during reading time suggested the possibility of attentional issues, but KM was extremely focused during math instruction. Her teacher considered her to be talented in math.

Prior to beginning testing, we had learned that KM was at risk for reading problems because of two factors: 1) low scores on kindergarten screenings that included phonological processing tasks, and 2) a family history of reading difficulty. At this point we still had unresolved questions about the possibility of attention deficit disorder and/or issues relating to the divorce.

DISCREPANCIES

Because there was a strong possibility that KM was dyslexic, we began the evaluation by asking her to read a word list from the WIAT in order to establish a discrepancy between IQ and reading ability. Her standard score on this test was 81, a standard deviation below the average range and more than three standard deviations below her IQ score. Because word reading is so idiosyncratic during first grade, we administered a second test to see if she might score higher on a different set of words. KM's standard score was 78 on the Word Identification test of the Woodcock Reading Mastery Test, with a large discrepancy between reading and IQ. We realized that we were basing a judgment on just a few words in both cases. However, we had confirmation of her very poor reading from her school's end-of-year standardized testing where she scored in the 7th percentile (roughly a standard score of 78) on a group administered reading achievement test, and from the less formal reading assessment we administered using her own books (see below).

To confirm our sense that KM was dyslexic, we wanted to see if spelling and nonsense word reading were especially low. KM's Woodcock Word Attack (nonsense word) standard score was 61. The pattern here was consistent with a diagnosis of dyslexia, with nonsense word reading significantly lower than word reading, which, in turn, was significantly lower than IQ. KM's spelling was also low; she scored 84 on the WIAT.

Because of possible attentional and emotional issues, it was important to establish reading as a specific rather than general academic discrepancy, so we wanted to see if reading and math were discrepant from each other. We like the Test of Early Mathematics Ability (TEMA-2; Ginsburg and Baroody 1990) for young children because it is interactive, uses manipulative materials, and includes follow-up probes for all items. Had KM's score not been so high we would have also administered the WIAT math tests to establish a discrepancy on tests normed on the same sample. With KM's score in the 99th percentile on the TEMA-2, this was not necessary; the discrepancy was clear. KM was quite talented in math and her disability was specific to reading.

PHONOLOGICAL PROCESSING
Phonological Awareness

Because phonological processing deficits are associated with dyslexia, we expected this to be a weak area for KM. Weakness here, together with the above discrepancies, would have made a strong case for the hypothesis of dyslexia. We were surprised to find that KM's phonological awareness skills were only moderately weak. She could blend phonemes into words on the Roswell-Chall Auditory Blending Test, scoring well above the first grade criterion level. On Rosner's Test of Auditory Analysis Skills she scored at the first grade level. She could delete many (but not all) initial and final consonant sounds from words. Keep in mind, though, that her school's kindergarten screening indicated initial weakness in this area. Her ability here was atypical. This relative strength in phonological awareness, together with our questions about ADD, made us question a diagnosis of dyslexia at this point.

Rapid Serial Naming

Our next finding, however, was consistent with a diagnosis of dyslexia. KM took an extraordinarily long time to complete serial naming tasks on the Rapid Automatized Naming Test (RAN). We knew from KM's school that she had done quite poorly at retrieving color names (the only subtest administered) when she took the RAN in connection with her school's kindergarten screening a year earlier. During our assessment KM scored in the average range on object naming, but was at least two standard deviations slower than age peers on each of the other subtests (colors, numbers, and letters). These results provided strong evidence that KM's reading difficulty was linked with slow retrieval rate. It explained the difficulty she had had in learning to say both letter names and letter sounds in kindergarten.

The discrepancies between reading and IQ, and between reading and math, as well as KM's slow retrieval rate pointed to a diagnosis of dyslexia, but we could not rule out ADD or emotional difficulties at this point.

INVENTORY OF STRENGTHS AND WEAKNESSES

Note that the following inventory is arranged into categories that ultimately became areas for remediation.

Letter knowledge

We began the final phase of the evaluation by taking an inventory of the letter sounds that KM knew. She could provide the appropriate sounds for almost all single consonants in isolation; exceptions were the sound of *v* and the soft sounds for *c* and *g,*. She was less secure on vowel sounds; short *a* was her only consistent vowel. Her letter sound knowledge was about that of a child entering first grade. Even though KM knew most consonant sounds she was quite slow to respond, which was consistent with her slow naming speed on the RAN. This was an area in which we wanted to provide remediation; KM needed to learn short and long vowels and she needed to increase response time on consonant sounds.

Spelling

We asked KM to write a story for us and she wrote the following, accompanied by a drawing of a brightly patterned Easter egg:

> This agg is aestrtagg
> a vere gudagg

This story seemed minimal when we consider that KM was a highly verbal child who had spent her kindergarten and first grade years in classrooms where writing was a daily event and where many children were prolific writers. Story writing was particularly hard for KM; her isolated spellings on the WIAT were easier to decipher. Several phonetically regular words were spelled correctly and the relationship between spoken and written language is clearer in her WIAT errors (below) than in her story.

lok	for	*look*
pay	for	*play*
rit	for	*right*
adt	for	*eight*

Right from the beginning KM had an easier time spelling and reading words in isolation. She seemed overwhelmed when asked to use several strategies at once in connected text. As with reading, we felt that she would need practice on letter-sounds to the automatic level before writing became comfortable. Vowel errors and omissions of consonants from consonant clusters in her spellings told us where to begin instruction.

Oral Reading

KM read passages from the Diagnostic Reading Scales (DRS) in order for us to establish the level of appropriate text that should be used for her instruction in school and in tutoring. We have transcribed the primer or beginning first grade passage on the left with KM's reading on the right. We introduced the passage by saying, "This is a story about a girl named Mary who is on her way to school."

Mary was on her way to school.	Milli was on her way to school.
She came to the corner.	She could to the church.
She saw a red light.	She saw a red all.
Then she saw the green light.	Then her science saw, said ... God! ... all.
Then she went on to school.	Then she was on to school.

Her performance here indicated that she was not ready yet to read primer level text, and that she was not self-correcting when text made little sense.

Because we wanted to see how KM handled more contextualized text, we used a book that she had brought with her from school. This was a picture book from New Zealand with just a few predictable and repeated words on a page. KM had memorized the text and *read* it without looking at the words. At no point, even when we modeled this for her, did she *fingerpoint-read*, or point at a word as she said it from memory. When she read incorrectly and we asked her to figure out another possible word, she looked around the room rather than at the printed word and became quite distracted. In fact, her attention span for any form of reading was short.

Probably the most striking thing about KM's reading was her failure to integrate appropriate reading strategies. Given text with little context, she used only letter cues and did not correct herself to make sense of what she had read. With familiar text, she used only prior knowledge of the content and failed to use letter cues at all to monitor herself. This dichotomy continued to characterize KM's reading for the first year of her remedial work with us. We hypothesized that retrieving letter sounds was so tedious for her that she had little energy to devote to other cue systems, and that if any other source of information was available, she used it instead.

UNANSWERED QUESTIONS

Diagnosing dyslexia is a complex process. KM's assessment left several questions unanswered. Her squirminess and short attention span during the evaluation (and during later tutoring) made us wonder if she had ADHD. Keep in mind that this was a suspected family pattern on her mother's side. We ended KM's evaluation report by stating that this was an unresolved issue and encouraged her family to follow up with a psychological evaluation.

When this was done during KM's second grade year, the psychologist confirmed KM's superior IQ score, stating that she was not especially low on those WISC-III subtests that are vulnerable to attentional issues. The psychologist concluded that KM's reading difficulty was not caused by ADHD or by issues related to the divorce. Her recommendation was for tutoring.

CONCLUSIONS

When we finished our evaluation we were convinced that KM was dyslexic based on the large discrepancy between IQ and reading and on her difficulty with rapid retrieval. While we needed a psychologist's opinion to ascertain possible need for either therapy or medication, we knew that in any event, KM would need specialized reading instruction.

The final chapter of this book describes the process of planning a tutoring program for KM based on these evaluation findings, and on the principles and techniques for remediation outlined in the chapters that follow.

II

Remedial Instruction

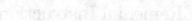

4

Principles and Techniques of Remedial Instruction for Dyslexic Students

Although we should not minimize the importance of understanding the nature of dyslexia, reading disabilities research has been justifiably criticized for focusing disproportionately on the search for causality and all but neglecting inquiry on correction or prevention of the problem (Bryant et al. 1980; Chall 1978; Lipson and Wixson 1986). The reading disabilities field has in fact been referred to as *deficit driven* (Poplin 1983). Rachel Gittelman, a psychologist at the College of Physicians and Surgeons, Columbia University, reviewing the research on the remediation of reading disorders, states "The literature on the treatment of children with reading retardation is full of opinionated practices devoid of even barely adequately controlled treatment research." (Gittelman 1983).

There are several plausible explanations for the relative lack of treatment research on dyslexia, the first being the effort and cost involved; the need for a remedy is usually urgent, therefore taking precedence over the need to plan for later evaluation. A second explanation is that many remedial programs began in the private sector where formal evaluation is not required for implementation as it is in many public school systems. Still another reason is that few of the more popular programs or techniques have been affiliated with a college or university where research is routinely conducted. Moreover, much of the research that does exist is methodologically flawed, as a task force of the Research Institute for the Study of Learning Disabilities at Columbia University Teachers College discovered in surveying the research literature (Peister et al. 1978–1980). Gittelman points out that small numbers of subjects in the sample population, lack of control groups, and failure to assign subjects randomly to treatment and control groups, are some of the design problems in the studies to date (Gittelman 1983).

Random assignment to treatment groups is particularly difficult to achieve, since dyslexic subjects are often already in treatment. The length of time needed to produce significant gains from remedial instruction, which is usually two years or more (Peister et al. 1978–1980), also tends to discourage practitioners from carrying out effective studies. Furthermore, as Gittelman notes, neither the duration nor the intensity of treatment is spelled out, calling into question any conclusions that may be drawn.

The Teachers College task force (Peister et al. 1978–1980) has drawn attention to the fact that even where control or comparison groups exist, the instruction applied in these groups often is not adequately described, making it difficult to determine which instructional components are actually being compared. The nature of choice of outcome measures frequently is not given adequate consideration in planning program evaluation or in interpreting findings from studies that have been carried out. As Gittelman (1983) points out, most standardized tests are not designed to pick up small gains over short periods of time; thus, with short-term or *one shot* studies the possibility of failure to detect treatment effects statistically where they exist is greatly increased.

DIRECT INSTRUCTION

Despite the lack of empirical support, there is remarkable consensus on the major principles to be applied in remedial treatment for dyslexic students (Bryant et al. 1980). One of the most often acknowledged principles is direct instruction. N. G. Haring and B. Bateman in their book, *Teaching the Learning Disabled Child* (1977), make the point that dyslexic children do not learn *by osmosis,* as other children seem to do. Rather, they need direct, intensive, and systematic input from, and interaction with, the teacher.

Three different models of direct instruction have been applied to dyslexic children: the tutoring model (Traub 1982), the small group model (Cox 1985; Enfield and Greene 1981), and the whole class model (Wolf 1985). Determining which of these models is most effective and most economically efficient is one of the critical challenges in the field of reading disabilities.

Nancy Karweit of Johns Hopkins University suggests that we judge the relative value of the different models of adaptive instruction in terms of *student use of instructional time* (Karweit 1985). This concept has been referred to alternatively as *academic learning time* (Berliner 1981), *academic engaged time* (Ysseldyke and Algozzine 1983), and *time on task*

(Otto, Wolf, and Eldridge 1984). In reviewing the drawbacks and advantages of different educational settings, Karweit adopts J. B. Carroll's definition of learning time as the ratio of time spent to time needed (when the two factors are equivalent, learning is maximized) (Carroll 1963). In the whole-class model, Karweit notes that the amount of active learning time varies widely with the size and heterogeneity of the class and the procedural demands on the teacher. However, in this model all teaching time can be devoted to direct instruction.

In the within-class grouping approach, instructional time for each group is divided between direct instruction and independent seat work. While reducing the amount of direct instruction for each student, this approach can place an excessive burden on a teacher, because he or she must monitor seat work in addition to working directly with each group. Looking at individualized instruction only within a classroom setting (a model, she notes, that is considerably less popular today), Karweit emphasizes the formidable management problems involved in distributing teacher time and the often large amount of time wasted in students' waiting for the teacher's attention. Although she does not attempt to confirm the superiority of one instructional model over another, Karweit provides an important perspective on classroom management.

Students with dyslexia need more time to learn than students without reading disabilities (Haring and Bateman 1977), and special educators have given considerable thought to the issue of academic engaged time. For example, Wayne Otto and his colleagues (1984) have concluded that this variable is the best predictor of academic achievement; James Ysseldyke and Bob Algozzine (1983) suggest that reading diagnosis should begin with an examination of student time on task. Ethna Reid (1986), in designing an instructional program to be used in classrooms to prevent reading failure, makes provisions for minimizing the length of teacher questions and student response latencies in order to maximize learning time. Unison oral response is incorporated in several programs (for example, DISTAR and Slingerland) to ensure that each student is fully involved in the lesson at hand. The use of teacher scripts (Calfee 1981-1984; Engelmann and Bruner 1983; Reid 1986) can be viewed as another approach to time management. These scripts are written formats provided to teachers to help structure their lessons. Scripts may be more or less specific; in the DISTAR program (see Chapter 18), for example, the scripts tell teachers exactly what to say and do during each lesson, when to call for responses, when to repeat statements for emphasis or correction, and so on, thereby controlling the pace of instruction.

Careful pacing of instruction is an essential feature of effective teaching for dyslexic students in order to prevent information overload, which occurs when the amount of information to be processed within a given time span exceeds the individual's capacity (Bryant et al. 1980).

N. D. Bryant and his associates (1980) have identified four processing problems that contribute to overloading: 1) slow speed of processing, 2) difficulty automatizing information learned, 3) failure to apply strategies, and 4) distractibility. The successful teacher or practitioner working with dyslexic students, regardless of instructional setting, must provide for this contingency in planning each lesson (Cox 1992; Gillingham and Stillman 1960; Slingerland 1976). Most established remedial methods and programs utilize a structured, hierarchical approach to learning, breaking down tasks into small units taught in order of difficulty (Bryant et al. 1980).

LEARNING TO MASTERY

Mastery is an extremely important factor in remedial or preventive instruction for disabled learners. Barak Rosenshine, who supports direct teaching, states that, to insure retention, mastery needs to reach levels of 70 to 80 percent when new reading skills are acquired; in independent practice, mastery should be 100 percent, especially for learners with disabilities (Rosenshine 1983). David Berliner, another strong advocate of direct instruction, maintains that younger and less able students need to achieve almost errorless performance on early learning tasks in order for later learning to be successful (Berliner 1981).

Gaining automaticity is a critical component of mastery learning in remedial reading instruction. Automatic processing at the word level frees up working memory to allow for more efficient processing at the sentence and passage levels of text (LaBerge and Samuels 1974; Perfetti 1985a; Stanovich 1984). As mentioned earlier, dyslexic readers in general are markedly slower at word recognition than good readers (Perfetti 1984; Stanovich 1980). Most of the established remedial programs for students with dyslexia, therefore, make ample provision for extended practice to attain automaticity beginning at the letter-sound level. Barbara Bateman in particular stresses the need for repetition with all new learning, a concept termed *overlearning* (Bateman 1979). However, as N. D. Bryant and his associates at Teachers College point out, practice needs to be carefully distributed over time, rather than massed. They suggest that massed practice reinforces short-term memory at the expense of long-term memory (Bryant et al. 1980). The majority of remedial programs for dyslexic students provide for systematic review of previously learned material at the beginning and end of each lesson.

Prompting techniques are often utilized in treatment approaches to decrease the possibility of errors and to help students to respond without overcontrolling their behavior (DeCecco 1968). Although there has not been much research on the subject, Bryant and his associates (1980) report on two studies that support the value of prompting in remedial instruction, which usually involves using picture or object cues as memory aids.

For example, remedial programs derived from the Orton-Gillingham approach (see Chapters 13 and 15) provide pictures to promote letter-sound associations. A picture of a pig, for example, could be considered a prompt for the sound of the letter *p*.

Academic feedback is another essential instructional component of learning to mastery (Berliner 1981). B. Rosenshine and R. Stevens (1984) cite immediate feedback from the teacher as one of the five most important contributive factors to academic achievement. They subdivide the feedback process into four instructional components: demonstration, guided practice, feedback, and independent practice. Although little research has specifically investigated the effects of this variable on students with dyslexia, some provision for feedback is incorporated in all established programs. It is not necessarily teacher driven, however, as in the classic Direct Instruction model exemplified by the DISTAR program (see Chapter 18; Engelmann and Bruner 1983). In some programs a *discovery* or *Socratic* method is used (Cox 1992; Lindamood and Lindamood 1975), albeit under careful teacher supervision to ensure correct responses. When working with older students, frequent performance assessment offers a way to inform them of their progress, thereby increasing motivation (Zigmond and Miller 1986). Providing standards against which to measure their performance also helps students to become self-monitors and take on more responsibility for their own progress (Bandura 1982).

Gaining pupil attention is particularly important in teaching children who are prone to distraction (Bryant et al. 1980) and often lack motivation due to previous failure (King 1985). Techniques to promote attending behavior have been incorporated into many instructional programs for these students. For example, the Alphabetic Phonics and Slingerland programs (see Chapters 13 and 15) require specific sitting positions to be assumed before reading and writing activities begin. Hand signals used to cue group response, as in the DISTAR program and Enfield and Greene's Project Read (see Chapter 17), also serve as attentional devices.

Monitoring and evaluating student progress is an essential component of successful academic treatment, although not all treatment methods for students with dyslexia include evaluation procedures. Naomi Zigmond and Sandra Miller (1986) report on studies that showed significantly greater academic gains for students whose teachers monitored student progress, as compared to students whose teachers collected no ongoing progress data. However, these reviewers emphasize that to be effective, progress evaluation must be frequent and systematic and teachers must use the data constructively to modify instruction when needed. Furthermore, a data-based approach has been found to be more effective in improving pupil achievement than informal observational procedures, though the data analysis need not be elaborate to provide adequate information on student progress. Note the daily record taking in Reading

Recovery (see Chapter 22) and the frequent curriculum-based evaluation in Alphabetic Phonics (see Chapter 13).

MULTISENSORY TECHNIQUES

The use of multisensory techniques in remedial intervention with children who are dyslexic is widespread and dates back to the 1920s with Grace Fernald who instructed students with reading impairment to trace letters or words while saying the names aloud (Fernald and Keller 1921). This procedure came to be known as the VAKT approach (visual, auditory, kinesthetic, tactile). Fernald maintained that VAKT reinforcement would help to produce a memory schema for the stimulus information. Samuel Orton's hypothesis that dyslexia is caused by incomplete cerebral dominance, resulting in reversal and sequencing problems, led to the adoption of multisensory teaching methods by his many disciples (Cox 1992; Gillingham and Stillman 1960; Slingerland 1971; Traub and Bloom 1975). The prototype of multisensory instruction for children with dyslexia was developed by Orton's colleague, Anna Gillingham, a psychologist, and is most often referred to as the *Orton-Gillingham approach*. Gillingham collaborated with Bessie Stillman, a remedial reading teacher, in writing a manual that describes this method (Gillingham and Stillman 1960).

Among these practitioners, the assumed rationale for multisensory remedial training has been that kinesthetic activities help to establish visual-auditory associations in learning grapheme-phoneme correspondences, as well as to establish left-to-right letter progression (Orton 1966). Aylett Cox, author of Alphabetic Phonics (see Chapter 13), a program derived from the Orton-Gillingham approach, refers to this learning procedure as *intersensory elaboration*. Other proposed benefits of VAKT or VAK techniques are that they encourage attention to details within letters or words (Gates 1927) and that they help in retrieving words from long-term memory (Slingerland 1971).

As the Teachers College task force (Peister et al. 1978-1980) has observed, there were considerable differences in specific techniques among the earlier practitioners of multisensory training. Orton, for example, stated that individual phonic sounds should be pronounced as the child traced a word; Gillingham believed that letter names should be said aloud; Fernald maintained that words should not be broken up artificially, and that whole words should be said aloud while tracing or writing. Today there is general agreement among practitioners of Orton-Gillingham derived methods that letter sounds are pronounced when reading words and letter names when spelling (Cox 1992; Enfield 1976). However, even among these programs there are variations in the degree of multisensory input incorporated in teaching procedures. For example, in order to emphasize precise speech sounds, Cox (1985) uses mirrors to demonstrate different oral positions in pronouncing these sounds, a technique derived from the speech therapy field. Charles and Pat Lindamood (Lindamood and Lindamood 1975) stress the importance of developing oral-motor awareness in children and adults with deficits in auditory conceptualization. Note that Patricia Lindamood's background is in speech/language therapy.

Despite the widespread inclusion of multisensory techniques in remedial programs for students with dyslexia and the almost unanimous conviction among practitioners using these techniques that they work, there is little empirical data to validate their effectiveness. We have substantial evidence that many of the programs incorporating these techniques are effective, but we cannot be sure that it is the multisensory factor that makes the significant difference, for in studies comparing multisensory instruction to an alternative remedial approach, the competing variables have not been well controlled.

There are in fact some practitioners who question the application of multisensory methods as a uniform treatment for all readers with disabilities. Doris Johnson and Helmer Myklebust of the Institute for Language Disorders at Northwestern University, for example, caution that some children with reading disability appear prone to sensory overload; thus the involvement of another sensory modality may serve only to confuse them (Johnson and Myklebust 1967). Unfortunately, these clinicians have not provided empirical data to support this contention, nor have they described in detail the children they have in mind. This research is from an era in which the distinction between readers with dyslexia and garden-variety poor readers was not made.

Susan Bryant (1979) has compared the effects of VA (visual, auditory) with VAKT procedures (visual, auditory, kinesthetic, tactile) on children with reading disability, keeping all other instructional variables constant. In doing so, she found no differing effects due to treatment between methods on either reading or spelling performance, despite the fact that the VAKT procedures demanded more student engaged time. However, because the intervention time in Bryant's study was only six days, efforts to generalize her results to actual clinical or classroom practice should be restrained. Conclusions drawn from one-shot experimental training studies such as Bryant's are always open to question.

After conducting an extensive review of the research on multisensory training, Bryant (1979) suggests two possible effects of multisensory instruction that are not sensitive to experimental manipulation and therefore may have gone undetected in the research thus far. The first is that multisensory methods may provide more feedback to the teacher and the child in initial learning, and the second is that multisensory activities allow for distributed and varied practice, thereby minimizing boredom.

Perhaps the most interesting research to date on the effects of multisensory instruction is that conducted by Charles Hulme. Seeking to understand the rationale for multisensory instruction with disabled readers by investigating the effects of tracing on visual recognition, Hulme (1981) finds that tracing letters significantly enhances the ability of disabled readers to remember letters they have seen and brings their recognition performance up to that of normal readers who have merely been shown the letters; however, tracing has little improvement effect on normal readers. With abstract shapes, on the other hand, tracing benefits both normal and disabled readers, and to a similar extent. Hulme maintains that these findings suggest that good readers have access to a phonological code, which is more efficient for storing verbal material than a visual code. In contrast, poor readers rely on visual memory which may be enhanced by kinesthetic input, such as tracing. Although this hypothesis appears to offer an explanation as to why multisensory teaching might benefit students with dyslexia, the fact that tracing in Hulme's experiments improved recognition of individual items only, but not of the sequences in which the items were presented, weakens, but does not totally invalidate, the credibility of this explanation. As Hulme himself points out, learning to read is dependent upon learning to recognize sequences of letters in words.

In attempting to understand the mechanisms underlying the effects of tracing on visual recognition, Hulme offers two competing hypotheses: 1) that tracing serves to direct attention to the stimuli to be remembered; 2) that tracing increases the information about the stimuli that may be stored in memory. Hulme questions the plausibility of the attentional hypothesis, citing the failure of similar attention-directing activities in previous research, such as haptic inspection of three dimensional objects, to enhance visual memory. Opting for the latter hypothesis, Hulme suggests that the primary effect of tracing is to provide information in memory about the movements made in tracing and posits the existence of a separate motor memory system which acts in conjunction with visual memory of the shapes of the items to be remembered. Lending support to this contention are Hulme's findings that visual interference during the experimental procedure disrupted memory for visually presented shapes but not for shapes that had been traced, whereas motor interference was most disruptive for recognition of shapes that had been traced.

Hulme asks a question more relevant to reading than to the research he conducted on visual memory: Does tracing enhance memory for verbal labels of visual configurations? Using children without reading problems, triplet shapes were paired with high frequency, high imagery nouns. Here, Hulme found that names were better remembered for the triplets that had been traced. He emphasizes the implications for these results for beginning and remedial reading instruction, which involves a similar form of visual-verbal paired-associate learning.

In another exploration of multisensory instruction, Hulme and Lynette Bradley (1984) used an Orton-Gillingham technique called *Save Our Spelling* (SOS)[1] in which a student reads a word and then copies it three times, saying each letter aloud as it is written. Both young normal readers and older poor readers learned to spell more words correctly using the multisensory SOS technique than when using a comparison technique in which lettered tiles were selected for spellings.

None of these studies identify the underlying mechanisms that produce effects for handwritten spellings. Whether or how information processed in one sensory modality can enhance the processing of information in another modality remains to be seen. Yet there is appeal in Hulme's hypothesis that multisensory processing establishes multiple memory traces that reinforce retention of information about spelling patterns. Hulme's conjecture that the benefits gained by disabled readers, but not good readers, from letter tracing are attributable to disabled readers' failure to employ a speech code to memorize letters (Hulme 1981) is credible in light of what is known about the phonological coding deficits in individuals with dyslexia.

Hulme's laboratory-based experiments are important as a way of understanding the underlying psychological processes involved in learning to read for children with dyslexia. Three recent studies designed to compare several treatments have all used some form of multisensory instruction and in all three cases this instruction was the regular school-based reading curriculum for these groups of children, with university-based researchers monitoring teacher training and collecting data periodically. Barbara Wise, who works with Richard Olson in Colorado, has incorporated Patricia Lindamood's Auditory Discrimination in Depth (ADD) program (see Chapter 14) into training that includes a computer-based practice component for young children with reading problems. Working with teachers, children are taught to recognize pictures of mouth positions that refer to the sounds made when their own mouths are in those positions (i.e., top teeth on lower lip producing the sound /f/). These new skills are then practiced on a computer program that incorporates both mouth movements and synthesized speech. ADD training is eventually extended into reading recognition training which also has a computer-practice component. Words that children cannot read can be highlighted for computer-based speech-synthesis production, segment by segment. The computer based segmentation training is called ROSS, or Reading with Orthographic and Speech Segmentation. Children in the ROSS group outper-

---

[1] The acronym SOS is used by Aylett Cox (1984) for two terms: Save Our Spelling and Simultaneous Oral Spelling (see Chapter 9). Both Cox (1984) and Hulme and Bradley (1984) base their procedures on Orton-Gillingham multisensory techniques. Hulme and Bradley use the technique with irregular words in this study. Note that when SOS is used with regular words, the model is auditory rather than visual; the teacher says the word rather than showing it to the child.

formed a control group trained in reciprocal teaching of phonological awareness and word attack skills after this multisensory training (Wise 1995).

Joseph Torgesen, Richard Wagner, and Carol Rashotte, at Florida State University, are also using Lindamood's ADD training. In their longitudinal study ADD is used in connection with a synthetic phonics instructional program in an intervention with first-grade children who are at risk because of poor phonological awareness skills. This intervention is called PASP, which stands for Phonological Awareness with Synthetic Phonics. Three additional treatment groups include: 1) implicit phonics instruction through the use of partially phonetically controlled basal-reader text, 2) one-to-one support for regular classroom instruction, and 3) regular classroom instruction alone. In contrast to the other treatments, there is indication in the preliminary data from the first year of this study that PASP, the multisensory, direct instruction, synthetic phonics model, is more effective than the other treatment models in terms of nonsense word reading, but not more effective, to date, in terms of real-word reading. On the latter measure, all three treatment groups were superior to classroom controls (Torgesen 1995).

Barbara Foorman, David Francis, and Jack Fletcher, of the University of Houston, are also using multisensory instruction as one of several treatment conditions being explored in a longitudinal study of 108 second- and third-grade children who are receiving resource room help because of poor reading skills. As with the two above studies, treatment is being carried out in the schools as part of the regular instructional program, in this case, by the resource room teachers. The first treatment, Alphabetic Phonics (see Chapter 13), is an Orton-Gillingham based, multisensory, synthetic phonics program. The Neuhaus Center in Houston provided training for teachers working with the Alphabetic Phonics group. The second treatment is a modified version of Recipe for Reading (see Chapter 16), also an Orton-Gillingham program with a multisensory approach, but one that utilizes both synthetic and analytic phonics activities. One modification to Recipe for Reading in this experiment includes training in onset-rime word segments rather than fully segmented phonemes. The third training condition is a whole-word program that involves visual discrimination between similar words and building memory for sight words. Preliminary results favor Alphabetic Phonics training (i.e., synthetic phonics) over both the modified Recipe for Reading training (i.e., analytic/synthetic) and the sight word training in terms of growth in phonological skills. In other words, using multisensory techniques to teach synthetic phonics provided an advantage in phonological skills. Contrary to expectations, however, children in the sight word group had higher scores on both spelling and broad-based reading measures[2] in comparison with the Recipe for Read-

---

[2] This was a composite reading score from the Woodcock-Johnson Tests of Achievement (Woodcock and Mather 1989b).

ing group (Foorman, Francis, and Fletcher 1995).

The authors of these three studies warn that their results are preliminary and that the children in their studies must be followed for several years before the effects of treatment are fully understood. The Texas and Florida studies are finishing the second year of federally funded five-year programs. Results are complex and will need to be interpreted over time, but initial results do support the use of multisensory synthetic phonics programs to increase ability in phonological skills for students at-risk for phonology-based reading deficits.

MODALITY SPECIFIC INSTRUCTION

Although the question of sensory modality preferences among reading disabled children seems closely related to the issue of multisensory training, it derives from a different theoretical perspective. Efforts to adapt instructional treatments to individual learners became prevalent in the 1960s, as information processing theory gained prominence in educational psychology. Helmer Myklebust and Doris Johnson, leaders in this movement, maintained that there are two types of dyslexic individuals, one type suffering from visual perceptual deficits, the other type from auditory processing deficits (Myklebust and Johnson 1962). Johnson and Myklebust (1967) recommended that visual dyslexics be taught by a synthetic phonics approach and auditory dyslexics by a whole-word or sight approach. Modality specific instruction was popular in the 1960s and early 1970s.

However, aptitude-treatment-interaction (ATI), as modality specific instruction came to be called, began to lose credibility as a viable concept during the 1970s, as accumulating research failed to demonstrate its effectiveness. Helen Robinson conducted an often cited study in which she tested 448 children after matching them for modality preference with either a phonics or sight approach to reading acquisition; she found neither method to be more effective with those children having the most notable differences in modality strengths (Robinson 1972). Two comprehensive ATI literature summaries (Cronbach and Snow 1976; Turner and Dawson 1978) have concluded that modality preference is not strongly related to achievement, teaching approach, or reading. As explanation for these findings, Sally Lipa, in a journal article on reading disability and its treatment, suggests,

> ...modality teaching failed to account for the fact that, regardless of mode of presentation, words must be learned linguistically, notably in the dominant language hemisphere. Teaching in a visual manner could not obviate auditory processing of words (Lipa 1984).

In other words, even if a reliable way to measure preferred modalities could be developed, and we don't have this technology, all children need to learn how to match visual letters with spoken sounds to read and spell. The demands of reading need to inform instruction. However, the efficacy of modality-specific teaching remains a commonly held notion in the popular literature twenty years after research began to make researchers question it.

5

Increasing Phonological Awareness

B oth phonics and phonological awareness are considered to be important aspects of remedial training programs. The word *phonics* is defined here as meaning a fairly low level, rote knowledge of the associations between letters and sounds. The term *phonological* is defined as pertaining to speech sounds and thus the term *phonological awareness* includes a range of higher level metacognitive understandings of word boundaries within spoken sentences, of syllable boundaries in spoken words, and of how to isolate phonemes and establish their relative locations within syllables or short words. This last step, the isolation of phonemes, is known as *phonemic* awareness. It appears to develop at about the time that reading instruction begins in normal readers, and both supports decoding and is supported by it. Both phonics and phonological awareness are key elements in decoding because together they help a child understand the relation between sounds in spoken words and letters in written words. As Joanna Williams explains:

> If the central task of the beginning reader is seen as learning to identify and use the correspondences between letter and sound, then phonemic analysis and blending are two fundamental component skills. To identify the correspondences it is necessary to be able to isolate the units, both in orthography and in the sound stream, such that appropriate mappings between orthography and sound can be made. (Williams 1986a)

Training in letter-sound knowledge and application of phonics skills in reading have been part of training in the Orton-Gillingham approach for many years (Gillingham and Stillman 1960). This has not been the case for phonological awareness. While evidence of the link between early phonological awareness and later reading was reported as early as the 1960s, it is only fairly recently that it has become common practice to include phonological awareness in training programs for children who are dyslexic or for young children as preparation for reading.

The following phonological awareness training studies have been arranged into a sequence with three levels (i.e., prereading, beginning reading, and remedial reading) and information has been included about the types of training tasks that have been used successfully at these levels.

TRAINING AT THE PREREADING STAGE

There is good evidence from a number of studies that early phonological training increases a child's level of phonological awareness prior to reading instruction. Before exposure to formal reading instruction, kindergarten children who are not at-risk, typically can match spoken words by rhyme and alliteration, can provide a rhyme at the end of a sentence in predictable text read aloud by the teacher, can clap out the number of syllables in multisyllable words, and can segment and represent beginning and ending consonants in *invented spellings* (e.g., LK for the word *like*). Some children can blend phonemes into words. A variety of training tasks have been used to increase ability in these areas.

Jerome Rosner trained prereaders to add, omit, substitute, and rearrange phonemes in orally presented words in sequenced exercises that are an elaboration of the TAAS tasks described in Chapter 3 (e.g., "Say *coat*. Now say it again but don't say /k/"). The program is described more fully in his training guide, *Helping Children Overcome Learning Difficulties* (Rosner 1975b). In Rosner's study, after 14 weeks of training the children were significantly better at these tasks than untrained children (Rosner 1974).

Richard Venezky's *Prereading Skills Program* (Venezky 1976) trained at-risk kindergarten children to associate sounds with pictures. Note that the sound is not the initial phoneme of the name of the picture but, rather, the sound that the object makes, such as /f-f-f/ for an angry cat. Then he successfully trained the children to blend the sounds into words.

Michael and Lise Wallach determined that disadvantaged urban kindergarten children have more difficulty than middle-class children in manipulating phonemes. Their readiness program used parents as tutors. Preliminary training involved asking children to isolate initial phonemes in orally presented words. Later, letter-sound associations were taught and blended in a traditional synthetic phonics approach (e.g., learning letter sounds and then blending these sounds into words). Posttesting after 30 weeks showed significant improvement in both word reading and sentence reading in comparison with controls (Wallach and Wallach

1979). This study was one of the earliest in which an effect was demonstrated directly on reading in kindergarten rather than on the level of phonological development.

Hyla Rubin has made important contributions in terms of playful tasks for teaching phonological awareness to kindergarten-age children as well as in terms of using this training successfully with young language-impaired children (Warrick and Rubin 1992; Warrick, Rubin, and Rowe-Walsh 1993). There is an entire suburban Connecticut school district that uses her training program with all of its kindergarten children, thus cutting down on referrals to special education programs in first grade. She trains kindergarten teachers to incorporate sound-play into jokes and games where sounds are manipulated (e.g., "I had Beerios for breakfast.") and into myriad formal and informal classroom activities. In a controlled study, 478 kindergarten children were trained in a three-part sequence: 1) rhyme and syllable analysis, 2) analysis of spoken words into phonemes, and 3) transfer activities such as invented spelling. By the end of the kindergarten year, children performing at the mean for this group could represent all sounds (e.g., medial vowels as well as initial and final consonants) in invented spellings. Descriptive studies in the literature indicate that most children can not do this until first grade. Performance on all tasks was significantly better than an earlier cohort of children in the same district who had not received intervention training (Rubin and Eberhardt in press).

Ingvar Lundberg and his Danish colleagues carried out a longitudinal study of 235 kindergarten children whose whole language classroom teachers provided phonological awareness training throughout the school year. Training involved rhyming stories and games, rhythmic moving to syllabic patterns, and phoneme segmentation practice. By the end of the year, these children were superior to controls on phonological awareness measures, with particularly strong effects for phoneme segmentation. The study is important because it followed these children to the end of the second-grade school year. While training was limited to sound analysis and did not involve reading, the trained children were superior to controls on reading and spelling measures two years after training ended (Lundberg, Frost, and Petersen 1988).

Lynette Bradley and Peter Bryant undertook what is considered a seminal study of phonological awareness training in England with four- and five-year-old children considered to be at-risk for reading failure because of low levels of phonological awareness (Bradley and Bryant 1983; 1985). The training involved practice in what they called *sound categorization*, which requires selection of the odd man out from a set of four pictures, three of whose names match in regard to alliteration (*bun, bus, rug, bug*), rhyme (*bun, hut, gun, sun*) or medial vowel (*hug, pig, dig, wig*). Training took place in 40 ten-minute sessions over a two-year period.

Toward the end of training, some of the children used plastic letters to segment and spell words. The sixty subjects were in four groups: 1) sound categorization, 2) sound categorization with letters, 3) categorization by concepts rather than sounds, and 4) controls. The group with a significant advantage in reading and spelling at the end of the study was the sound categorization group whose training included plastic letters, and this advantage held two years after the study ended (Bradley and Bryant 1985).

This leads to the question of whether or not to include letters in phonological awareness training. Linnea Ehri's work suggests that this should be done. She trained kindergarten children to segment with both blank tokens and with letters. Her results indicated that using letters for segmenting produced superior ability in both segmenting and blending (Hohn and Ehri 1983). In a later study (Ehri and Wilce 1987b), kindergarten children were taught to read using segmentation in combination with letters. These children had a significant advantage over controls who were trained in letter sounds but not in segmenting words. Ehri makes the point that spelling (segmenting using letters) leads into reading.

Benita Blachman, who studied with Liberman, later worked with her own student, Eileen Ball. They used both phoneme segmentation and letter-sound training with kindergarten children and taught them to segment phonemes, and, as a consequence, to read and spell better than a letter-sound–only group and a control group by the end of the kindergarten year (Ball and Blachman 1991). The training involved groups of five children, for 20 minutes, four times a week for seven weeks. They used a *Say it and move it* activity similar to Elkonin's pictures and tiles (e.g., saying a word in response to a picture, saying each sound in that word, and sliding a token down for each sound). This was done first with blank tiles and later with a mix of blank and lettered tiles. Other activities included a sound–sorting task based on the one used by Bradley and Bryant (1985) and training in letter–sound associations. Blachman has used this treatment again in a recent study with kindergarten children (Blachman et al. 1994) and includes it in a reading program for first graders (see below).

Brian Byrne, working with colleagues in Australia, used a program called *Sound Foundations*. Children were taught that different words can share common sounds through the use of brightly colored posters, some with objects beginning with the same word, and others with end sounds in common. They were also taught letter-sound associations. At posttest the children were taught to read word pairs (e.g., *sat*, *mat*) and then tested for transfer of knowledge (e.g., "Does *sow* say 'sow' or 'mow?'"). Trained children had a distinct advantage in development of phonemic awareness (Byrne and Fielding-Barnsley 1991). In a follow-up study of these children at the end of the first-grade year, Byrne found that those who had entered first grade with the highest levels of phonemic awareness were the most successful readers (Byrne and Fielding-Barnsley 1993).

TRAINING DURING BEGINNING READING INSTRUCTION

Around the time that children are exposed to formal reading instruction in first grade, there is an increase in ability to segment phonemes in spoken words. Whereas invented spellings in kindergarten usually involve more consonants than vowels, early in first grade there is often a dramatic increase in ability to represent the presence of vowels. Ability to separate vowels from consonants and, then, consonants from each other within consonant clusters, are the important phonemic segmentation milestones during the early primary grades.

One of the first procedures designed to promote phonemic awareness in beginning readers was used by D. B. Elkonin and his colleagues in the 1960s and 1970s in what was then the Soviet Union. Their training tasks used pictures to help a child remember the target word and boxes to help a child conceptualize the sound structure of a spoken word. Small tiles were moved from the picture to the boxes as the word was said aloud one phoneme at a time. See the illustrated example provided here.

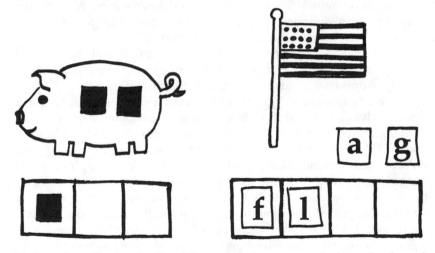

Elkonin-type boxes with unlettered and lettered tiles to move into boxes to represent the phonemes in spoken words.

As training progressed, colors were used to differentiate vowels from consonants, and later on, hard from soft consonants. Eventually, letters were provided on the tiles, beginning with vowels. With the introduction of vowels, an activity known as *word changes* was added to the basic segmentation exercises. An English equivalent would involve changing the word *cat* to *cut* by exchanging the *a* tile for a *u*. Consonants were added later and the word-changing exercises continued. Word-changing is an especially effective way to teach children awareness of consonant clusters (e.g., clap–lap–cap–clap; sit–slit–split–spit–pit). Several training studies by various Russian researchers are described briefly by Elkonin and reported as successful in the translated reviews of this literature, but none of the research methods is described in detail (Elkonin 1963, 1973).

Benita Blachman includes phoneme segmentation in a five-part lesson she has used in several studies of beginning reading in inner-city schools. The lesson includes these five components: 1) letter-sound practice, 2) segmenting and blending activities similar to Elkonin's *word changes* using letters in a pocket chart, 3) reading phonetically regular words and sight words, 4) reading from phonetically controlled readers as well as trade books, and 5) writing from dictation. Two research studies have reported a significant advantage in reading for children who were trained, in comparison with controls (Blachman 1987; Blachman et al. 1994).

We have used segmenting and spelling training in a school setting with 22 first graders (a mix of at-risk and normal readers). Using a sequence of c–v–c (e.g., *map, hit*) and c–c–v–c–c words (e.g., *flap, milk, blast*), the children were taught to segment with blank blocks and later with lettered blocks, to type these words into a computer from dictation, and to play computer spelling games with these words. All activities stressed analyzing phonemes in spoken words. Elkonin-type *word-change* activities were used to teach consonant clusters. After seven months, these first graders had a significant advantage over controls on a variety of reading skills with the most dramatic difference being in phonetic reading of nonsense words (Uhry and Shepherd 1993a).

We have found this training to be effective in a clinical setting as well. Twelve first and second graders were trained in an after-school tutoring center. Note that KM was one of these children (see Chapters 3 and 24). The children were considered to be at-risk because of poor phonological awareness skills, family history of dyslexia, and, in the case of the second graders, failure to acquire reading. After-school tutoring twice a week included letter-sound training, segmentation and spelling training, and guided reading in both phonologically controlled and narratively controlled text. Over a five-month period, they made significant gains in phonological awareness, and in standard scores on word reading, nonsense word reading, and spelling tests. Although remediation was not complete at the end of this initial training period, the anticipated discrepancy between word reading, viewed in the literature as remediable, and nonsense word reading, viewed as a chronic deficit, did not develop. In fact, after training, nonsense word reading was stronger than word reading for the group as a whole and for 8 of the 12 children when considered individually (Shepherd and Uhry 1993).

Patricia and Charles Lindamood were early advocates of phonological awareness training. Their program, Auditory Discrimination in

Depth (ADD), is described more fully in Chapter 13. It begins with an emphasis on oral-motor awareness of sound production. Descriptive labels are used to refer to the mouth action used in producing different sound categories. For example, the term *lip poppers* is used for sounds such as /p/ and /b/. Once students are proficient at associating these pictures with sounds, training moves to exercises involving the manipulation of markers representing phonemes in spoken words (see Elkonin 1963, 1973). These exercises also incorporate the descriptive labels mentioned above. One research study of this method reports that second- through fifth-grade scores rose over a five-year period for children who began this training in first grade (Howard 1982). The program can be used with prereaders as well as much older students.

Currently, two large-scale studies are in the second year of federally funded five-year grants to study treatments for reading disability. One of the grant teams, headed by Joseph Torgesen (1995), is using the Lindamoods' ADD program as one component of a prevention program for young, at-risk readers (see Chapter 14). This longitudinal research should provide a clearer picture of the effects of the Lindamood program.

TRAINING IN CONNECTION WITH REMEDIAL READING

As with beginning reading programs, remedial reading programs are rarely based on phoneme segmentation training alone. It is more usual to find it included as one component of a total program. This makes it hard to isolate the specific effect for phonological training.

Joanna Williams was an early advocate of phonemic awareness training. Her *ABD's of Reading* (analysis, blending, and decoding) was used with older learning-disabled students in New York City public school special education classes (Williams 1980). The program began with auditory syllable analysis, followed by phoneme analysis using only nine phonemes, in an adaptation of the Elkonin technique. At the next step the phonemes, which were represented by wooden squares, were blended into bigrams and trigrams. Later, letters were introduced on the squares and the children manipulated the squares to form words. Eventually, six more letters were added to the original nine, and practice on c-c-v-c and c-v-c-c words was introduced. Williams reported significantly greater improvement in phonemic analysis and blending skills for these children in comparison with controls. Skill transfer was noted in superior ability to read nonsense words.

Much of the research on the Lindamood program involves studies of its use in regular classrooms. However, it is widely used in remedial programs with older children. A team working with Joseph Torgesen in Florida used the Lindamood program, Auditory Discrimination in Depth (ADD), in an after-school tutoring program to train ten dyslexic children (Alexander et al. 1991). This successful project is reported in more detail in Chapter 14. Of particular note was the dramatic growth in nonsense word reading, contrary to the widely held opinion that poor nonsense word reading is an enduring and hard-to-remediate characteristic of the reader with dyslexia. The program is distinctive in that it initially teaches sounds without letters, even with older children and adults.

In a year long study, three bright fourth-grade children with dyslexia were trained using segmenting and spelling techniques to see whether increasing phoneme awareness could help them become more skilled with vowel digraphs and trigraphs (e.g., *au*, *igh*). Using a single-subject design with multiple measures taken over baseline and treatments, several different traditional phonics-based training conditions failed to produce improvement in ability to generalize vowel patterns to nonsense words. The improvement in generalization to nonsense words was dramatic only when spelling-based phoneme analysis training was used (Uhry 1993b).

Overall, the evidence from training programs suggests that phonological awareness training should begin as early as kindergarten and should be continued until children can decode with accuracy. Studies by Bradley and Bryant (1985), Byrne and Fielding-Barnsley (1993) and Lundberg, Frost, and Petersen (1988) indicate that training carried out with pre-readers can have an impact on later reading skills. Work by Bradley and Bryant (1985) and Ehri (Hohn and Ehri 1978; Ehri and Wilce 1987b) indicates that using letters, even right from the beginning, increases levels of phonemic awareness. Work with at-risk and dyslexic children indicates that the characteristic deficit in nonsense word reading can be remediated in children with dyslexia (Alexander et al. 1991; Shepherd and Uhry 1993; Uhry 1993b).

This sort of training is beginning to be a standard part of both remedial and regular classroom training programs, but there are few systematic, long-term programs that take children through a sequence of strategies. Teacher training programs have not focused on this area so that many teachers are lacking in an understanding of the complexity of the processes involved here. To compound the problem even more, many teachers do not have well-developed phonological awareness skills themselves. Louisa Moats provides evidence of this in a study in which she surveyed the phonological awareness skills of 89 experienced teachers (e.g., classroom teachers, reading teachers, speech/language pathologists, and special education teachers). She found that many of them were lacking in phonemic and morphemic knowledge and were unable to segment words into phonemes (Moats 1994). This is an area in which there is clear and strong evidence that a particular sort of training can have effective results and it is crucial that this training be built into teacher-training programs as well as into both remedial and regular reading programs.

6

Phonics Instruction

Among reading theoreticians, there is almost unanimous agreement that phonics instruction should be part of the reading curriculum for all school children (Adams 1990; Anderson et al. 1984; Chall 1983a; Liberman 1984; Resnick 1979; Venezky and Massaro 1979; Williams 1985). Furthermore, despite the fact that the research on effective reading methods has been fraught with methodological problems (Pflaum et al. 1980), the general findings suggest that early and direct teaching of sound-symbol relationships produces better decoding skills than later and less explicit phonics instruction (Adams 1990; Chall 1983a). Since decoding ability has been shown to contribute to reading comprehension (Gough and Tunmer 1986; Lesgold and Resnick 1982; Perfetti and Roth 1981; Stanovich, Cunningham, and Feeman 1984), phonics instruction seems pedagogically justified. Unfortunately, as indicated in Chapter 1, this conclusion has not generalized broadly to classroom practice where basal reader and whole language philosophy programs predominate. Most of these programs place emphasis on teaching whole words; children are expected to apply knowledge from learned words to new words, thus learning by analogy.

Failure to teach the phonological features of the alphabet systematically is particularly detrimental to children with dyslexia who seem not to acquire phonics knowledge naturally, nor to apply phonological strategies spontaneously (Gough and Tunmer 1986; Olson et al. 1985; Liberman et al. 1983; Mann 1986; Perfetti 1985a; Vellutino 1983). Among

83

reading specialists who work with dyslexic children and are aware of these deficiencies, phonics instruction is fundamental (Bateman 1979; Cox 1992; Enfield 1976; Liberman and Shankweiler 1979; Slingerland 1971). However, it is important to specify how phonics should be taught to these children.

Two distinct alternative approaches exist: the *explicit phonics* approach (also termed synthetic phonics instruction) and the *analytic phonics* approach (also referred to as the functional, incidental, or intrinsic approach). Explicit phonics instruction, as the name implies, explicitly teaches individual grapheme-phoneme correspondences before they are blended to form syllables or whole words. For example, the letter-sound /ph/ is taught in isolation before children are expected to read this grapheme in a word. Usually, the letters are presented first on a small card for practice. For example, in Alphabetic Phonics (see Chapter 13) the digraph *ph* is presented on a card with a picture of a phone to help children remember the sound. A child practices by responding with the phoneme /ph/ when shown the card by a teacher or tutor. Once the letter-sound correspondence has been practiced in isolation, the grapheme, in this case the digraph *ph,* is synthesized, together with other already-learned letters, into a word for reading. In contrast to the synthetic method where words are built up from known parts, the analytic approach introduces whole words first and encourages children to deduce letter-sound relationships as they appear in those words. The analytic method differs from the basal method only in that the words presented are selected for their phonemic elements, which are introduced systematically, rather than for their prevalence in children's vocabularies, as in basal series.

Although most remedial specialists espouse the synthetic or explicit phonics approach, some theorists contend that it places undue demands on sound blending abilities, which can be weak in children with poor phonological awareness skills (Lyon 1985; Olson et al. 1985; Siegel 1985; Vellutino and Scanlon 1986). Despite the possible lessening of blending difficulties, there is reason to question the effectiveness of an analytic approach with students who are dyslexic. Analytic training methods, as Joanna Williams observes (Williams 1985), have proven least successful with poor readers. A training study conducted with normal and dyslexic fifth-grade students found that the latter group needed extensive training in generalizing, as well as in analogy strategies, in order to produce analogue words for nonsense words (Wolff, Desberg, and Marsh 1985).

Another important point that needs to be made is that an analytic approach, to be used effectively, necessarily requires extensive reading in order to develop a broad basic knowledge of exemplar words against which to compare newly encountered words. The very fact that children with dyslexia read less than normally achieving students would seem to put them at a disadvantage in applying analytic decoding strategies. These caveats, in addition to the evidence that individuals with dyslexia do not spontaneously learn the phonological code, are persuasive reasons to recommend explicit phonics instruction for most of these students, albeit with provision for extensive blending practice. Initial results of a longitudinal comparison of these two methods support the use of synthetic rather than analytic phonics for children with phonological deficits (Foorman, Francis, and Fletcher 1995; see Chapter 4).

EXPLICIT PHONICS INSTRUCTION
ORTON-GILLINGHAM APPROACH

The Orton-Gillingham approach, mentioned in Chapter 4, was designed for one-to-one instruction. In 1960, Anna Gillingham and Bessie Stillman published an instruction manual for remedial tutors, along with instruction materials. Since then, the method has become the basic model upon which multisensory remedial intervention programs for dyslexic children have been built. Alphabetic Phonics, the Slingerland Program, Recipe for Reading, Enfield and Greene's Project Read, and the Wilson Reading System, which are all described in Part III of this book, and Preventing Academic Failure, described at the end of this chapter, are all based on the Orton-Gillingham approach.

June Orton, the wife of Samuel Orton, summarized the three most important distinguishing features of the Orton-Gillingham approach as follows:

1. It is a *direct* approach to the study of phonics, presenting the sounds of the phonograms orally as separate units and then *teaching* the process of blending them into syllables and words.
2. It is an integrated, total language approach. Each unit and sequence is established through hearing, speaking, seeing, writing it. Auditory, visual, and kinesthetic patterns reinforce each other and this also provides for individual differences among the students. It is a circular, multi-sensory process.
3. It is a systematic, step-by-step approach, proceeding from the simpler to the more complex in orderly progression in an upward spiral of language development. (Orton 1964, p. 11).

As Gillingham and Stillman (1960) described it, the method is built on the close association of visual, auditory, and kinesthetic aspects of language to form what they called the *language triangle*. In strong contrast to an analytic phonics method, the Orton-Gillingham approach teaches letter sounds and the blending of these sounds into words. It should never be used, according to its authors, as a supplement to sight or basal reader approaches. Furthermore, any reading outside of Orton-Gillingham material is discouraged. Complying with this restriction obviously presents a problem, and tutors using this method have had to deviate to some extent from the method with any child who remains in a regular classroom. Gillingham and Stillman placed considerable emphasis on the need for older children to break old habits. In order to *establish the alphabetic principle* among these children, words must no longer be viewed "as ideograms to-be-remembered as wholes" (Gillingham and Stillman 1960), and all guessing must be eliminated.

In the Orton-Gillingham approach, letters or phonograms are introduced as visual symbols printed on cards. First, the letter name (or names, in the case of digraphs) is taught. The tutor says the name, the child repeats it. Then the tutor asks what letter it is, and the child gives the name. When this is secure, the letter sound is taught in the same manner. The association between visual and auditory characteristics of letters is made in this way. Then *auditory-to-auditory* association is established—the tutor says the letter sound and asks the pupil for the letter name. This is followed by *visual-kinesthetic* and *auditory-kinesthetic* associations. The tutor writes the letter, carefully explaining its formation and orientation, and the student traces the letter, then copies it, then writes it from memory, and finally writes it from memory with eyes averted. This last step is to internalize the visual and kinesthetic image of the letter. For auditory-kinesthetic reinforcement, the tutor gives the letter sound and asks the student to write the letter that makes that particular sound. When writing, however, the student always says the letter name, not the sound, a procedure that is called *Simultaneous Oral Spelling (SOS)* (see footnote on page 71).

The introduction of letters and letter combinations is carefully sequenced. Initially, ten letters are taught: two vowels (*a, i*) and eight consonants (*f, h, b, j, k, m, p, t*). Each letter is introduced with a *key word*, for example, *i-igloo*. When the a card is exposed, the student's response should be "/a/-apple-*a*." The difference between vowels and consonants is taught, drawing the student's attention to the open and closed positions of the mouth in pronunciation, and reinforced using different colored cards for vowels and consonants. These cards are used to bring learning to mastery in drill exercises. Once letter names and letter sound knowledge are secure, reading begins. Three letter cards are laid out (for example, *b-i-t*), and the student is asked to produce each sound in succession, repeating them with increasing speed and smoothness, until able to pronounce the word. The same associations are established with words as with letters; the child traces, copies, and writes each word. Printed cards for each word, provided in a file box referred to as the *Jewel Case*, are used in word recognition drill exercises. Recognition speed is encouraged through use of a stopwatch or egg timer, and the tutor keeps a progress graph for words learned. In this way, the student builds his reading lexicon.

Orton-Gillingham lessons are intended to be conducted within 40- to 60-minute periods. A guide for developing a daily routine is provided in the teacher's manual. New phonograms are introduced gradually, usually not more than two in one lesson, and must be taught in invariant order to match the word cards and other materials provided.

In the Orton-Gillingham approach, reading of text begins only when the student is able to read c-v-c (consonant-vowel-consonant) words perfectly (presumably to a highly automatic level), as well as phonetic four-letter words with digraphs such as *th* and *ph*. Stories containing words the student has learned are printed in the teacher's manual. Nonphonetic sight words, which the student has not previously encountered, are underlined and told to the student by the teacher. The student reads each sentence silently first, asking for help if needed. In oral reading, he is encouraged to read with inflection. Gillingham and Stillman contended that the pleasure children derive from finally being able to read justifies the bland contents of these phonetically controlled texts. The same stories are used for dictation exercises.

Syllabication is taught to all students and particularly encouraged for those who previously used a whole-word approach. Practice begins with students reading words with syllables separated, followed by their rearranging jumbled syllables to form real words. They are taught to place stress marks on accented syllables.

Additionally, the Orton-Gillingham approach describes the evolution of written language. As an introduction to remedial instruction, the dyslexic student is given a brief history of the development of written language, from pictographs to ideographs to alphabets, which helps him to understand the concept of an alphabetic system. For teachers, a brief history of the English language is provided to increase their understanding of word derivations. The information is intended to help teachers develop a knowledge of spelling patterns, and thereby transfer this knowledge to their students.

TEACHER TRAINING IN THE ORTON-GILLINGHAM APPROACH

A number of sites for training in the Orton-Gillingham approach are listed in the Resource and Teacher Training Guide at the end of this book. Many of them can supply information about tutoring and evaluation resources for children and adults with dyslexia. The Reading Disabilities Unit at Massachusetts General Hospital in Boston has provided this training for many years. Teachers (or college graduates) can begin training at Massachusetts General in either the early summer or the fall. Training includes both lectures and practical work. The program was started by Dr. Edwin Cole, a neurologist who was also instrumental in starting the Carroll School in Lincoln, Massachusetts. This school for children with dyslexia uses the Orton-Gillingham method and also serves as a training site. Barbara Wilson, author of the Wilson Method, trained at Massachusetts General (see Chapter 23).

EVALUATION OF THE ORTON-GILLINGHAM APPROACH

Although it has been used extensively with children and adolescents who are dyslexic, until recently little research has been conducted to validate the effectiveness of the Orton-Gillingham approach, as defined by Gillingham and Stillman (1960). Probably the primary reason for the lack of systematic data collection is that the method has been used almost exclusively in tutorial, one-to-one situations and, to a large extent, in private practice. In addition, it is almost impossible to know to what extent tutors are complying with the instructions provided in the teacher's manual, in other words, how representative of the approach the tutoring actually is.

ANALYTIC PHONICS INSTRUCTION
THE GLASS-ANALYSIS FOR DECODING ONLY

The Glass-Analysis for Decoding Only method was developed by Gerald and Esther Glass (Glass and Glass 1976). Unlike the Orton-Gillingham synthetic phonics approach, the Glass-Analysis method presupposes a basic knowledge of grapheme-phoneme correspondences. The term for decoding only refers to the fact that word meaning and comprehension are de-emphasized in order that complete attention be placed on analyzing the orthographic structure of words. The student is taught to recognize phonemic units within words. These units are not morphemes, but rather, letter clusters. The clusters are never isolated, but always shown to the student within the context of words. The authors of this method have identified 119 letter clusters and placed them in two sets of words, arranged in order of apparent difficulty. These words are called service words, their major purpose being to provide a medium in which to foster perceptual conditioning for letter clusters.

Five procedural steps for the instructor to follow are listed in the Glass Analysis manual:

1. Identify the whole word and ask for the word to be repeated.
2. Give the sound(s) and ask for the letter(s).
3. Give the letter(s) and ask for the sound.
4. Take away letters and ask for the remaining sound.
5. Ask for the whole word (Glass and Glass 1976).

This method resembles some phonemic training procedures described in the previous section. The teacher is advised never to separate letter blends or digraphs. A problem arises, however, with suffixes that may overlap letter clusters taught as units, as for example, the er in spider, a word containing the cluster ide. In this case the teacher is told to ask,

"What letters say 'sp'? What letters say 'ider'? What letters say 'ide'?" and then to ask for the sounds those particular letter clusters make, but to ignore the suffix *er*. The authors claim that their intent is to teach letter clusters that can be generalized and to avoid "esoteric linguistic concerns about the dropping of the final e before adding the suffix."

The teacher is urged to work as fast as possible, because the authors believe fast response is important for habituating decoding patterns. Fifteen minutes should be allotted for each instructional session, plus additional time in the *Follow Through Practice Books*, which are designed for what they call *oral at-sight reading*. In oral reading the teacher intervenes whenever a word containing a common letter cluster is missed and tells the student what letters to attend to. If it is an irregular word, called a *Nix* word, the teacher simply voices the word and has the student repeat it. Carefully chosen basal readers may also be used for this purpose.

The Glass–Analysis method was not specifically designed for readers with disabilities, although the manual mentions its use with students with severe learning disabilities. In an effort to address the needs of students having, as they expressed it, "a handicapping condition affecting learning," Glass and Glass published the *Easy Starts Kit* (Glass and Glass 1978a) containing twelve *cluster packs* of word cards that represent some of the more basic letter clusters found in c-v-c words (*at, in, et, ad, it, an, ap, un, op, en, ab, and*). They have also provided *Follow Through Practice Books* for oral reading of short sentences containing these cluster words. Words appearing in these sentences that are not cluster words are termed *preview words* and are taught as sight words before the sentences are read.

Realizing that many students do not have secure letter-sound knowledge and that this knowledge is a necessary prerequisite for the Glass–Analysis method, Glass and Glass developed a program to teach the alphabet, which they called *Quick and Easy* (Glass and Glass 1978b). The program consists of *Alphabet Cards* (one letter to a card), *Word Cards* (c-v-c words with basic letter clusters), *Mixed Letter Cards* (eight different letters on each), and a consumable student workbook, the *Program Book*, which also contains directions for the teacher. Letter identification begins at the word level: as the teacher holds up a word card, for example, *hat*, she asks the students to locate the word on their workbook pages. The teacher next points to the first letter, *h*, says its name, and has the students say the name aloud several times. She then asks the students to circle this letter where it appears on their workbook pages. The remaining letters in the word *hat* are taught in the same way. A *Letter Starter* exercise is followed by *Do-More* exercises which provide practice both in identifying letters as the teacher names them and in naming letters as the teacher points to them. Mastery tests are provided in the back of the book to be administered informally and individually.

"ong" cluster

(For every word, say the whole word and ask that the word be repeated.)

song

[From sound to letters]

[From letters to sound]

This word is *"song"*. What is the word?
•*In the word, "song", what letter makes the* "sss" sound?
What letters make the "ong" sound?
•*In the word, "song", what sound does the letter* /s/ make? What sound does o/n/g make?
•If I took off the /s/ what sound would be left?
•What is the whole word?

longest

[Sound to letters]

[Letters to sound]

[Combine two]

[Take off letters or sound]

•*In the word, "longest", what letter makes the* "lll" sound? What letters make the "ong" sound? What letters make the "long" sound? What letters make the "est" sound? What letters make the "ongest" sound?
•*In the word, "longest", what sound does the* /l/ make?
What sound does the o/n/g make?
What sound does the l/o/n/g make?
•*In the word "longest", what sound does* e/s/t make?
What sound does o/n/g/e/s/t make?
•If I took off the l/o/n/g, what sound would I have left?
If I took off the "est" sound, what sound would be left?
•What is the whole word?

[Remember, to end off, always tell the word and ask for its repetition]

stronger

[Ask for letters first]

[Then ask for sounds]

[Take off]

•*In the word, "stronger", what letters make the* "st" sound?
What letters make the "ong" sound?
What letters make the "rong" sound?
What letters make the "strong" sound?
What letters make the "er" sound?
•*In the word, "stronger", what sound does* s/t make?
What sound does the o/n/g make?
What sound does the r/o/n/g make?
What sound does the s/t/r/o/n/g make?
In the word, "stronger", what sound does the e/r make?
The o/n/g/e/r?
•If I took off the s/t, what sound would be left?
If I took off the e/r what sound would be left?
•What is the whole word?

EVALUATION OF THE GLASS-ANALYSIS METHOD

A study investigating the effectiveness of the Glass-Analysis method for teaching word decoding, oral reading skills, and spelling skills was conducted (Barger 1982) with 154 reading disabled children. Pre- and post-test analyses indicated gains in decoding and significant gains in spelling, which is particularly noteworthy as spelling instruction is not a component of this method. Glass-Analysis training did not increase fluency or accuracy in oral reading, however. Unfortunately, because this training was provided as a supplement to a basal reading program and because there was no control group of subjects who did not receive the training, it is not possible to determine the extent to which the basal program or the Glass-Analysis method contributed to the results.

Lydia Poe investigated the effects of Glass-Analysis instruction, which she referred to as segmentation training, with first grade children who were unable to segment oral words or to read segments of words (Poe 1983). A control group of untrained children was included in the study. After four weeks of instruction it was found that oral segmentation ability, but not decoding of segments, was enhanced for the experimental group.

Thus the research so far on Glass-Analysis training has produced somewhat conflicting results. For children with dyslexia, the Glass method serves no purpose until their letter-sound associations have been secured. However, once that point is reached, the Glass method can be used to increase automaticity in word recognition, as it encourages the student to look for orthographic patterns in words. One major shortcoming of the method is its disregard for morphemes, such as suffixes, which bear meaning and therefore play a critical role in fluent reading and comprehension of text.

THE STERN STRUCTURAL READING SERIES

The Stern Structural Reading Series, developed by Catherine Stern and Toni Gould (Stern and Gould 1965) is a beginning reading program designed to promote learning by insight and thus might best be described as an analytic phonics method. The Stern method presents whole words and draws a child's attention to particular elements within those words. The program begins at a readiness level, which teaches phonemic awareness. The child learns to listen to and distinguish the initial sounds in orally presented words. Once letter sounds are familiar, the child learns sound-symbol correspondences through the presentation of pictures representing words beginning with the letter to be taught; the letter appears next to the picture. The child says the letter *sound*, not the name, and then copies the letter formation. The child also learns the difference between a vowel and a consonant at this pre-reading level (a vowel has a prolonged sound — it can be sung; a consonant, instead, is "blown, mumbled or hissed," and has a clear sound only with an accompanying vowel).

In first grade, teaching begins with spoken, not written, words. The child is shown pictures representing consonant-vowel-consonant words, all having the same vowel, for example, *man, cat, hat*. The teacher says one of the words, emphasizing its letter sounds, but always pronouncing the initial consonant with the accompanying vowel, and the child points to the word. Then the child says the word in the same way. In the author's view,

> The structure of the word *hat* is not revealed by adding up, in piecemeal fashion, the single elements, /h/ plus /a/ plus /t/; the word is divided structurally into a main part /ha/ and an ending /t/. The salient point in our method is this

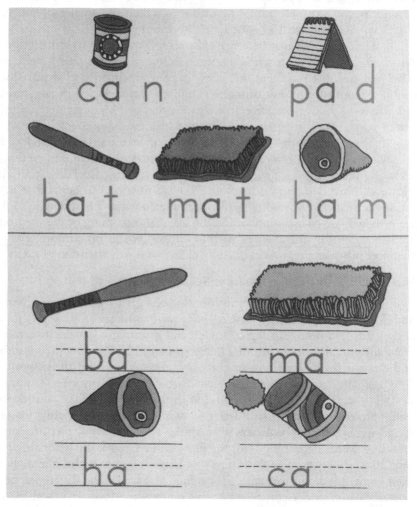

Workbook Page from Structural Reading: We Discover Reading *by Catherine Stern, Toni S. Gould, and Margaret B. Stern. (Reproduced with permission from Random House, Inc., New York, NY. Copyright 1984.)*

emphasis on giving the child insight into the way spoken words break naturally (Stern and Gould 1965).

Note that there is research (e.g., Goswami 1986; Treiman 1985) suggesting that the more natural break point in a word for a beginning reader is between the onset (i.e., *h-*) and the *rime* (i.e., *-at*), rather than as presented by Stern and Gould. In the Stern method, words for reading are color coded to emphasize the vowels and later the digraphs, final silent *e*, and suffixes. All reading is reinforced with writing using manuscript letters.

Stern and Gould stress meaning at all levels of their program, first in pictures, then in individual words with picture counterparts, then in sentences, and finally in stories. Newly encountered words are taught individually beforehand.

In the beginning stages of the program, reading beyond the program is discouraged in order that children do not adopt a whole word, or sight, approach before learning the individual sound-symbol correspondences. Once the basic foundations of structural analysis have been laid, Stern and Gould suggest that children be given a diversity of reading material in addition to the readers and workbooks provided in the program. The authors contend that, in their experience, many children are so adept at sounding out words that they are able to read nonphonetic irregular words without help.

Reading and spelling are taught simultaneously in the Stern program, and reading vocabulary expands through the systematic introduction of increasingly more sophisticated common word elements. Spelling rules and first grammatical concepts — singular and plural noun and verb forms and simple verb tenses — are also included in the Stern curriculum.

EVALUATION OF THE STERN PROGRAM

Research on the effectiveness of the Stern program is limited, particularly in regard to its use with readers who are dyslexic. The program was developed for use in regular classrooms with children in kindergarten through second grade. Its authors, however, maintain that it is readily adaptable for remedial instruction. In the back of their book, *Children Discover Reading*, Stern and Gould provide data showing the effectiveness of their program in regular classrooms. They claim success with over one hundred students who experienced difficulty learning to read. Although they provide no empirical evidence to support this claim, they describe four successful tutoring cases, each involving a five-year-old child evidencing initial reading difficulties. It must be acknowledged that while the Stern method may be appropriate for readers with mild disabilities, its utility for children with dyslexia has not been verified.

THE MERRILL LINGUISTIC READERS

The Merrill Linguistic Readers (Wilson and Rudolph 1986), like the Stern series, is intended as a beginning reading program for regular classroom use and, like the Stern, is sometimes used in remedial intervention. It also aims at teaching letter-sound correspondences within the context of real words instead of as isolated individual units. The Merrill program emphasizes word endings (often called *word families* in other situations; *man, can, Dan*, etc.), in contrast to the Stern program, which presents variation in both initial and final consonants in words with only the vowel held steady (*fox, rod, hog*, etc.). Note, too, that in the Stern series the break point for segmenting is just before the final consonant (e.g., /ma/-/n/) and that the Merrill series uses the onset-rime break (e.g., /m/-/an/). In the Merrill readers the child is taught to direct his attention to word endings and to note the varying initial consonants, applying the principle of minimal contrasts. Letter recognition is a readiness requirement. The child is taught to attend to the special visual features that identify each letter and distinguish it from others similar in shape. Letter names, but not letter sounds, are taught, and emphasis is placed on left-to-right progression.

The program consists of eight readers and workbooks. Before beginning each chapter, all new *words in pattern* which are included in the chapter are introduced on the chalkboard, the first being c-v-c words with short *a*, as well as any high frequency words not falling in that pattern. These words are also listed in the readers at the beginning of each new story. Pictures are excluded from all books, in order not to distract from strategies utilizing the printed words. Pupils read the text silently

---

A Cat on a Mat

Is a cat on a mat?

A cat is on a mat.

Is the cat fat?

The cat is fat.

Is the cat Nat?

The cat on the mat is Nat.

Excerpt from The Merrill Linguistic Reading Program: I Can *by Rosemary G. Wilson and Mildred K. Rudolph. (Reproduced with permission from Charles E. Merrill Publishing Co., Columbus, OH. Copyright 1980).*

first. Scripted comprehension questions are provided in the teacher's guide. Because of both phonemic and semantic redundancy, the texts in the early books tend to be bland; the entire first book is based on short *a* words.

EVALUATION OF THE MERRILL PROGRAM

The Merrill is one of ten or more linguistic readers on the market. The basic rationale for using any one of these linguistic programs with disabled readers has been that a linguistic approach, with its onset-rime break, makes blending easier and enables reading by analogy. Usha Goswami's research indicates that even very young children can read through analogy (Goswami 1986). Keep three things in mind in considering a reading series like the Merrill. First, the linguistic approach provides no direct instruction in letter-sound correspondences, which children with dyslexia need. Second, research suggests that analogy reading is enhanced by prior phonics knowledge (Ehri and Robbins 1992). Third, for children who already have this knowledge, the series provides the redundancy necessary for adding words to a lexicon of sight vocabulary words.

In our clinical practice with children with dyslexia at the Child Study Center at Teachers College, Columbia University (see Chapter 24; Shepherd and Uhry 1993, Uhry 1994) we have used the Merrill readers, but not with beginners. We prefer to start with a synthetic approach, together with spelling-based phonological awareness training, until children have completely internalized the left-to-right, letter-by-letter strategy and have a repertoire of mastered sounds. We use the Merrill readers later on, once children have mastered letter-sound correspondences for short vowels and basic consonants and can read and spell c-v-c words and nonsense words accurately but slowly. We find that reading whole pages of words with the same rime unit helps children *chunk* these units for greater automaticity.

Phyllis Bertin and Eileen Perlman have designed an Orton-Gillingham based curriculum, *Preventing Academic Failure* (Bertin and Perlman 1995), which combines synthetic phonics instruction with use of the Merrill Linguistic Readers. The program is used in both mainstream and special classes in public schools in White Plains, New York and at the Windward School, an independent school in White Plains for children with learning disabilities. A guide and several student handwriting workbooks are available through Educators Publishing Service.

7

Training in Automaticity and Fluency

TRAINING IN AUTOMATICITY

The theory that fast, as well as accurate, word recognition is related to proficient reading was first proposed in 1974 by David LaBerge and S. Jay Samuels (see Chapter 1). Charles Perfetti and Thomas Hogaboam (1975) elaborated upon this hypothesis by suggesting a *limited capacity mechanism* within children's information processing systems to account for differential performance in reading comprehension. Similarly, Charles Perfetti and Alan Lesgold (1979) contend that poor decoding hampers comprehension by creating a *bottleneck*; the more time and effort required for decoding, the less processing capacity available for comprehension. Perfetti (1985a) refers to this hypothesis as a *verbal efficiency theory*. Using multiple regression analysis, Keith Stanovich and his associates provide substantial support for the verbal efficiency hypothesis by determining that decoding speed is the highest contributing variable to reading comprehension (Stanovich, Cunningham, and Feeman 1984).

There is, therefore, a theoretical rationale for instruction in rapid word decoding, most particularly with disabled readers whose major weakness seems to lie in this area. Unfortunately, research so far has failed to provide direct evidence that such instruction does, in fact, improve reading comprehension. For example, Linda Fleisher, Joseph Jenkins, and Darlene Pany carried out two automaticity training studies with fourth- and fifth-grade children who were poor readers, the first involving single words, the second involving phrases (Fleisher, Jenkins, and Pany 1979). Although such training increased the subjects' speed of single word decoding, it had no effect on their comprehension of passages containing these words. Similarly, in a training study with below-average readers, Mary Strother was unable to increase comprehension of text by increasing speed and accuracy of word recognition. She concludes that subskills of reading are "mutually facilitative," that they develop through "levels of proficiency," and that "insufficiently developed subskills prevent development of higher-level" skills (Strother 1984).

Despite the failure of experimental studies to demonstrate a causal relationship between decoding speed and reading comprehension, reading experts are paying increasing attention to automaticity training and to new methods of providing it. Recently, efforts have been made to apply computer technology toward this purpose. Such training is generally referred to as *computer assisted instruction (CAI)*. J. F. Frederiksen and his associates have designed microcomputer activities for use with high school students who are poor readers (Frederiksen 1983). These activities focus on developing three reading subskills: 1) perception of multiletter units within words; 2) efficient phonological decoding of orthographic information in words; 3) use of context frames in accessing and integrating meanings of words in context. Computer assisted criterion tasks have revealed significant effects of training in the three subskill areas, as well as evidence of transfer to other componential skills of reading. As far as comprehension is concerned, the investigators maintain that increased reading speed on an inference task produces no decrement in comprehension. One of the most helpful features of the microcomputer as a training medium is its ability to provide immediate corrective feedback that can be acted upon.

Steven Roth and Isabel Beck have also investigated the effects of microcomputer automaticity training of reading subskills on reading comprehension (Roth and Beck 1984). In contrast to earlier studies with small subject samples and short-term laboratory-type intervention, Roth and Beck's training was administered in three fourth-grade classrooms over an eight-month period. A unique aspect of this training was the use of speech, provided by recording, both for corrective feedback and assistance when needed. The major emphasis of the training was on teaching knowledge of orthographic patterns in English words. Practice conditions, intentionally designed to be semantically meaningless, forced the subjects to focus attention solely on the orthographic patterns in English words. Rapid response rates were encouraged, but for the purpose of creating a *game-like atmosphere*, rather than as a means to promote better comprehension. The study comprised two principal activities, the first, called *Construct-a-Word*, involved subjects' constructing real words from sets of subword letter clusters; the second, called *Hint and Hunt*, required subjects to attend to subword letter clusters during word recognition.

Two types of pre- and posttests were administered in the Roth and Beck study (1984): 1) achievement tests measured subjects' decoding and comprehension skills relative to national norms, and 2) laboratory tests measured accuracy and speed of word recognition as well as understanding of word meaning. Based on pretest data, subjects were split into three ability groups. Posttest analysis indicates that training benefitted only those subjects in the low ability group. Almost two years gain was made on the reading vocabulary subtest of the California Achievement Test by the low ability subjects, suggesting, the investigators maintain, that decoding rather than vocabulary deficits penalize these students. Although their reading comprehension improved at the sentence level, no gains were evidenced at the passage level, paralleling findings from earlier investigations.

Roth and Beck (1984) concluded that perhaps direct training with multisyllable words, which had not been provided in their training programs, was necessary to enhance proficiency with text, since many syllables that appear in longer words are not common in one-syllable words or may be pronounced differently. In addition, they caution that this type of computer instruction may not be appropriate for beginning readers who are not yet able to differentiate between real and nonsense words.

Joseph Torgesen and Kay Young stress several additional advantages of CAI activities for students with reading disabilities (Torgesen and Young 1984). One is that by providing a variety of formats for extensive practice or overlearning, computer-based instruction lessens the boredom that usually accompanies traditional teacher-based practice activities and hence increases sustained attention. A second important advantage is that CAI programs can accurately measure response times and, through game formats, encourage faster responses.

TRAINING IN FLUENCY

Instructional efforts to increase reading fluency have entailed methods such as *repeated reading*, in which the student reads short meaningful passages several times until reaching a satisfactory level of fluency. Although both speed and accuracy are measured, the former is emphasized over the latter. The method is to be used as a supplement to developmental reading instruction, according to S. Jay Samuels, who is probably its leading advocate. He compares repeated reading to developing musical or athletic abilities which require practicing basic skills until they can be performed with adequate speed and smoothness (Samuels 1979).

Samuels (1986) suggests several techniques for implementing repeated reading. One technique is the *use of audio support*, in which a student reads silently while listening to a tape-recorded narration of the passage. Another technique is to have the student read for one minute and count the number of words read in that time and then record that number on a graph; after criterion level is reached, the student moves on to another passage. *Paired reading*, having two students read alternately and record for each other the number of words read, is yet another approach.

William Henk, John Helfeldt, and Jennifer Platt suggest several additional variations of the repeated reading model, one being *imitative reading* — the teacher reads a segment of text aloud while the student follows along silently before reading the segment himself, imitating the teacher's intonation and phrasing (Henk, Helfeldt, and Platt 1986). This technique is appropriate for the most disabled readers, according to Henk and his associates. *Radio reading*, in which the student, acting as announcer, reads a script aloud to the rest of the class, can avoid embarrassment, since only the student and the teacher share the script. *Chunking*, or reading in phrases, is another method suggested by these educators to promote fluency. A multisensory technique, referred to as *neurological impress* (NIM), involves the teacher and student simultaneously reading a passage aloud. The teacher forces the pace with her voice and by moving her finger along under the text, refusing to allow any pauses. Group use of this technique resembles the audio support method suggested by Samuels, but has not been found to be as effective as the one-to-one system, according to Henk and his colleagues.

Samuels (1986) reports on research that has shown repeated reading to be an effective instructional tool with disabled readers, particularly those with decoding problems. A theoretical explanation for this finding is proposed by Peter Schreiber, who suggests that repeated reading helps students learn to listen for the prosodic cues, such as intonation and pacing, not found in print (Schreiber 1980). Carol Rashotte investigated the question of whether repeated or nonrepeated reading of passages by learning disabled students produces greater fluency and comprehension and whether degree of word overlap between passages is an influential factor (Rashotte 1983). Results of her study indicate that repeated reading is more effective than the equivalent amount of nonrepeated reading only when a large number of words is shared across passages.

Rashotte and Torgesen have studied the effects of *computer administered repeated reading* of passages on learning disabled fourth-grade students (Rashotte and Torgesen 1985). They find that students enjoy this activity because they receive immediate feedback on their improved reading speed and take pleasure in their ability to read the passages with increasing fluency. The major effect of this practice, however, has been to enable students to identify individual words in the passage with greater speed. Particularly encouraging is the finding that learning to read words in context seems to generalize to reading these words out of context.

The Slingerland program, one of the remedial language arts programs for children with dyslexia described in Part III of this book (Chapter 16), encourages fluency in round-robin reading by having children first practice reading words and phrases from the chalkboard before encountering them in the basal stories.

Deficits in automaticity and fluency are the symptoms of older individuals with dyslexia that are the most difficult to correct. Additional research on training methods in this area is needed.

8

Reading Comprehension Instruction

The topic of reading comprehension instruction raises the issue of the definition of dyslexia. Remediation in this area should differ, logically, depending on whether one is talking about dyslexia with oral language intact, other than the specific linguistic deficits associated with dyslexia, or whether one is talking about dyslexia in connection with more global oral language disorders. The latter requires a reading comprehension program linked to an oral language comprehension program designed by a language specialist. Unfortunately, much of the existing research literature on comprehension does not differentiate between learning disabled readers with poor listening comprehension and children who are poor decoders and good comprehenders. The programs described here are appropriate for children with comprehension difficulties associated with decoding problems. Many of these programs are also appropriate for children without special needs. It is beyond the scope of this short chapter to present a complete review of the literature on reading comprehension instruction. For this, readers are refered to more comprehensive reviews (e.g., French, Ellsworth, and Amoruso 1995; Pearson and Fielding 1991; Maria 1990; Oakhill and Garnham 1988; Stothard 1994). It is our intent here to present just a few representative approaches that might be appropriate.

HISTORICAL PERSPECTIVES

Historically, children with dyslexia have received little training in reading comprehension (Maria 1987). For many years reading instruction for these children focused almost exclusively on decoding, with minimal attention directed toward reading for meaning. Most children with dyslexia were not taught how to think critically while reading (Baker and Brown 1984; Harste 1985).

The reasoning behind this has been that if dyslexia is a disorder at the word reading level, then remediation should focus on decoding. The unspoken assumption is that if comprehension rests on decoding and decoding is remediated, then comprehension skills will follow. This reasoning seems faulty. Keith Stanovich's *Matthew effects* theory is an argument for the phonological core deficit as an initially specific problem that causes a global problem. Although comprehension may have been a secondary, reactive problem at the onset, it can become a real and enduring one for children with dyslexia. Because they cannot decode, they are cut off from developing reading comprehension strategies and need this instruction in addition to decoding instruction (Stanovich 1986b).

A number of studies of older children with reading disabilities have found specific comprehension deficits. For example, in a recent study, Joanna Williams found that older children with reading disabilities, when matched by comprehension level with younger readers, are more apt to overuse idiosyncratic background knowledge and thus to struggle in identifying themes in stories (Williams 1993).

The point needs to be made here that while children with dyslexia may have difficulty with comprehension (and not all do), this difficulty is not the primary problem. These children should respond to the same sort of reading comprehension instruction that is appropriate for all children.

One reason for the omission of comprehension instruction for children with dyslexia is that until the 1980s there was little focus on comprehension in either regular education classrooms or in reading research. When the first edition of this book was published, Diana Clark wrote, "Reading comprehension instruction has an abysmal record, not just for reading disabled students, but for all learners" (Clark 1988, p. 79). She cited Dolores Durkin's study in which fewer than 50 minutes were spent on comprehension instruction out of 17,997 minutes of classroom observation time (Durkin 1978-1979). David Pearson and Linda Fielding make the point that until 1981 there simply were no reviews of research on comprehension (Pearson and Fielding 1991).

By 1984, in the first edition of the *Handbook of Reading Research*, Robert Tierney and James Cunningham were able to report a dramatic increase in research on comprehension (Tierney and Cunningham 1984). By 1991, when the second volume of the *Handbook* was published, Pearson and Fielding refer to the recent *explosion* in comprehension research and begin with a review of recent reviews. In the 1990s there are a great many choices of approaches to reading comprehension instruction.

SPECIFIC SKILLS APPROACH

One approach to instruction in reading comprehension has been conceptualized as a bottom-up or specific skills approach in which comprehension is broken down into skills that typically are pretaught in short exercises before they are practiced in text. Skills are taught at both the vocabulary or word comprehension level, and the sentence or text comprehension level.

VOCABULARY INSTRUCTION

In a review of research on vocabulary instruction with poor readers, Joanne Carlisle distinguishes between *definitional approaches* to vocabulary, in which new words are learned in isolation, and several other approaches in which new words are learned in the context of meaningful reading (Carlisle 1993). She cites research to make the point that comprehension instruction needs to be a good match for a particular type of reading problem. For example, students with low verbal ability lack the conceptual base to learn new words through definitions alone, and benefit from contextually based instruction.

On the other hand, poor readers with high verbal ability lack access to vocabulary because of their poor decoding. They have difficulty extracting meanings for new words when they read because their decoding is so slow. For these children, Carlisle suggests embedding vocabulary instruction in lessons in which the teacher reads stories aloud. She also suggests learning vocabulary through instruction in which decoding and word origins are taught together, such as the phonics component of Robert Calfee's Project READ, described in Chapter 20. In this approach Anglo-Saxon words are taught before ones derived from Romance languages, with initial emphasis on letter-sound associations for decoding words with short and long vowels, followed by syllable division, and then morphemic knowledge of roots and affixes. Thus connections between letter patterns and word meanings are built into instruction (Henry 1988).

SPECIFIC SKILLS IN TEXT READING

At the text level, skills often include getting the main idea, finding facts, detecting the sequence, and making inferences. Often these skills are taught through drill in reading short passages and then answering questions. The Barnell Loft Specific Skills Series (Bonig 1982) is typical of what is commercially available for this type of instruction. Each skill-type is available in a series of graded texts with a monitoring system that can be carried out by the student as well as by the teacher. A package of these materials allows a classroom of children to work independently on a variety of specific skills at many different reading levels.

Probably one of the most systematic deliveries of this specific skills approach involves computer-assisted instruction (CAI). One example of such application is the program described by Judith Boettcher (1983) which was developed by Control Data Corporation and is known as the Reading Comprehension System. It is structured around a five-by-six matrix that enables the teacher to select appropriate lessons for a student depending on instructional needs; there are five levels of difficulty applied to short reading passages written at six vocabulary levels. Each passage includes ten comprehension questions, two for each of the following five comprehension areas: word meanings, syntax, word relationships, inferencing, and interpretations. Students receive immediate feedback on their answers, and continue working until the computer judges them to be at mastery level on each skill.

Boettcher conducted a study of the effectiveness of the Reading Comprehension System with 28 students with learning disabilities in self-contained fourth- and fifth-grade classrooms. After nine weeks of 45 minutes of instruction a week, these students had made about a year's gain on the Vocabulary and Comprehension subtests of the California Achievement Tests. Boettcher acknowledges considerable variance in individual gain scores, and the lack of control group. Despite these short-comings, she concluded that the gains were impressive (Boettcher 1983).

The specific skills approach to teaching comprehension has received criticism on several counts. In a review of comprehension instruction for children with learning disabilities, Katherine Maria questions the notion of specific skills instruction, noting difficulty in defining what is meant by *main idea*, for example, and in making decisions about which skills to teach (Maria 1987).

Another criticism of a specific skills approach is that many of the available materials for this instruction represent something closer to a test than to real instruction, as Dolores Durkin points out (Durkin 1978-79). In other words, instead of breaking a skill into component parts and pro-viding guided learning experiences with each part, instruction is apt to involve exercises in which students are expected to perform a task over and over without any special guidance.

A notable exception can be found in the research of Joanna Williams who uses task analysis and step-by-step teaching to break com-prehension down for children with reading difficulty. Her work on main idea identification with children with learning disabilities represents an innovative approach to comprehension skills instruction (Williams 1986). Acknowledging that there is considerable controversy over the definition of the term *main idea*, Williams avoids it altogether and borrows instead the labels *general topic* and *specific topic of discourse* from Walter Kintsch and Teun van Dijk's theory of text processing, in which the general topic is the title subject of an essay or story, and the specific topic of discourse is the topic sentence or implicit main idea in each paragraph (Kintsch and van Dijk 1978). Williams contends that the ability to select main ideas from text requires basic classification skills. Thus, she provides students with initial instruction in categorizing objects and pictures, which is later related to text organization.

When first working at the paragraph level, students are asked, "What is this paragraph about?" (i.e., "What is the general topic?") and then required to circle the word referring to the general topic. The next question is, "Does this paragraph tell us everything about __?" followed by, "What is the specific topic?" In this way students learn to identify topic sentences within paragraphs. Later they learn to determine the main ideas in paragraphs that do not contain topic sentences, the more common type of paragraph, according to Williams (1986). All work is carefully sequenced from simple to complex, from choosing titles, for instance, to writing summaries.

Investigating the effectiveness of this approach with 11-year-old students with learning disabilities, Williams found that they produced better paragraph summaries than did controls who had not received this training. However, performance at posttest was far from optimal, leading Williams to conclude that the length of training time needs to be extended for these children (Williams 1986).

INSTRUCTION IN COMPREHENSION STRATEGIES

In a recent research review, Janice Dole and her colleagues described the difference between what they call traditional instruction in comprehension *skills* and a newer approach that involves *strategy* instruction (Dole et al. 1991). They view skills as being a rather passively learned set of routines whereas strategies are viewed as cognitive processes requiring decision making and critical thinking. Indeed, cognitive theory has played a major role in the development of recent comprehension instruction. Pearson and Fielding summarize some of the new findings as follows:

> Singer called it active comprehension (1980), Wittrock and his associates (e.g., Doctorow et al., 1978) have labeled it generative learning, Pearson and Johnson (1978) called it relating the new to the unknown. But whatever the label, the principle seems clear: Students understand and remember ideas better when they have to transform these ideas from one form to another. Apparently it is in the transformation process that *authors'* ideas become *readers'* ideas, rendering them more memorable (Pearson and Fielding 1991, p. 847).

Several concepts from the field of cognitive psychology have contributed to this new view of both reading and the reader (Maria 1987). One concept is *schemata*, or psychological frameworks that develop out of an individual's cultural experiences (Rumelhart 1980). According to this view, the reader must fit new facts into an existing mental schema for a particular idea, or if necessary, adjust the schema. Schema theory led to an awareness of the importance of the reader's background knowledge to understanding and interpreting text.

Another concept that has had tremendous influence on reading comprehension research is *metacognition*, defined by Linda Baker and Ann Brown as "the knowledge and control the child has over his or her own thinking and learning activities." By knowledge, they refer to the awareness of the processing demands of a particular task, and by control, the ability to check, plan, monitor, or evaluate one's own activities while reading (Baker and Brown 1984). Isabel Beck and Margaret McKeown make the point that many of the strategies now being labelled as metacognitive skills were formerly taught as study skills, the difference being that under the metacognitive label, the rationale for the application of these strategies is explained to the student (Beck, Omanson, and McKeown 1982).

A third concept that has gained prominence in the reading comprehension literature is the notion of interaction between student and teacher in the learning situation. This concept developed out of L. S. Vygotsky's theory of guided learning, in a social context within a student's *zone of proximal development* which he defined as:

> . . . the distance between the actual developmental level as determined by individual problem-solving and the level of potential development as determined through problem-solving under adult guidance or in collaboration with more capable peers (Vygotsky 1978).

Reuven Feuerstein's theory of *mediated learning* has also contributed to our understanding of the teacher–student interaction. Feuerstein maintains that early learning is shaped by interactions in which a parent models problem solving that eventually allows a child to solve problems on his own (Feuerstein 1979).

The three concepts just discussed—schema theory, metacognition, and mediated learning—have led researchers to a new conceptualization of the instructional conditions thought to promote optimal learning. Katherine Maria, for example, conceptualizes reading instruction as an interaction between reader, text, and teacher. The reader brings decoding ability, oral vocabulary, and background knowledge to the text. The text is no longer perceived as having a single meaning for all students; rather, meaning is constructed through this interaction. The teacher is viewed as a manager and facilitator who provides direct instruction in strategies but who also encourages independence (Maria 1990). Linda Baker and Ann Brown offer a particularly apt description of the way guided learning theory has been applied in this new wave of reading comprehension:

The current interest in dynamic learning situations has seen a move away from experimenter-controlled or teacher-controlled instruction of the traditional kind towards a concentration on interactive processes. It is through interactions with a supportive, knowledgeable adult that the student is led to the limits of her own understanding. The teacher does not tell the student what to do and then leave her to work on unaided; she enters into an interaction where the child and the teacher are mutually responsible for getting the task done. As the child adopts more of the essential skills initially undertaken by the adult, the adult relinquishes control (Baker and Brown 1984, p. 382).

Jerome Harste claims that most direct instruction models, in assuming that only the teacher can teach, do not allow for internalization, nor do they provide opportunity for students to learn from their peers (Harste 1985).

Michael Pressley and his colleagues review and describe some of these strategies (Pressley et al. 1989b). They view *summarization* as a collection of strategies (e.g., deleting unimportant details, selecting a topic sentence). These strategies appear to have characteristics in common with Joanna Williams' techniques for task analysis of main idea. Another strategy for constructing and remembering information from a reading passage is *mental imagery,* which can involve *representational images* (i.e., mental pictures of details described in text) and *mnemonic images* (i.e., idiosyncratic images consciously constructed in order to remember text that is not familiar to the reader). Pressley points out that there is evidence in the research literature that this strategy can be effective for children past the age of 8. Training in *knowledge of story grammar* (e.g., character, setting, problem, resolution) has been found to increase comprehension in poor readers who do not appear to grasp this structure without direct instruction. Instruction in *self questioning* strategies can increase comprehension of factual detail, and if carried out over a longer period of time, it can increase comprehension of inferences as well. Pressley and his colleagues also review comprehension strategies that involve a commitment to long-term instruction. For example, teaching children to activate prior knowledge in order to make inferences can be a lengthy process.

There are a number of different methods for teaching these strategies. *Reciprocal teaching,* an instructional model designed by Annemarie Palincsar and Ann Brown, is an example of an interactive approach to teaching metacognitive strategies that has been used successfully with students who are poor readers. This model contains two major components. The first is a sequence of four strategies: 1) generating questions about the text prior to reading, 2) summarizing portions of the text, 3) predicting what will happen next, and 4) clarifying and evaluating after reading the text. The second component of reciprocal teaching is an interactive dialogue between teacher and students, and eventually, between the students themselves, about the text and the strategies used in processing it (Palincsar 1986; Palincsar and Brown 1983, 1985).

Reciprocal teaching instruction begins with a teacher-led discussion about the kinds of problems readers may experience in comprehending what they read. It introduces the four strategies, each on a separate day, and explains why they are helpful. Instruction usually begins at the paragraph level, but can involve single sentences for readers who are more disabled. The discussion aims at stimulating metacognitive awareness so that students learn to guide and monitor their own comprehension. Once students have caught on to the four strategies, the teacher turns over her role to one of the students, who leads the activities and calls on other students. This peer teaching provides the reciprocal teaching component. The teacher subtly guides and provides feedback to the student-as-teacher. After the activities are mastered, they are applied to classroom texts.

Palincsar and Brown conducted several evaluations of their techniques and report significant improvement in students' comprehension, as measured daily on reading passages. This improvement was maintained over eight weeks following treatment (Palincsar and Brown 1983, 1985). Moreover, effects carried over into other subject areas, such as science and social studies (Brown, Palincsar, and Armbruster 1984).

Michael Pressley has worked with research colleagues and with teachers to develop teaching methods that he calls *transactional strategies* instruction. Pressley views this instruction as Vygotskian in that compre-

---

Aquanauts

Student 1: My question is, what does the aquanaut need when he goes under water?
Student 2: A watch
Student 3: Flippers
Student 4: A belt
Student 1: Those are all good answers.
Teacher: Nice job! I have a question too. Why does the aquanaut wear a belt, what is so special about it?
Student 3: It's a heavy belt and keeps him from floating up to the top again.
Teacher: Good for you.
Student 1: For my summary now... This paragraph was about what the aquanaut need to take when they go under the water.
Student 5: And also about why they need those things.
Student 3: I think we need to clarify "gear."
Student 6: That's the special things they need.
Teacher: Another word for gear in this story might be equipment, the equipment that makes it easier for the aquanauts to do their job.
Student 1: I don't think I have a prediction to make.
Teacher: Well, in the story they tell us that there are "many strange and wonderful creatures" that the aquanauts see as they do their work. My prediction is that they will describe some of these creatures. What are some of the strange creatures that you already know about that live in the ocean?
Student 6: Octopuses.
Student 3: Whales?
Student 5: Sharks!
Teacher: Let's listen and find out. Who will be our teacher?

A Reciprocal Reading Teaching Script. (Reproduced with permission from the author, Annemarie Palinscar.)

hension develops as the result of social interactions between students and teacher. Students are provided with direct instruction in a number of comprehension strategies and are encouraged to talk about and choose a strategy for understanding as they read. Teachers model their own thinking aloud and encourage students to do this for each other. Students are provided with positive reinforcement when a strategy is successful, and are encouraged to attribute success to use of the strategy. Thought processes are valued more than product. Pressley compares transactional strategies instruction to whole language instruction in some regards (e.g., process over product) but comments that whole language is more based in philosophy than in cognitive psychology. Teachers using transactional strategy instruction tend to step in as coaches whereas whole language teachers tend to be in favor of noninterventionist learning. Pressley differentiates it from other strategy instruction models that use direct explanation by the degree to which this model becomes part of the texture of every aspect of school life over a very long period of time (Pressley et al. 1992).

Irene Gaskins of the Benchmark School is a collaborator of Pressley's. Benchmark is an independent school outside of Philadelphia for elementary and middle school children with reading problems. Teachers at Benchmark have been actively involved, together with a team of researchers, in the development of transactional strategy instruction. Research on this instruction has involved extensive teacher interviews indicating a high level of enthusiasm and involvement among faculty (Pressley et al. 1991). Pressley makes use of detailed and extensive transcriptions of teacher–student interactions to document this instruction (Pressley et al. 1992).

Both the Palincsar and Brown model and the Pressley model make use of principles believed to be related to effective instruction for children with reading difficulties: carefully sequenced lessons, direct instruction, and opportunity for practice over a long period of time.

COMPREHENSION AND DYSLEXIA: SPECIAL CONSIDERATIONS

While a number of the programs described above have been found to be effective for children with dyslexia, none of them is specifically designed to be used in programs for this population. In addition to use of the techniques described above, several modifications to comprehension instruction come to mind for children with specific decoding ability. According to information processing theory, working memory is overtaxed by decoding in children with reading disorder, leaving little processing space for understanding (LaBerge and Samuels 1974). The logical course to take here is to provide very easy text for reading comprehension in combination with listening comprehension instruction using text at the child's intellectual level. Text can be read aloud by the teacher or the child can listen to Books on Tape. Tapes of any necessary educational materials are provided free of cost by the Library of Congress to children and adults with vision impairment. Children with dyslexia are entitled to the same free services.

Providing listening experiences to increase comprehension is fairly standard practice in the remediation of children with dyslexia, but is not documented in the research. Another solution is to use computers that can *read* difficult text aloud for the child.

COMPUTER ASSISTED INSTRUCTION (CAI)

Bookwise, a Xerox Corporation computer-delivered literature program is an example of computer assisted instruction (CAI) that takes advantage of current technology, presenting print on a screen while speaking the words. Speed is adjustable and the vocalized sentence is highlighted. Vocabulary words can be defined by the computer's voice, and text can be scrolled backwards and forwards. In a recent study, Jerome Elkind and his colleagues used Bookwise with middle school students in a California school for children with dyslexia (Elkind, Cohen, and Murray 1993). These children were already engaged in multisensory decoding instruction using the Slingerland method. It should be noted that not all of the 28 subjects had deficits in reading comprehension, but 70 percent were at least a grade level below grade placement in this skill. Treatment involved half an hour using the computer and half an hour discussing the literature each day. Controls read the same books and discussed them within a comparable time frame. Each of the two classes served as control to the other during the two semesters of treatment, so that each child's, and each class's, gains could be compared with and without CAI. Results were mixed: 70 percent of the students made a year's worth of growth in the CAI semester, and 40 percent made as much as five grade-levels of growth. A few subjects actually lost ground, probably because of kinesthetic-motor problems with the computer.

COMPREHENSION THROUGH INDUCED IMAGERY

Some children with dyslexia are believed to have better-than-usual spatial ability or ability with imagery. This is a claim made, for example, by Aylett Cox about children she saw for remediation using the Alphabetic Phonics approach (see Chapter 13). Advocates of Howard Gardner's (1983) theory of multiple intelligences suggest using imaging techniques with these children because the techniques build on what may be areas of strength. The following represent brief descriptions of a few programs.

Induced Imagery is a technique for increasing students' comprehension through guiding the generation of images from text. This literature is reviewed by Robert Tierney and James Cunningham who conclude that, "inducing imagery is likely to increase learning from text for selected students (those who can learn from pictures) in and above grade 3" (1984, p. 622). Nanci Bell, who works with Patricia Lindamood at Lindamood–Bell Learning Processes in San Luis Obispo, California, has developed a program called Visualizing and Verbalizing for Language Comprehension and Thinking (V/V) for use with individuals with comprehension problems (Bell 1986). Bell uses this program to correct what she believes is a cognitive processing disorder that she calls *Concept Imagery Disorder* (CID). Note that many of Bell's subjects have adequate word reading and phonemic segmentation skills, and thus cannot be considered dyslexic. The program, however, is a good example of a highly structured and explicit comprehension model. There are specific, sequenced steps to V/V, in which students move from describing pictures with feedback, to developing images for increasingly complex language, beginning at the word level, and moving to sentences, paragraphs, and finally, pages of text. Text, level of questioning, and feedback become more abstract as the V/V program progresses. Evaluation of Bell's program with reading-impaired children has focused on pretest-posttest improvements in individuals in a remedial laboratory setting; these gains have reached statistically significant levels on a number of measures of oral directions and reading comprehension (Bell 1991).

COMPREHENSION IN WHOLE LANGUAGE CLASSROOMS

There have been positive changes in reading comprehension theory and practice since the time of Durkin's studies. Children with dyslexia in the mid 1990s are lucky to have available so many models of comprehension instruction. Although the advent of whole language has brought complaints from dyslexia specialists about the lack of explicit instruction in decoding, whole language classrooms present an opportunity for improved reading comprehension instruction; it tends to be interactive, to focus on the integration of decoding and comprehension strategies right from the start, and to use meaningful text at the child's level, rather than independent practice in skills-oriented workbooks.

9

Spelling Instruction

PRINCIPLES OF SPELLING INSTRUCTION

Some of the most important pedagogical issues related to spelling instruction are brought to light by Margaret Stanback and Marylee Hansen in their review of the literature on spelling instruction (Stanback and Hansen 1980). One of these issues, which has been referred to as the *generalization controversy* (Yee 1966), concerns the question of whether or not the sound–symbol correspondence of English orthography is sufficiently regular to warrant teaching rules and regularities. This question has provoked a number of studies aimed at determining the amount of regularity in the English spelling system. Ernest Horn, the staunchest opponent of teaching generalizations in spelling, states that over a third of the words in a standard English dictionary have more than one pronunciation, that more than half of these contain silent letters, that most letters—particularly vowels—have more than one sound, and that unstressed syllables are hard to spell (Horn 1960). Horn advocates teaching only those rules that apply to a very large number of words and have few exceptions. In contrast, Paul Hanna and his associates, after conducting a computerized analysis of 17,000 English words, conclude that only 3 percent required rote memorization, falling into the category of *demon* words (Hanna et al. 1966).

Whereas Horn and Hanna and his colleagues examined only the phonemic regularity of English words, Richard Venezky has analyzed

20,000 words, taking into consideration morphemic features as well. As a result of his findings, Venezky recommends three categories of spelling patterns: 1) predictable, 2) unpredictable and frequent, and 3) unpredictable and rare, rather than the standard two category regular/ irregular classification (Venezky 1970).

Although research on the instructional implications of the generalization controversy has apparently produced ambivalent results, Stanback and Hansen cite two studies that imply that direct instruction in spelling generalization was beneficial to slower learners. They conclude that there may not be one best way to teach spelling, but observe that

> ... in the light of analyses such as Venezky's, the phonology and orthography are seen to be closely related, especially when certain morphological principles are understood. For example, the past tense marker *ed* is consistently spelled, no matter that it is pronounced in three different ways, e.g., /id/ in *landed*, /d/ in *planned*, and /t/ in *rushed*. In fact, the morphology is highly dependable for spelling, as there are few exceptions. Prefixes and suffixes, inflectional and derivational, are added to roots by fixed and dependable rules (Stanback and Hansen 1980).

Another important instructional issue is whether spelling should be taught *systematically*, as a relatively independent subject, or whether it is best taught *incidentally* in the context of other subject areas. Here again, there is no definitive empirical support for either approach; however, as Stanback and Hansen point out, research indicates that the hundred most frequently misspelled words are among the most frequently occurring words in text, and therefore it seems clear that repeated exposure to a word in reading does not ensure spelling knowledge of that word.

The frequency of testing in spelling instruction, the type of practice provided (distributed versus massed), and the number of spelling words presented in a lesson have been found to have differing effects on good and poor spellers. According to Stanback and Hansen, these variables have only minimal influence on good spellers, but poor spellers do better with frequent testing, with distributed rather than massed practice, and with fewer numbers of words per lesson. This point is made, as well, in a more recent research review that suggests teaching as few as three new words in any single lesson (Gordon, Vaughn, and Schumm 1993).

Roderick Baron maintains that poor readers are more likely to use an orthographic approach (attending to spelling patterns) to reading and a phonological approach (attending to letter sounds) to spelling, but that good readers are able to apply either strategy as needed (Baron 1980). Therefore, he advises teaching both strategies and cautions that too much emphasis on one or the other strategy might encourage overspecialization of that strategy.

MULTISENSORY METHODS OF REMEDIAL
SPELLING INSTRUCTION

Multisensory teaching has probably had its greatest impact in the area of remedial spelling instruction, the two best known approaches being the Orton-Gillingham and the Fernald methods. As previously described in Chapter 4, the Orton-Gillingham approach teaches spelling as the inverse of, in conjunction with, and as reinforcement for, reading. Learning progresses from small units (phonemes and syllables) to larger units (words and sentences). Enormous emphasis is placed on the alphabetic principle and phonetic regularity of the English spelling system. All learning is carefully sequenced. Inconsistent spelling patterns are only gradually introduced, and optional spelling patterns representing similar sounds are taught as separate units. Irregular spellings are not taught until the student becomes comfortable with phonetic spellings. Although considerable practice with syllables is provided, inflectional endings, as well as prefixes and suffixes, are treated as morphemes and taught by the rule. The technique applied to studying spelling is called *Simultaneous Oral Spelling (SOS)*, wherein the child pronounces the word, spells it orally, and then writes the word, saying the letter names as she writes.

In contrast to the Orton-Gillingham approach, the Fernald method (Fernald 1943), while also multisensory, teaches spelling with whole words of a student's own choosing, rather than word units following an orderly sequence. The Fernald procedure closely resembles the *neurological impress* method described in Chapter 7. It focuses on the student's development of a distinct visual image of the word and automaticity for the motor pattern for writing the word, both processes being mutually reinforcing. The technique involves having the student say the word while looking at it, with the teacher underlining each syllable as it is pronounced. The student then repeats the word slowly, tracing each syllable as it is pronounced. The next step requires the student to write each syllable while saying it slowly so that individual letter sounds may be heard. Finally, the student writes the whole word from memory (while pronouncing it) on the reverse side of his paper. With some students the tracing stage may be bypassed. However, words are never copied. Fernald's approach is based on the rationale that putting all modalities into play compensates for weaknesses in visual perception and visual memory.

Another multisensory approach to spelling is Bannatyne's method which shares some of the features of the two methods just described while differing from them in several respects (Bannatyne 1971). Alexander Bannatyne is primarily concerned with the sound blending problems demonstrated by many learners and stresses the need for disabled spellers to hear their "phonemic vocal inner language" in order to master the sequencing aspects of spelling. Bannatyne's technique requires a student to first pronounce the spelling word slowly, then to pronounce it separating the phonemes, then to study the word in print visually, separating the graphemes that represent the phonemes, then to pronounce each phoneme in sequence as a teacher points to the corresponding grapheme, then to write the graphemes while articulating the phonemes as a rhythmic sequence, and finally, to practice this technique until the word is learned. Tracing and copying may be involved if necessary. Multisyllable words are introduced only when the student can spell at the syllable level; with multisyllable words, the syllable, rather than the individual phoneme, becomes the articulated unit.

The Childs Spelling System (Childs and Childs 1971, 1973) is one of several variations on the Orton-Gillingham approach to remedial spelling instruction. Sally and Ralph Childs, the authors of this method, reorganized and simplified many of the Orton-Gillingham generalizations and rules, classifying spelling words into three groups: *sound-words*, which can be sounded out, *think-words*, which require individual study, and *see-words*, which require memorization. Multisensory techniques are not applied, however, in the Childs system.

The Slingerland Multisensory Approach to Language Arts for Specific Language Disability Children (Slingerland 1971), which was developed for classroom use, incorporates a *simultaneous, auditory-visual-kinesthetic approach* intended "to strengthen inter-sensory associations" (Aho 1967) and begins with handwriting instruction (see Chapter 15).

Slingerland classifies spelling words into three categories which are similar to those in the Childs' system. *Green-flag words*, or short vowel, purely phonetic words, are studied by having the teacher dictate the word, the student repeat the word and then give the vowel sound. The student then names the vowel while forming it in the air, then spells the word orally, writing each letter in the air as he names it, and then says the word. Finally, the student writes the word on paper and traces it for further memory reinforcement.

In *red-flag words*, which are nonphonetic or irregularly spelled, the difficult parts are stressed, but the word is studied as a whole, involving primarily the visual and kinesthetic modalities. The student copies the word from a model, the teacher checks spelling and letter formations, the student traces over the word, naming each letter, and then when ready, closes his eyes and writes the word in the air.

Yellow-flag words are words containing ambiguous spelling patterns, or patterns representing sounds that can be spelled in more than one way (e.g., *ai, ay, a-e, eigh* all pronounced as the long /a/ sound), and are introduced only after vowel digraphs, diphthongs, and phonograms have been taught. By third grade, students should be able to recall all of the possible spellings for phonograms and to select the correct one for particular words (Aho 1967). Considerable practice with morphographs, syllables, and spelling rules is provided in the Slingerland program. All learning is reinforced by writing from dictation, first at the letter, then the word, and then the sentence level.

In *Alphabetic Phonics*, Aylett Cox incorporates the Orton-Gillingham principles but has reorganized the Orton-Gillingham spelling generalizations and rules (Cox 1984, 1992). She brings spelling instruction to a considerably more complex and sophisticated level, as is reflected in the subtitle (*Formulas and Equations for Spelling the Sounds of Spoken English*) of her teaching manual, *Situation Spelling* (Cox 1977). The term *situation spelling* refers to the fact that the spelling of a particular speech sound tends to vary with its position in a particular word. In this manual, Cox states:

> By studying systematically each sound and its most likely symbols in every significant position in monosyllabic and multisyllabic words, the student can eventually incorporate all of his knowledge of spelling the separate sounds in base words into his reflexes (Cox 1977).

Cox's remedial program, which has reportedly been successful with children and adults who are dyslexic, in tutoring, clinical, and small class settings, presents a challenge to instructors as well as students because of its level of sophistication. Multisensory techniques, such as SOS, are incorporated into teaching at all levels of the program, as well as instruction in the situation rules.

Sister Marie Grant has developed an instructional program for at risk first graders using a combination of several multisensory elements including: 1) a linguistic approach, 2) a modified version of Cox's situation spelling techniques, and 3) spelling instruction that precedes reading instruction. The unique aspect of Grant's remedial approach, though, is the introduction of hand motions to introduce sounds. The procedure for spelling the word *be*, for instance, involves the student's learning the hand motions for its two phonemes or letter sounds, pronouncing the phonemes, and then blending them before writing the word on the chalkboard ("for more muscular perception") and then on a piece of paper. After four years of instruction these at-risk children had markedly higher spelling scores than controls receiving traditional instruction (Grant 1985). While Grant has provided empirical support for her program, her study has not identified the aspect(s) of this complex treatment that most affected spelling growth.

In their program, *Auditory Discrimination in Depth (A.D.D.)*, Charles and Pat Lindamood emphasize that, in order to spell, contrasts in spoken language must be perceived before contrasts in written language can be understood (Lindamood and Lindamood 1975). They maintain that many children do not naturally acquire the degree of

SHORT VOWEL SOUNDS

(ă) Voiced

I.   REGULAR FOR SPELLING   Example

     A.   Initial or Medial Position in a Base Word

          (ă) = a (in a closed syllable)   apple*

     B.   Final Position in a Base Word - never in English words.

Formula:	Application:
Sound Situation = Symbol	Pronunciation = Spelling
1^+syl b.w. $_{(ă)c}$ = 1^+syl b.w. $_{ac}$	(ă'p'l) = apple

Etymology: The letter a is never doubled in English words.

Pronunciation: The speech sound (ă) is in the middle of the scale in tone. The production opens the speaker's mouth wider than does (ĕ) and less wide than (ŏ). The student can associate tone, mouth shape, and kinesthetic memory for spelling reinforcement if he practices while watching his own mouth in a small mirror.

II.   IRREGULAR FOR SPELLING (rare):   Example

     A.   Initial or Medial Position in a Base Word

          (ă) = au (in a very few words)   laugh

     B.   Final Position in a Base Word - never in English words.

Formula:	Application:
1^+syl b.w. $_{(ă)}$ = 1^+syl b.w. $_{au}$	(lăf́) = laugh、

Learned Words

au	Misc.
laugh	plait
aunt	morale
etc.	

A Lesson from Situation Spelling by Aylett R. Cox. (Reproduced with permission from Educators Publishing Service, Inc., Cambridge, MA. Copyright 1977.

phonological knowledge, or auditory-perceptual skills, needed for proficient spelling or reading. After working for many years with dyslexic individuals, Lindamood and Lindamood conclude:

> The one factor common to all these students was their lack of auditory-perceptual skills, with its attendant problem in self-monitoring their production of specific

sounds and sequences while pronouncing words, or monitoring and integrating sound-symbol identities and sequences during reading and spelling activities (Lindamood and Lindamood 1975, *Book 1*).

Spelling instruction in the Lindamood program begins with auditory conceptualization. A distinctive and important feature of this program is the attention brought to bear on sound production and the labeling of all letter sounds according to the real movements involved in articulating these sounds. The sounds /b/ and /p/, for example, are called *lip poppers*; /f/ and /v/ are called *lip coolers*. A student is taught to discriminate sounds in nonsense words by manipulating cards with pictures representing these sound labels. She then progresses to working with colored blocks that represent the sounds (the colors have no specific relationship to the letters but serve only to differentiate one sound from another). Once she can perform this task proficiently with single syllables, the student is given letter symbols to manipulate in spelling activities. Spelling instruction progresses from single to multisyllable words, starting in each case with nonsense words and moving to real words.

Chapters in Section III describe spelling instruction in several multisensory programs (Alphabetic Phonics, Auditory Discrimination in Depth, Slingerland). These chapters include research on their success in teaching both reading and spelling. Although there is substantial evidence that these and other multisensory programs work with children with learning disabilities, additional research is needed to determine what aspects of these programs are most influential and why. Most evaluations of multisensory programs have collected end measures on reading and spelling, but have not attempted to control for the possible contributions of various components of the programs.

British researchers Lynette Bradley and Charles Hulme have been interested in issues of multisensory instruction (Bradley 1981; Hulme 1981). They have used the Orton-Gillingham SOS technique in which children choose a word that interests them and practice spelling it by saying each letter as they copy it. Handwritten spellings were contrasted with practice in which subjects chose plastic letters for spellings. As reported in Chapter 4, multisensory instruction with handwritten spellings of irregular words was more effective than instruction with plastic letters (Hulme and Bradley 1984).

Anne Cunningham and Keith Stanovich replicated this study with first graders but added a keyboard condition. They found that handwritten spellings were more effective for teaching both reading and spelling, but wondered if the results weren't affected by the children's unfamiliarity with the keyboard (Cunningham and Stanovich 1990). Sharon Vaughn responded to this work with a training study involving writing, tracing, and typing spellings into a computer. Vaughn found that all three methods worked equally well with children with and without learning disabilities. (Vaughn, Schumm, and Gordon 1993).

NATURALISTIC SPELLING METHODS

There is current worry among practitioners about children with dyslexia in whole language classrooms employing the writing process and basing instruction on invented spelling. With this technique, children are encouraged to represent sounds as best they can and to focus on meaning in their stories. Practitioners worry that without direct instruction in spelling patterns, children with dyslexia will retain their own misspellings. Rebecca Treiman's book *Beginning to Spell* (1993) documents the developmental spellings of children in a whole language classroom over the course of their first-grade year, much in the tradition of Charles Read's work (1971, 1986) and Glenda Bissex's *GNYS AT WRK* (1980). However, Treiman entered these invented spellings into a special computer program designed to analyze frequencies of phoneme spellings under different orthographic conditions. Treiman draws several conclusions from analysis of her data: 1) invented spellings do not become permanent misspellings in first graders, and, in fact, they encourage children to think about the relationships between sounds and letters, and 2) the process of inventing spellings helps children acquire the alphabetic principle. That spelling can lead into reading is in keeping with Frith's stage theory (Frith 1985, 1986), but Treiman feels that exposure to print influences spelling as well. Treiman adapts a connectionist model of spelling:

> In such models, there are connections from phonological units to orthographic units. Learning to spell involves modifying the weights on the connections to reflect the relations between sounds and spellings in the words to which the person has been exposed (Treiman 1993).

Treiman cites a study with similarly encouraging results that is described in detail in Marilyn Adams' book (Adams 1990). First grade Canadian children instructed through invented spellings wrote more prolifically and spelled more accurately than children taught to spell correctly (Clarke 1988). We need to keep in mind that Treiman and Clarke worked with normally achieving children. What works for most children may not be explicit enough for children with dyslexia.

Chapter 22 describes spelling procedures used in the Reading Recovery approach. Within the context of writing a story based on interest in a book a child has read, a tutor encourages the child to listen for sounds in words which the child cannot spell. Reading Recovery takes advantage of the connections between phoneme segmentation and spelling with Elkonin-type boxes used for writing letters as these words are sounded out with support from the tutor (see Chapter 5,

Increasing Phonological Awareness). This is a modification of invented spelling, with a tutor providing cues for a child to use in self-correcting. With words that the child wants to use but that are beyond her developmental spelling level, the tutor simply provides the letters for her to copy. Thus the child has the advantage of sounding out invented spellings that are within what Vygotsky would call the *zone of proximal development* without the disadvantage of seeing her own misspellings later in the lesson when these words are used for reading instruction. Research on Reading Recovery has tended to focus on reading rather than spelling so that we cannot be sure of the effect of this instruction on the spellings of these young children who are at risk for reading failure.

10

Handwriting Instruction

B eatrice Furner characterizes handwriting development as a perceptual learning process in which the learner must actively participate in order to internalize the procedures for letter formations (Furner 1983). An important aspect of perceptual learning is the ability to discriminate characteristic features. She criticizes most existing instructional programs for placing too much emphasis on tracing and copying procedures and not enough on active learning. Although there is a place for these procedures in early writing instruction, in and of themselves they do not force children to discriminate between letter shapes and to note the distinguishing characteristics of each letter.

When compared with tracing, copying seems to promote better learning (Askov and Greff 1975; Hirsch and Niedermeyer 1973); the explanation has been that copying involves a greater degree of visualization and attention to detail (Askov and Greff 1975). Joanna Williams (1975) has found that both copying and letter discrimination training contribute to handwriting development but in different ways; discrimination training, as in a matching-to-sample procedure, tends to generalize to new letters, whereas copying does not (each letter has to be learned individually). However, when compared to demonstration of letter formations or verbal description of rules for these formations or a combination of these two techniques, copying is found to be the least effective technique (Kirk 1981). C. Jan and Joan Wright designed flip-books, one for each lowercase letter which they gave to first-graders to use during independent practice (Wright and Wright 1980). When children flip a book, a letter appears as if being written, much as in animated cartoons. This innovative method has proved more successful than copying from static models; not only do the flip-books serve to demonstrate formational procedures, but the children enjoy using them, which adds a motivational factor.

Furner maintains that both discrimination and production are important processes in handwriting development, though they are useful for different reasons, and urges that demonstration and verbalization of letter formations replace the copying and tracing that predominates in handwriting instruction. In her own work, Furner combines perceptual learning principles with problem-solving methods, using questioning and discovery techniques, and she reports data supporting this approach (see Furner 1983 for a list of these principles). Although her research, as well as the research she reviews, deals with normal kindergarten and first-grade children, there is no reason to believe that it should not apply to children with dyslexia.

Regina Cicci, in addressing the writing problems of students with dyslexia, lists seven forms of handwriting difficulties that may accompany dyslexia: incorrect pencil grasp, excessive tension in pencil grasp, incorrect position of paper, inappropriate size and spacing of letters and words, poor visual memory for letter formations, slow rate, and poor fine-motor coordination, or dysgraphia[1]. She suggests compensatory modifications to help children and adolescents with dyslexia cope in the regular classroom; such modifications include using parents as scribes and proof readers, accepting taped or oral reports, and reducing length of written assignments (see Cicci 1983 for a complete list). Keep in mind that these seven difficulties are concomitant to dyslexia, and not symptomatic of this reading disorder.

Many of the instructional principles advocated by Furner may be found in remedial handwriting programs for children with dyslexia, most particularly those programs based on the Orton-Gillingham approach. For example, Alphabetic Phonics (Cox 1992) and Slingerland (1971) incorporate teacher demonstration, combined with verbal directions for particular letter strokes which a student repeats while forming the letters. *The Johnson Handwriting Program* (Johnson 1977), which Cox advocates for her students once they have received her own training in cursive writing, teaches three *control strokes* as the basis of all cursive letter

---

[1] The term *dysgraphia* is used by Cicci to denote handwriting difficulty associated with poor fine-motor control. There is little agreement as to a single meaning for this word. Others in the field use it to mean a range of problems. Orton used the term *agraphia*, which he considered a separate issue from spelling-related writing difficulties, which are symptomatic of dyslexia. (Uhry and Shepherd 1993b).

formations: the *drop stroke*, the *anchor turn* (made directly on the base line), and the *release stroke*. Cox adds a fourth classification, the *approach stroke* which she breaks down into four subcategories—*swing-under-up-stop*,—for the initial approach into a letter formation.

The Cox and Slingerland programs, as well as that of Diana King (1985), which is designed specifically to teach writing skills to adolescents, all require extensive tracing and copying. However, the inclusion of such practice is not arbitrary, as Furner implied it may be in some classrooms, but rather is considered an essential component of the multisensory training espoused by the authors of these programs. Other multisensory activities include King's prewriting exercises, such as *the wind tunnel*, a series of circular scribbles that are done with eyes closed to develop rhythm, relaxation, and comfort in the handwriting situation, and Cox's and Slingerland's *sky writing* techniques, which require whole arm (i.e., gross-motor) movements in the air prior to forming letters on paper.

Correct sitting posture and paper position are stressed in these programs, the latter differing for left- and right-handed students. Left-

Perceptual Patterns Desk Card, The Johnson Handwriting Program. *(Reproduced with permission from Educators Publishing Service, Inc., Cambridge MA. Copyright 1977.)*

handers are not allowed to hook their wrists in writing. Cox (1992) claims that handwriting retraining for dyslexic students who are not identified early is more difficult and time consuming than reading remediation. King (1985), who works mainly with adolescents, states, however, that true dysgraphia is extremely rare, despite the fact that the diagnosis is frequently made. She maintains that it is always worth the effort to develop good handwriting, and further, that with intensive retraining older students often make remarkable progress in a relatively

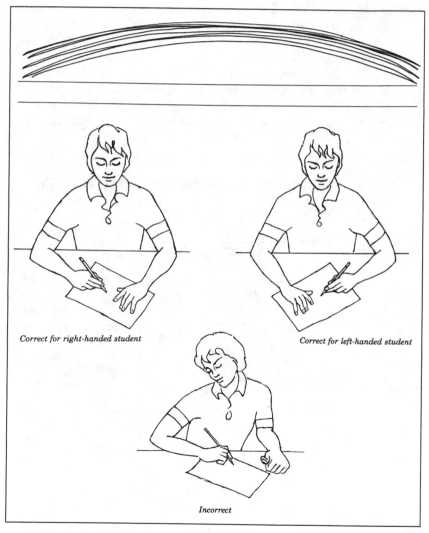

Correct for right-handed student

Correct for left-handed student

Incorrect

From Writing Skills for the Adolescent *by Diana Hanbury King. (reproduced with permission from Educators Publishing Service, Inc., Cambridge, MA. Copyright 1985.)*

short period of time. King and Cox both urge that students with dyslexia learn to type, in addition to, but not in lieu of, developing handwriting skills.

King has in fact written an instructional manual called *Keyboarding Skills* (King 1986) to teach typing to students with dyslexia in any grade. She describes her method as teaching "an alphabetic sequence with simultaneous oral spelling." The student learns by saying each letter aloud while typing it, which King believes establishes a conditioned reflex. She claims that many students can master the entire alphabet in less than an hour.

Whether to teach manuscript or cursive writing initially to children with dyslexia has been a controversial issue over the years. Cox (1992) and King (1985) insist that cursive writing be used exclusively by students with dyslexia. According to Cox, cursive writing reinforces left-right directionality, reduces reversals because the pencil is not raised off the paper, promotes rhythm and flow in letter formation, and eliminates the need to learn two writing systems. Furthermore, she contends, cursive letters are unique letter shapes and not mirror images of other letters. Beth Slingerland (1971) and Romalda Spalding (Spalding and Spalding 1986), on the other hand, advocate manuscript writing in order to conform to general school practices, as well as to avoid confusion with the manuscript formations in the child's readers. Cursive writing, in their programs, is not introduced until late second or third grade.

Nina Traub's *Recipe for Reading* (Traub and Bloom 1975) begins with manuscript produced on special paper, available from Educators Publishing Service, with each line delineating spaces with names based on the high and low areas of a color coded *little red house* (e.g., the term *cellar* is used for areas below the base line in letters such as *j* and *f*). Both manuscript and cursive are produced on this paper accompanied by a series of verbal directions that help in motor planning, as with other Orton-Gillingham based programs. Traub's manuscript formations include a follow-through stroke with some letters. Inexperienced readers can have problems differentiating mirror-image *ball and stick* letters such as *b* and *d*. Traub's manuscript letter formations avoid this problem.

There are benefits to both the manuscript and cursive points of view, which teachers and clinicians need to weigh before deciding which form of writing to teach.

11

Composition Instruction

Donald Graves, a leading authority on teaching writing, contended in 1978 that instruction in expressive writing is given short shrift in the education of American children. For many children in schools where teachers have been encouraged to use Graves' *writing process* approach, this contention has changed dramatically since 1978. Simulating the process used by adult writers, children are encouraged to brainstorm ideas, write, share work for feedback, and revise for content, with mechanics corrected prior to *publication* in a final draft. Substantial time is spent writing in these classrooms (Calkins 1983; Graves 1983; Graves and Stuart 1985; Hansen 1987)

For many children, however, especially young and disadvantaged children, writing instruction still involves little more than spelling tests and occasional chances to copy a set piece from the board. This has tended to be the case for children with reading deficits. Historically, writing has been overlooked in texts for teachers of children with learning disabilities (Silverman et al. 1981) and little time is devoted to writing in special classrooms. An investigation of eleven classrooms for children with learning disabilities reveals that only ten percent of the school day is spent in any sort of writing activity, and that 75 percent of this instruction involves copying (Leinhardt, Zigmond, and Cooley 1980).

Edna Barenbaum points out that the omission of composition instruction with children who have dyslexia or other learning disabilities has been mainly intentional, deriving from Helmer Myklebust's theory of language development. Myklebust (1965) hypothesized that language abilities follow a hierarchical progression from Oral Receptive (listening) to Oral Expressive (speaking) to Written Receptive (reading) to Written Expressive (writing); in his view a child is not ready to write until able to read. Thus, students with dyslexia frequently do not receive instruction in written expression until at least the late elementary grades, and then the instruction tends to be in grammar and mechanics (Barenbaum 1983).

ORTON-GILLINGHAM BASED WRITING INSTRUCTION

A second influence on delayed composition instruction is the belief of Samuel Orton (1937) and his associates Anna Gillingham and Bessie Stillman (1960) that spelling and other mechanics constituted the major writing difficulty in children with dyslexia. Fearing that free writing would reinforce these problems, they advocated that children dictate ideas to tutors and wait until high school to begin written composition. Orton's theory has influenced programs such as Alphabetic Phonics (see Chapter 13) in which early writing instruction focuses on handwriting, spelling, and phonetically controlled tutor-dictated words and sentences. Historically, Orton-Gillingham instruction focused on discrete skills, in a classically bottom-up approach, in the belief that handling all of these components at once overloads a student who is dyslexic. While the Orton-Gillingham tutor or teacher provides linkages between, for instance, spelling and handwriting, the student is not expected to integrate these skills in writing on her own.

Diana King's writing program, *Writing Skills for the Adolescent* (1985), is based on Orton-Gillingham principles and is intended to be used with Orton-Gillingham reading instruction. This is probably the most comprehensive writing program developed to date for students with dyslexia. It deals with handwriting, spelling, and composition. It is intended as a tutoring program for college-bound adolescents many of whom have been diagnosed late as having dyslexia. King's approach is exceedingly pragmatic, most likely because time is of the essence with these students. Rebuilding confidence is an important element of this program for older students, with competence achieved through much drill and practice. The program involves extensive retraining in handwriting, as well as remediation of spelling, mechanics, and formulation.

King's curriculum begins with having students write single words and then sentences, paragraphs, and essays. Early composition is linked with spelling instruction. Lists of spelling words are used as the basis of sentence composition. Once simple sentences can be written with some facility, grammar instruction begins. In her guide, King points out that grammar is important for college-bound students and she informs students that they can learn all they need to know about grammar in just a few months. Grammar is taught by having students compose sentences rather than completing workbook exercises, and involves a progression from parts of speech to various types of clauses, to what King calls *verbals*, by which she means participles, gerunds, and infinitives.

King calls paragraph construction "an exercise in logical thinking." Instruction begins with generating ideas and sentences, moves on to composing a topic sentence from this material, and then ends with weaving all of the sentences together. Several paragraph types are taught (e.g., *definition, narrative, process*). Essay writing follows this pattern of instruction. The student is taught to compose an introductory paragraph with a thesis statement, followed by paragraphs each containing a topic sentence, and ending with a concluding paragraph. King supports her method with a series of convincing case histories including before-and-after writing samples (1985).

OTHER INSTRUCTIONAL MODELS

King's program is a good example of a writing instruction model which George Hillocks (1984) identifies as a *presentational mode* or *skills approach*. In this model the teacher presents specific, skills-oriented assignments and provides most of the feedback on student performance. In an oft-quoted meta-analysis of research on composition instruction undertaken at the University of Chicago, Hillocks identifies three additional models. In the *natural process mode* popularized by Graves, the teacher acts mainly as a facilitator whose primary role, as Hillocks puts it, is "to free the student's imagination and promote growth by sustaining a positive classroom attitude." This model incorporates many of Graves' interests such as choosing topics of interest, sharing results with peers for feedback, editing and revising. The students learn by doing rather than by studying or copying stylistic models.

Hillocks' *environmental mode* combines aspects of both the *presentational* and *process modes* and in many ways appears a compromise between the two. Objectives are clearly stated and assignments selected by the teacher. A high degree of structure is used as small groups work through an idea together. Later children work on their own with teacher support. Hillocks comments that the *environmental* model "brings teacher, student, and materials more nearly into balance and, in effect, takes advantage of all resources of the classroom."

The last model, the *individualized mode*, involves one-to-one instruction that tends to involve use of *environmental* and *presentational modes* and varies too much in content for inclusion in Hillocks' analysis. His comparison of the three group-instruction models indicates that the *environmental mode* (the combination model) is nearly three times as effective as either the *presentational* or *process* models. Furthermore, the most widely used approach, the *presentational mode* was the least effective group model. Some of the other outcomes from Hillocks' meta-analysis are worth noting: 1) instruction through presentation of grammar does not improve the quality of writing and can actually lower it, 2) sentence combining, or the practice of building more complex sentences from simpler ones, has a positive effect, 3) establishing criteria for peer critiques has a positive effect, and 4) a problem solving approach, which Hillocks calls *inquiry*, in which students are presented with sets of information and asked to take a position or develop an argument, has an extremely positive effect on writing quality. Keep in mind, in thinking about the implications of this meta-analysis, that the subjects in these studies were not dyslexic or even learning disabled.

Carol Sue Englert and her colleagues at Michigan State University have developed a model of writing instruction for use with children with learning disabilities that might be characterized as an example of Hillocks' *environmental model*. She refers to Vygotsky (1978) and the importance of social interaction in learning when expectations are a little beyond the student's level of mastery. In a summary of several studies, Englert (1990) describes what she calls *Cognitive Strategy Instruction in Writing* (CSIW), a process-oriented approach to expository writing that uses many of the strategies found in Graves' model but within a more teacher-directed framework in the early stages. Englert has based CSIW on extensive research, her own and that of others, describing the writing characteristics of children with learning disabilities (e.g., Englert et al. 1989; Englert and Thomas 1987). This research suggests that children with learning disabilities have deficits in analyzing text structure in reading and in using it effectively in writing expository text. These children have little knowledge of the vocabulary of the writing process and are poor at self-regulating the writing process steps. They tend to see writing as outer-directed and teacher regulated, and they have little sense of purpose for writing or of audience. Keep in mind that Englert's studies looked at meta-cognitive skills. Doris Johnson and James Grant, in a comparison of the writing of children with and without learning disabilities, found differences specific to spelling, handwriting, and syntax, factors more typically assessed in the traditional literature (Johnson and Grant 1989).

Englert's CSIW instructional model uses the acronym POWER (*Plan, Organize, Write, Edit/Editor, Revise*) for a series of structured steps including *think sheets* to fill in at each new stage in the process. At the *Plan* step, students are encouraged to consider their audience, their purpose for writing, and their own background knowledge of the topic. At the *Organize* step, they categorize and sequence their ideas and consider text structure. At the *Write* step, they write a first draft on colored paper, reserving white paper for the final draft. The teacher models explicit use of key phrases to provide cues to the reader about the text structure being used. Teachers encourage students to elaborate on ideas at this stage. At the *Edit/Editor* step, think sheets are available for both the author, who self-edits, and the peer editor, who reads the work and makes suggestions. Note (above) that Hillocks reports that this has benefits for the peer editor as well as the author. The teacher provides *think aloud* conversations during further editing conferences before the student begins to prepare a final draft. The *Revise* think sheet suggests putting a check mark next to any editing suggestions that the student intends to use. Sharing the final product is an integral part of the process and of the life of the classroom. Englert refers to the creation of "a literacy community of writers and readers," using rhetoric familiar to advocates of Graves' writing process.

Englert emphasizes that the POWER steps must be supported by three important contributions from the teacher: 1) *dialogue* during the writing process which should include the teacher modeling aloud the thinking process she uses when she composes 2) *scaffolded instruction* with graduated prompts provided by the teacher until the student is successful, as well as *procedural facilitation* in which prompts remind the student to use learned strategies, and 3) *teaching for generalization* during which the teacher provides fewer and fewer dialogues and prompts and encourages increasing amounts of self-talk until the student can work independently, without even the support of think sheets. CSIW is described more fully in an article by Raphael and Englert (1990).

CSIW is intended for use in either classrooms or resource rooms serving children with learning disabilities. Several studies have demonstrated the effectiveness of CSIW (e.g., Englert et al. 1989). Reports include extensive use of before-and-after writing samples as well as transcriptions of dialogues. One study demonstrated that socially mediated instruction increased ability to talk about writing processes in upper-elementary-age children with and without learning disabilities in comparison with controls, and that this involved both reading and writing achievement. This form of writing instruction had a particularly positive effect on the sense of self-regulation in children with learning disabilities (Englert, Raphael, and Anderson 1992).

Englert and King offer two methods for remediating the writing problems of students with dyslexia. Each is theory driven and each provides a structured, workable approach. There are advocates of using the third of Hillocks' models, the *natural process* approach for remediating writing. First-grade children in Reading Recovery (see Chapter 22), who are lagging behind in reading but have not been diagnosed as dyslexic, usually are exposed to the Graves' approach in their regular classrooms. This begs a comparison of their response to process writing in comparison with children who are stronger readers, but at this point there is no conclusive documentation.

Despite the limited amount of research on teaching writing to children with dyslexia, there are a number of instructional principles and procedures that seem to be important. The first among them is the need to begin this instruction early rather than waiting for reading or spelling skills to reach a certain level (Barenbaum 1983; Silverman et al. 1981). Graves stresses the importance of daily writing and of a working studio atmosphere in which individuals write with the teacher's presence felt as a support. Barenbaum emphasizes the need for a safe environment, that is positive and reinforcing. The finished work of all children should be displayed and valued. One-to-one conferences are important in the revision process. Donald Graves makes four suggestions about correcting errors during these conferences: 1) identify revision elements in order of importance with a meaningful story line or exposition higher up on the hierarchy than mechanics, 2) choose only one point for revision at a given time, 3) focus on specific writing problems as the need arises, and 4) provide more than one experience to solidify new learning (Graves 1983). Diana King cautions against discouraging students by focusing on errors. In her program, tutors are prohibited from placing red marks on student papers for at least a year after remediation has begun and are advised never to correct all errors on a page. One method that makes sense involves expecting children to correct only those spelling patterns that have been directly taught. A major hurdle in beginning work with children with dyslexia is simply getting them to write at all.

WORD PROCESSORS IN WRITING INSTRUCTION

Another debate in the remediation of writing, in addition to approach, is the issue of whether or not to use computer word processors. The surge of interest in the writing process during the 1980s, with its emphasis on revisions and multiple drafts, has coincided with a surge in the educational use of computers in schools. The computer is an ideal vehicle for the writing process, eliminating tedious copying-over, and for children with spelling problems, the computer spell-check provides a release from the tedium and uncertainty of proofreading for misspellings. The facilitative power of computers in regard to spelling is an especially important advantage for children with dyslexia. This can make a difference in the mechanics of the finished product so that the focus can shift to content. Of equally great importance, it can also make a difference in terms of willingness to write.

The use of word processing programs for writing instruction has great appeal. However, there is only a relatively small body of research that has investigated its use with students who are either learning disabled or dyslexic. Some of the observed advantages of computerized word processing for these students include: the ability to produce a neat, easy-to-read, printed copy which provides the student with feedback on his writing and may also increase his motivation; the ability to edit and revise without tedious recopying; the ability to type which can compensate for poor handwriting (MacArthur and Schneiderman 1986). A major advantage from the teacher's standpoint is that computers provide a record of the process of writing if various drafts are saved. Computers encourage collaborative writing activities which can facilitate improvement in both the quality and quantity of written work (Morocco and Neuman 1986).

Word processing may or may not lead to greater quantities of writing than does handwriting. Some researchers contend that writing on a computer produces much longer pieces than does writing with paper and pencil (e.g., MacArthur and Schneiderman 1986; Steeves 1987) while other studies do not replicate this finding (e.g., MacArthur and Graves 1988).

A nationwide survey on the use of computers with students with special needs found that computers tend to be used, not for drafting revisions, but only for typing out final copies (Mokros and Russell 1986). Another study suggests that instead of encouraging greater focus on content, as opposed to mechanics, word processing induces students to spend more time correcting minor mechanical errors.

The role of the teacher is a key factor here. The teacher's choice of whether to employ a skills approach or a process approach to writing will influence the way computers are used for composition. For example, MacArthur and his colleagues at the University of Maryland have designed a writing curriculum that encourages emphasis on "meaningful writing in a social context." The Computers and Writing Instruction Project (CWIP) curriculum combines use of a computer, a writers' workshop or process approach to writing, and metacognitive strategy instruction. Using methods MacArthur describes as similar to those of Lucy Calkins, children write daily and receive regular support and advice from peers. Metacognitive strategy instruction involves detailed and structured steps for planning, writing, and expanding their work, much as Englert does in her curriculum. MacArthur has used the CWIP curriculum with children with learning disabilities in special classes in grades four through six. He describes several studies indicating that children in CWIP classrooms outperformed controls in overall quality of writing (MacArthur, Schwartz, and Graham 1991).

In the first edition of this book, Diana Clark wrote that there is no single word processing program deemed best for dyslexic students. This continues to be the case, and choices have become even more difficult since 1988 because of the many new options available to support students with writing disabilities. There are word processing programs that have the capability to check spelling, grammar, and capitalization, and provide mini-lessons on errors. Some can find synonyms to expand a student's vocabulary. Speech synthesis is available to *read* aloud what has been written. Some word processors can suggest topics at the planning stage and then illustrate the finished story. Portable computers can be taken to class for note taking by older students. A recent and thorough review of these features ends with this advice:

> The possibilities increase only to the degree that teachers are informed consumers of the technology available and are able to make sound instructional decisions relative to the needs of their students (Hunt-Berg, Rankin, and Beukelman 1994, p. 178).

12

The Reading-Writing Relationship

The relationship between reading and writing has captured the attention of a number of respected theorists who believe that reading and writing are mutually facilitative skills. These theorists have questioned the standard classroom practice of delaying writing activities until reading skills have been acquired, and have advocated that, at the very least, reading and writing should be taught together.

Maria Montessori (1964) was perhaps the first educator to suggest that writing precedes reading developmentally and that it is thus more natural for children to begin reading instruction by composing their own words, rather than by attempting to read the words of others. One of the strongest proponents of Montessori's view has been Carol Chomsky (1971, 1979) who feels that when children start school they are better able to apply their own language to encode meaning than to decode meaning from formal printed language. Chomsky believes, as did Montessori, that building an awareness of the communicative purposes of written language is one of the primary advantages of having children write before teaching them to read. In addition, she maintains that this approach enhances phonological awareness. From her observations of children composing self-generated stories as part of their first grade schooling. Chomsky concluded:

> The invented spellers, during the months that they engage in their writing activities, are providing themselves with excellent and valuable practice in

139

phonetics, word analysis and synthesis, and letter-sound correspondences (Chomsky 1979).

Uta Frith has proposed a developmental model of reading acquisition that concurs with Chomsky's conclusion (see Chapter 1; Frith 1985, 1986). Following acquisition of the beginning or *logographic* strategy, in which reading precedes and facilitates spelling, children acquire the *alphabetic* strategy in the inverse order; alphabetic spelling leads into alphabetic reading. Paraphrasing Frith, Sylvia Farnham-Diggory cites the advantages of early writing activities: "... the writing process requires segmenting and sequencing and thus sets up the conditions for the discovery of the alphabetic principle." (Farnham-Diggory 1986a).

One of the major concerns raised about this approach is that it may perpetuate incorrect spellings. This is the position held by most Orton-Gillingham trained teachers who work with dyslexic children. As mentioned earlier (see Chapter 11), these remedial educators do not introduce free writing activities until their pupils have mastered basic phonics skills, although copying and practice in writing from dictation forms a substantial portion of their curriculum. However, Chomsky, as well as Charles Read (1971, 1975, 1986) and Glenda Bissex (1980), in observations of kindergarten and first-grade children without dyslexia, have found that invented spellings are gradually replaced with orthographically conventional ones as the children gain reading experience. Note that this is consistent with Frith's notion that orthographic reading precedes and leads into orthographic spelling. That is, seeing words in print eventually influences spellings. These investigators also noted remarkable consistency in the patterns of spelling approximations among the children (e.g., the letter *H* is frequently used to represent the sound of the letters *ch*; the letter *J* is used to represent the sound of the letters *dr* as in *drum*). These children appeared to be constructing a set of rules for spelling by linking the names of letters and the sounds of phonemes.

Note that in Linnea Ehri's reading model there is an additional stage between Frith's *logographic* and *alphabetic* stages (see Chapter 1). At this stage children read only some salient features of a word, reading *look* as "like," for example. In the early stages of invented spelling, both of these words might be spelled as "LK." An argument could be made that as children become aware of medial vowels and begin to segment and spell the word *like* as "LIK" they will be more apt to look for a vowel when they read the word *look*, and to recognize that it is not a match for the lexically stored word *like*.

A second concern about the writing-before-reading approach to teaching is that children may be confused by the differences between their own spellings and the printed words they encounter when they begin to read. This is not a problem, according to Chomsky (1979). Reporting on Read's observations (Read 1970), she claims that children appear to have no difficulty making the distinction between their spellings and conventional spellings and that they tend, in fact, to view writing and reading as completely separate tasks, a conclusion that Lynette Bradley and Peter Bryant also reach in their research (Bradley 1985; Bradley and Bryant 1979).

Timothy Shanahan investigated the reading-writing relationship with second- and fifth-grade students, by applying multivariate statistical analysis to scores attained on various reading and writing tasks (Shanahan 1984). He found that, despite a significant relationship between the two skill areas, the degree to which skill in writing influences skill in reading and vice versa is no more that 40 percent. In a second analysis (Shanahan and Lomax 1985), he attempted to determine the direction-ality of the relationship by constructing three theoretical models (i.e., reading-to-writing, writing-to-reading, and an interactive model) to represent the flow of influence. Results of the analysis indicate that read-ing has a stronger facilitative influence on writing than the other way around, but that the relationship is best represented by the interactive model. Furthermore, within the interactive model, the interaction between writing and reading is more significant at the word level than at the passage level and appears stronger in second grade than in fifth grade. Similarly, Connie Juel and her colleagues (Juel, Griffeth, and Gough 1985) find the relationship to be greater at the word level and stronger with younger (first-grade) than with older (second-grade) chil-dren. Shanahan and Lomax suggest that these findings reflect the fact that considerably greater amount of instructional time is devoted to reading than to writing in our schools. These results might not hold in schools where this is no longer the case.

In an early effort to explore the effects of writing on reading in children with reading disability, Lee Dobson took eight first graders who had failed to learn to read by mid-year and provided them with daily half-hour free-writing sessions. The children were encouraged to draw pictures and then write stories to accompany them. The teacher acted only as facilitator, never correcting their spelling errors, and when help was requested, deferring to the other children for their input rather than immediately providing the answer. Although he collected no quan-titative data, Dobson maintains that notable progress was made in both writing and reading ability as a result of this activity. Many of the mis-spellings eventually dropped out, though admittedly after a longer period of time than might be expected for normally achieving children. An especially important treatment outcome, Dobson believes, is the improved motivation among these children who had earlier met with failure (Dobson 1985).

Another line of research leads to an explanation that can be found in reading processes rather than in increased motivation. This research links spelling with phoneme segmentation. Keep in mind, that in Frith's model it is the alphabetic stage of reading at which children with dyslexia fail to read. The phonological processes that are necessary for skilled alphabetic reading are the very ones that are poorly developed in these children. Much of this research has been described earlier in greater detail. In brief, Ehri and Wilce found that kindergarten children trained for a few weeks in spelling exercises in which orally presented words were segmented and then spelled with lettered tiles had an advantage over controls in reading new words with these letters (Ehri and Wilce 1987b). Bradley and Bryant found that preschool children, at risk for reading failure because of poor ability in sound-matching, read and spelled better than controls after two years of training in matching oral words by rhyme and alliteration and in segmenting and spelling these words with plastic letters (Bradley and Bryant 1983, 1985).

We have found that first graders in whole language classrooms could read and spell better than controls after seven months of segmenting and spelling on the computer (Uhry and Shepherd 1993a). This finding held when the progress of students in this study who were at risk for dyslexia was documented in brief case studies (Uhry 1989). It also held true for fourth-grade children with dyslexia; these children read more nonsense words correctly after segmenting and spelling their real-word analogues on the computer, in comparison with several other treatments including phonics-oriented reading instruction (Uhry 1993a). As Linnea Ehri puts it:

> Spelling might be expected to contribute to reading skill because, in learning to spell, children are taught some of the elements of decoding skill. They learn to divide pronunciations of words into their constituent sounds. They learn to represent sounds and words visually by converting sounds into letters. Both of these elements, phonemic awareness and letter-sound knowledge, are thought to be important components in reading words (Ehri and Wilce 1987b, p. 48).

The Spalding Method is a beginning reading program for classroom use that starts with spelling and writing. The teacher's manual, developed by Romalda Spalding, is called *The Writing Road to Reading* (Spalding and Spalding 1986). Sylvia Farnham-Diggory is a psychologist and professor at the University of Delaware and also runs the Reading Study Center at the university. In the introduction to *The Writing Road to Reading*, she states that she has used the Spalding Method with remarkable success for both beginning and remedial instruction, though she acknowledges the need for further documentation of its effectiveness with disabled readers (Farnham-Diggory 1986).

Romalda Spalding was trained in the Orton-Gillingham approach by Orton and then went on to develop a language arts program that could be used with a whole class. Thus, the Spalding Method incorporates many of the Orton-Gillingham principles, including an emphasis on integrating the various sensory modalities involved in learning to read. However, it differs from the earlier method in many respects, most particularly by teaching writing before reading and by introducing first the most commonly used English words, many of which are not phonetically regular. The Orton-Gillingham approach focuses primarily on words that have phonetic spelling patterns and introduces any that do not, as exception words.

The Spalding Method teaches the set of phoneme-letter units or phonograms selected by Anna Gillingham in developing the Orton-Gillingham program: the twenty-six letters of the alphabet and forty-four combinations of two, three, or four letters that make a single sound (e.g., *ai, igh, ough*). Students are first taught to spell and write fifty-four of these phonograms and later, 150 of the 1,700 most frequently used words. Teachers follow a general lesson script that involves saying the word to be learned, asking how many syllables it has, asking what is the first sound, and having students write the letter as she writes it on the chalkboard. The procedure continues until the word has been written.

Students write all words in notebooks which they add to as they proceed through the program. These spelling books serve as their major reference source. Manuscript writing is taught, primarily so as not to confuse students when they encounter print, but instruction in cursive writing usually begins by the middle of second grade. Twenty-nine spelling rules are taught in the program; students write these in their books along with examples of application. In addition, students are taught a marking system to help them identify and remember phonogram spellings and pronunciations: phonograms are underlined and, for those having more than one sound, numbers are used to identify which sound a phonogram represents in a given word. Farnham-Diggory maintains in her introduction to the program manual that knowing the seventy phonograms and these twenty-nine rules enables anyone to spell 80 percent of all English words (Farnham-Diggory 1986b).

Reading in the Spalding Method begins after students have mastered 150 words, that is, they can spell them aloud, write them from dictation, and read them. Rather than using a basal program, students read trade books from the beginning; Spalding has provided a list of suggested books for five grade levels in the program manual appendix. According to Farnham-Diggory, reading in this method is never taught; children "simply pick up a book and start reading" (Farnham-Diggory 1986b). She adds that the Spalding Method exposes them early to good literature and furthermore, encourages them to write their own stories, plays, and poems.

Several more recently developed programs include an oral spelling activity to enhance reading. Benita Blachman includes a segmenting and spelling activity in a program for at risk beginning readers using a pocket chart with letters for spelling orally presented words (Blachman 1987; Blachman et al. 1994). Patricia and James Cunningham use a technique that they call *making words* in regular primary level classrooms to enhance the relationship between invented spelling and decoding (Cunningham and Cunningham 1992). A restricted set of letters on cards is used to build words from oral directions in an activity that is something like the Elkonin *word changes*. Children are asked, "Now, change just one letter, and change *sing* to *ring*. Now we will make a five-letter word. Add a letter to change *ring* to *rings*." Each child works with a set of his or her own letters and then each word is spelled with large letters for the whole class to see. Note that this gives children a chance to correct their invented spellings. A range of words, employing two to five letters, provides instructional opportunities for children with a range of abilities.

Whether or not a writing-before-reading approach is an effective way to teach children with dyslexia is a question that calls for further exploration. Having children write words that they may not have learned by sight draws their attention to the sounds in those words and thereby enhances phonemic awareness. Writing also gives children a feeling of empowerment and ownership over the words they learn, increasing their motivation to learn more. The Writing to Read program (see Chapter 21; Martin and Friedberg 1986), which contains a word processing component aimed at promoting reading acquisition among kindergarteners and first graders, may be a step in this direction.

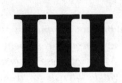

III

Reading Programs for
Students with Dyslexia

The chapters that follow provide information on special instructional programs that serve as alternatives to regular classroom programs for teaching reading, writing, and spelling skills. Many of these programs were designed for children who are dyslexic or who might be at risk for reading failure. Some derive from the Orton-Gillingham multisensory approach for teaching beginning reading skills. These include *Alphabetic Phonics*, the *Slingerland Program*, *Recipe for Reading*, and *Enfield and Greene's Project Read*. The *Wilson* System is an Orton-Gillingham program for adolescents and young adults. It has become available since this book was first published in 1988. The Lindamoods' *Auditory Discrimination in Depth* uses multisensory techniques derived from remedial instruction in the field of speech remediation.

DISTAR is a direct instruction beginning reading program, and *Corrective Reading* is its upward extension for grades four through twelve. They were originally developed for culturally or economically disadvantaged children, but are included here because of their subsequent use with children classified as learning disabled, many of whom might be considered dyslexic.

Calfee's Project READ and *Writing to Read* were not designed specifically for children with reading disability. They are included here because they represent a significant departure from the traditional classroom approach to reading instruction and incorporate many of the instructional principles and teaching methods that research has shown to be effective with students with dyslexia.

Reading Recovery was added to this edition because it is a widely used and well documented program for first grade children who are behind their classmates in beginning reading. *Reading Recovery* is quite different in design from the other programs described here, but its use is supported by well controlled experiments.

Each program is described in terms of its basic rationale, or theoretical perspective, its curriculum and instructional method, its teacher training requirements, and where information is available, its effectiveness. The descriptions should be taken as overviews rather than comprehensive investigations. There is no attempt to compare the effectiveness of the programs or to single out the one "best" program. Instead, readers are encouraged to use the theoretical framework provided in the earlier chapters of this book to develop judgment about the relative value of the programs.

The final chapter, *Curriculum Planning: A Case Study*, outlines the process by which an individual remedial plan can be designed from assessment results for a student with dyslexia.

13

Alphabetic Phonics

BACKGROUND AND RATIONALE

Alphabetic Phonics is an "organization and expansion" (Cox 1985) of the Orton-Gillingham multisensory approach for teaching children with dyslexia from elementary school through high school. The program was started in the mid 1960s at Texas Scottish Rite Hospital for Children in Dallas as a collaboration between Sally Childs (a colleague of Anna Gillingham) Lucius Waites (a pediatric neurologist who established the Child Development Division at the hospital), and Aylett Royall Cox (a teacher who organized and published the Alphabetic Phonics Curriculum together with the Dyslexia Laboratory staff). The program was developed and revised over a ten-year period during which over 1000 children with dyslexia came daily to Waites' clinic for remedial instruction. In order to meet the needs of the number of children referred, teaching at Scottish Rite was expanded at that point from tutorials to small group remediation.

The Alphabetic Phonics curriculum (Cox 1984, 1992) is built upon Samuel Orton's theories, and uses multisensory activities to build linkages between the visual, auditory, and kinesthetic senses. It is an assumption of this curriculum that the majority (80 percent) of the 30,000 most commonly used English words can be considered phonetically regular and therefore predictable, once rules have been learned. The term *alphabetic phonics* refers to "a structured system of teaching students the coding patterns of the English language" (Cox 1985). To this theoretical framework, the program has added a discovery approach to learning. Hierarchically sequenced rules for letter sounds are discovered, articulated, practiced toward mastery, and used to build words through a synthetic approach to reading.

CURRICULUM AND INSTRUCTION

The Alphabetic Phonics curriculum is described in a guide for teachers, *Foundations for Literacy: Structures and Techniques for Multisensory Teaching of Basic Written English Language Skills* (Cox 1992), a revision of the earlier guide, which was titled *Structures and Techniques* (Cox 1984). In addition, there are two companion guides, *Situation Reading* (Cox 1989) and *Situation Spelling* (Cox 1977), student workbooks, drill cards, and wall cards, all available from Educators Publishing Service.

Progress is documented through use of what Cox calls *Benchmark Measures*, or post-instruction measures coordinated with the *schedules* or steps in the sequenced program. These curriculum-based instruments are designed to measure letter knowledge, alphabetizing skills, reading, spelling, and handwriting.

The curriculum is extremely comprehensive in that it covers many aspects of language acquisition, including listening skills, and extends from basic skills such as letter recognition to sophisticated levels of linguistic knowledge, such as coding polysyllabic words after breaking them into syllables. Students are taught an extensive vocabulary to use in their language learning (e.g., "The word *fight* is a one syllable base word with the trigraph *igh* in medial position"). Judith Birsh, an Alphabetic Phonics teacher trainer, refers to this terminology as a "meta-language," a language for talking about language (Birsh 1988).

As its name implies, Alphabetic Phonics stresses the unique characteristics of written English, most particularly phonology and letter sequence. The term *situation learning* is applied to both reading and spelling, and refers to the fact that the sound of a letter may vary depending on the situation. For instance, *one-one-one* words have one syllable and one short vowel followed by one consonant. A striking feature of the program is the time spent teaching students how to code words using diacritical marks, as used in Webster's 2nd edition, for the 68 graphemes which represent 44 sounds in 98 different situations. For example, the digraph *ck* is underlined to indicate that the two letters make a single sound, and the *c* is diagonally slashed to indicate that it is silent. The demands placed on the student are substantial.

The structured daily lesson takes an hour to complete, with 11 activities typically lasting 3 to 10 minutes each. The standard activities with suggested times are outlined below. Each is followed by examples from observations of demonstration lessons by master teachers working with one, two, and three children during training sessions at Teachers College, Columbia University during the summer of 1994.

1. *Language* (5 min.) This activity is intended as an orientation to the English language. One teacher showed children a globe and gave a brief lesson on the spread of the alphabet around the shores of the Mediterranean by the Phoenicians.

2. *Alphabet* (5 min.) This activity emphasizes sequence and directionality, and leads to alphabetizing and dictionary use. During the observed session, two students touched the letters A and Z on an alphabet strip as they recited "My left hand is my *before* hand. My right hand is my *after* hand. *A* is the initial letter of the alphabet. *Z* is the final letter of the alphabet. All the letters between *A* and *Z* are the medial letters." Then they used the left index finger to point at and read each letter *A-M*, with the right hand finishing up *N-Z*.

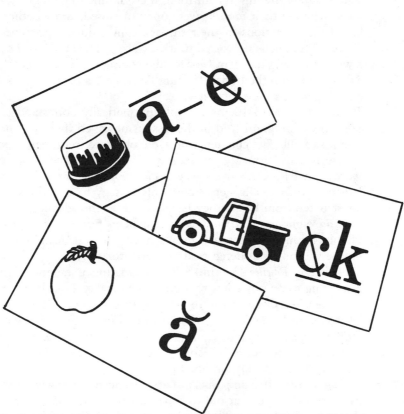

Initial Reading Deck by Aylett R. Cox. (Reproduced with permission from Educators Publishing Service, Cambridge, MA. Copyright 1971.)

3. *Reading Decks* (3 min.) These drill cards (Initial and Advanced Decks) provide practice in responding automatically to letters for reading. A teacher was observed showing beginning students a few Initial Reading Deck cards which had been introduced in prior lessons. Students responded with the name of the letter, the name of the object (key word), and the phoneme or letter sound.

4. *Spelling Decks* (3 min.) During the observed session, the teacher said the above mentioned phonemes aloud, one at a time, and the students echoed the sounds and then said the letter names. A set of teacher hand signals was used to prompt the student to listen, echo the phoneme, say the letter name, and finally, write the letter. This is a particularly effective technique; trained teachers mentioned spontaneously using the hand signals in other teaching situations as prompts.

5. *New Learning* (5 min.) In this observation, two students had been taught short *i* in a prior lesson, and were introduced here to the sound of short *a* through the use of a discovery activity . They watched their mouths in a mirror as they said the sound. The teacher asked whether their mouths were open or closed, and whether they could feel vibrations in their throats. One student spontaneously offered, "It's open and voiced so it's a vowel." They practiced coding a written *a* using the term *breve* for the coding mark and were shown a flash card from the Initial Reading Deck with a picture of an apple and an *a* with a breve over it.

6. *Reading Practice.* (5–10 min.) Only phonetically controlled text is used in the program, and in the lessons observed there was no use of books at all. The children who were observed in the introductory course had had roughly ten lessons. They read *instant words* (sight words) on flash cards (e.g., *they, could, people, no*) and they used a left-to-right, letter-by-letter blending strategy to sound out words constructed from letters they had studied. In the advanced training class an eight-year-old boy, who had been tutored in Alphabetic Phonics for nine months, was given sentences to code prior to reading, but he was not considered ready to read stories yet.

7. *Handwriting Practice* (5 min.) Cursive writing is taught from the beginning to reinforce left-to-right directionality. Four basic strokes are taught (see Chapter 10). In one observed session, an introductory level student learned to say, "The name of the letter is *s*. Swing up. Stop. Curve out around. Come in to close. Stop and release," while drawing an *s* in the air (a technique called *skywriting*), on the board with chalk, and finally, on lined paper.

8. *Spelling Practice* (10 min.) Spelling was practiced in the advanced class by asking an eight year old to spell two vowel sounds (short *a* and short *u*) using printed letters called *ice tray letters* after the tray used for their display and storage. After this preparation he spelled *bag*,

bug, *tag*, and *tug* using *Simultaneous Oral Spelling* (SOS). He listened, echoed the word, *unblended*[1] the word while looking in a mirror, spelled the letters aloud and then pulled printed letters into place to spell the word. To check himself, he coded the word using a small piece of macaroni for the breve mark and then read the word aloud.

9. *Verbal Expression* (2-10 min.) In a beginning level lesson, the teacher wrote out a sentence and read it aloud, and then used parts-of-speech cards (e.g., *noun*, *article*) from the Winston Grammar Program, asking the child to cover words with them. Parts of speech that had not yet been taught were covered with "mystery cards" or blank cards used as place holders These activities differ from teacher to teacher.

10. *Review* (5 min.) In all sessions, index cards were prepared by the teacher with mnemonic clues for reviewing new learning at the end of a lesson.

11. *Listening or Reading Comprehension* (5 min.) In an advanced training session the teacher read four Shel Silverstein food poems aloud and asked the student how the poems were all alike. Material is chosen on the student's intellectual level rather than reading level, in order to develop comprehension skills.

Most of the materials either have been designed specifically for the program or are teacher made. Reading materials vary from site to site but are always phonetically controlled (e.g., *Let's Read*, Bloomfield, Barnhart and Barnhart; *Learn to Read Books*, Gould and Warnke; *J and J Language Readers*, Sopris West; *MTA Readers*, Educators Publishing Service).

TEACHER TRAINING

Training is based on the need to fill three gaps in teacher education: 1) knowledge of the structure and history of written English; 2) knowledge of the science of phonetic spelling; and 3) a carefully structured and hierarchically sequenced curriculum (Cox 1985). Presently there are at least 14 Alphabetic Phonics teacher-training centers in the United States, all listed in the Resource and Teacher Training Guide at the back of this book. This is over twice the number reported in the first edition of this book (Clark 1988). Many of these centers are directed by teacher trainers who originally trained under Aylett Cox or Connie Burkhalter in Texas.

Training for teachers of Alphabetic Phonics is extensive and demanding. It includes a minimum of 150 instructional hours followed by 700 hours of supervised practice with students. Teachers are required

---

[1] The term *unblending* in Alphabetic Phonics refers to segmenting, or saying each phoneme in isolation.

to attend a three-to-four-week introductory summer course and a two-week advanced course the following summer. During the school year between these summer workshops they are required to tutor children under supervision and to attend periodic seminars. Daily training sessions during the workshops last for seven hours and include lectures, demonstrations, and practice teaching. In addition, substantial readings and projects are assigned. Trainees become Alphabetic Phonics therapists once they have completed two years of training.

Several introductory and advanced-level summer training sessions were observed at Teachers College, Columbia University during the summer of 1994. The 25 beginners and 12 advanced trainees were classroom and resource room teachers, tutors, and graduate students in special education. They met with master teachers early in the morning in small groups to talk about goals for the tutoring session they were about to view. Trainees then watched through a one-way mirror as a master teacher tutored a child or small group of children for an hour. By the second week of the introductory session each trainee was assigned a small portion of the lesson. Feedback was provided immediately afterwards by the master teacher and by the rest of the group, who then worked together to plan the next day's session. Over the course of training, more and more responsibility for planning and teaching the lesson was assigned to trainees. During the rest of the day, lectures and discussions focused on specific aspects of the program as well as on broader issues such as research. After the day's session trainees were expected to read assignments and to prepare lessons to teach the next day.

EVALUATION AND IMPLEMENTATION

When this book was first published in 1988, Diana Clark reported that several evaluation studies of Alphabetic Phonics had been conducted during the 1980s (e.g., Brightman 1986; Frankiewicz 1984, 1985; Roy 1986). These four studies indicated gains in reading for children with dyslexia instructed in Alphabetic Phonics in either individual tutorials or small groups. None, however, used control groups, so that it could not be claimed that training in Alphabetic Phonics was responsible for the gains.

Since 1988 there have been new studies, most designed, again, to measure gains in standard scores after training, but without the use of controls. For example, Hutcheson, Selig, and Young (1990) describe a collaboration between the Neuhaus Education Center and the Houston public schools in which 126 resource room teachers were trained in Alphabetic Phonics. Later 252 elementary and secondary students described as learning disabled were tested before and after remediation in resource rooms and were found to have made significant gains in reading and spelling.

ADAPTATIONS OF ALPHABETIC PHONICS

The Multisensory Teaching Approach (MTA) is an adaptation of Alphabetic Phonics intended for whole classroom use. It was designed by Margaret Smith and Edith Hogan, both former Alphabetic Phonics teacher trainers, for use in regular classrooms or as a remedial program for children with dyslexia. Smith and Hogan have developed a series of kits that contain the essential instructional manuals and materials needed for teaching the program. The manuals provide more specific instruction for teachers than do the original Alphabetic Phonics manuals, and they include actual lesson scripts. The MTA kits are distributed by Educators Publishing Service. The kit is considered an excellent resource for any Alphabetic Phonics teacher. Training is offered by Edmar Educational Services in Dallas, Texas. MTA teachers take a two-week basic course, and academic language therapists take this course plus two years of practicum (four advanced workshops and six individual consultation/demonstrations), followed by an additional two-weeks of training.

A four-year evaluation of MTA was conducted in Texas where the program was used in regular public school classrooms as well as in remedial classrooms (Vickery, Reynolds, and Cochran 1987). Children receiving MTA instruction in grades three through six were compared with traditionally taught students in the same classrooms in previous years. California Achievement Test (CAT) scores indicated significantly greater gains in reading and spelling for the children instructed in MTA during grades three, five, and six, but not during grade four. Gain sizes tended to increase with additional years of the program.

The Dyslexia Training Program (DTP) is another adaptation of the Alphabetic Phonics curriculum. In 1987 DTP introduced videotaped lessons for schools without access to trained therapists. It was developed by Lucius Waites, Anna Ramey, and the staff of the Dyslexia Lab at Texas Scottish Rite Hospital for Children in Dallas, Texas. The tape version of DTP is a two year program, involving 350 one-hour videotapes, for students with dyslexia and those at risk for dyslexia. It is currently in use in over 400 school districts in Texas and in over 30 states. The major advantage of the program is that it is relatively cost effective. The classroom teacher, called a *proctor*, learns the program from the teacher's guides and from watching the tapes with the students. A second set of videotapes, the Literacy Program, has been developed at Scottish Rite for adolescents and adults who read poorly for a variety of reasons. This consists of 160 hour-long tapes that can be completed in a school year, or in community-based adult literacy programs. Guides, student workbooks, and the Bloomfield-Barnhart *Let's Read* readers are available from Educators Publishing Service. The videotapes must be ordered directly from the Scottish Rite Hospital.

A report issued by Texas Scottish Rite Hospital for Children and dated 1992, chronicles the progress of 2,037 public school children trained using video tapes in the Dyslexia Training Program. The data was generated by a training project intended as a method for helping classroom teachers provide children with dyslexia with appropriate materials as they moved through the program. The children ranged from 2nd grade through middle school. Reading, writing, spelling, and alphabet skill levels are reported in terms of criterion-referenced curriculum levels on the seven schedules (or levels) of the program.

A recent DTP evaluation study involves the use of controls and was initiated in 1991 by a group headed by Jeffrey Black, Medical Director of the Child Development Division of Texas Scottish Rite Hospital for Children. In a short summary (Black et al. 1994) the group reports a comparison of progress made over a two-year period by 22 elementary age children with dyslexia in two DTP instructional programs with that of 26 controls who received school-based reading instruction without a phonics emphasis. In comparison with the school-based controls, the two DTP groups made more progress in decoding over two years, and more progress in comprehension during the first year. Note, however, that only 7 of the 26 school-based controls received any special reading services. Within the two DTP groups the 12 children receiving taped DTP instruction made as much progress as the 10 children in the live instruction DTP group, which is encouraging in terms of the effectiveness of taped instruction. Neither DTP group made significant progress in spelling.

14

Auditory Discrimination in Depth

BACKGROUND AND RATIONALE

Auditory Discrimination in Depth (ADD) was developed by Charles and Patricia Lindamood, the former a linguist and the latter a speech pathologist. ADD is a preventive, developmental, or remedial program designed to teach auditory conceptualization skills basic to reading, spelling, and speech. The program is intended to complement any reading program. It can be used with kindergarten children to bolster the development of auditory-perceptual awareness as well as with children and adults who fail to read and spell successfully because of failure to acquire phonemic analysis skills.

The Lindamoods (1980) draw attention to the importance of self correction for language learning and literacy acquisition and to the fact that this skill requires auditory conceptualization judgment, which they define as "the ability to perceive the identity, number, and sequence of speech sounds in spoken patterns, and to perceive *how* and *where* patterns are different." In a recent report (Lindamood, Bell, and Lindamood 1992) this component of phonological awareness is referred to as the *comparator function* or the ability to hold two phonological structures in memory for comparison. The Lindamood Auditory Conceptualization Test measures this ability by asking the student to use colored blocks to represent nonsense words with items such as, "If this (yellow-red-yellow sequence of blocks) says *pip*, show me *ip* (red-yellow)." The student is

155

expected to make a judgment about how and where the words are different based on this auditory comparison and then to represent the new word by changing the blocks.

This ability has been found to be significantly correlated with word reading in grades 1 through 12 (Calfee, Lindamood, and Lindamood 1973). The Lindamoods' research led them to conclude that for over half the population auditory conceptualization matures naturally and is fully developed for single-syllable words by fourth grade, but that for a substantial segment of the population this skill does not develop spontaneously and remains deficient into adulthood. The Lindamoods claim to have found a surprising number of adults, involved in many professions (banking, engineering, medicine, teaching, etc.), with hidden deficits in this area. They have called these individuals *closet illiterates*. Regardless of the age of an individual, however, the Lindamoods contend that auditory conceptual function can be developed through direct, multisensory instruction.

CURRICULUM AND INSTRUCTION

The ADD program contains five developmental levels. The first level, called *Setting the Climate for Learning*, introduces the concept of auditory perception and how we can aid our learning by making it consciously multisensory. Optional activities include identifying environmental sounds, comparing sounds, and sequencing sounds.

The second curriculum level encourages students to identify and classify speech sounds. All sounds have been categorized and labelled on the basis of the shape and position of the lips, teeth, and tongue when

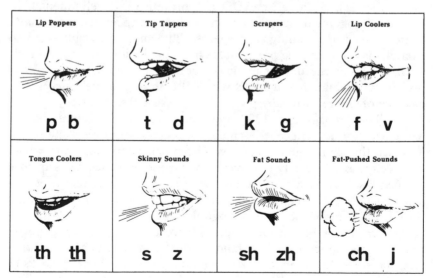

Letter Sound Labels. The A.D.D. Program: Auditory Discrimination in Depth *by Charles H. Lindamood and Patricia C. Lindamood. (Reproduced with permission from PRO-ED. Copyright 1976.)*

the sounds are produced. Sixteen of the consonant sounds have been grouped in unvoiced/voiced pairs. For example, the phonemes /p/ and /b/ are paired and labeled *lip poppers* with /p/ the *quiet brother* and /b/ the *noisy brother*. For vowels, which have more subtle characteristics in pronunciation, students are taught to "associate the physical sensation of making each sound, the appearance of the mouth when the sound is made, and the sound they hear" (Lindamood and Lindamood 1975, Book 1). Students are asked to think of the vowels as falling on a half circle moving from the front to the back of the mouth, depending upon placement of the tongue when a vowel is pronounced. The short /i/ sound, for instance, is produced with the tongue placed high in the front of the mouth.

At the third level, students learn to distinguish and name the various sound categories, using colored blocks to represent sounds. Later they learn to track sounds in nonsense words. Colored blocks are used here to distinguish phonemes. For example, the teacher says, "If that says *zab* show me *zat*." and the child removes the yellow block in a red-blue-yellow sequence to replace it with any other color. In this way, simple syllables (CV, VC, CVC) and complex syllables (CCV, VCC, CCVC, CVCC, CCVCC) are conceptualized.

Not until students have become proficient at encoding nonsense words in this manner are letter symbols applied to spelling and reading.

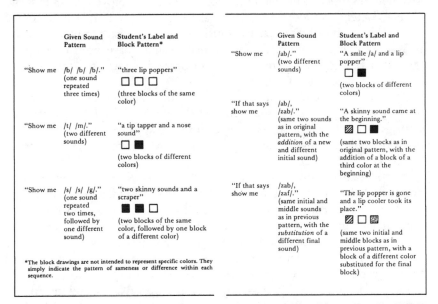

Given Sound Pattern	Student's Label and Block Pattern*		Given Sound Pattern	Student's Label and Block Pattern
		"Show me	/ab/." (two different sounds)	"A smile /a/ and a lip popper"
"Show me /b/ /b/ /b/." (one sound repeated three times)	"three lip poppers" (three blocks of the same color)			(two blocks of different colors)
		"If that says show me	/ab/, /zab/." (same two sounds as in original pattern, with the *addition* of a new and different initial sound)	"A skinny sound came at the beginning." (same two blocks as in original pattern, with the addition of a block of a third color at the beginning)
"Show me /t/ /m/." (two different sounds)	"a tip tapper and a nose sound" (two blocks of different colors)			
"Show me /s/ /s/ /g/." (one sound repeated two times, followed by one different sound)	"two skinny sounds and a scraper" (two blocks of the same color, followed by one block of a different color)		"If that says show me	/zab/, /zaf/." (same initial and middle sounds as in previous pattern, with the *substitution* of a different final sound)	"The lip popper is gone and a lip cooler took its place." (same two initial and middle blocks as in previous pattern, with a block of a different color substituted for the final block)

*The block drawings are not intended to represent specific colors. They simply indicate the pattern of sameness or difference within each sequence.

Color-Encoding Isolated Sounds. The A.D.D. Program: Auditory Discrimination in Depth *by Charles H. Lindamood and Patricia C. Lindamood. (Reproduced with permission from PRO-ED. Copyright 1976.)*

Color-Encoding Sounds in Syllables. The A.D.D. Program: Auditory Discrimination in Depth *by Charles H. Lindamood and Patricia C. Lindamood. (Reproduced with permission from PRO-ED. Copyright 1976.)*

At this fourth level of the curriculum students first use letters printed on tiles for spelling activities and then progress to writing letters themselves. Real words are introduced at this level along with commercially available spelling programs. Students learn to sort out phonetically regular, or dependable, words from nonphonetic words. This allows them to concentrate on the irregular features of the latter type, according to the Lindamoods, and reduces the number of words that must be memorized.

Reading is taught at the fifth or highest level of the program, which overlaps to some degree with the spelling level. Note that this is consistent with Uta Frith's (1985; 1986) model in which spelling leads into reading (see Chapter 2). Reading instruction at this level follows much the same sequence as spelling instruction, beginning with lettered tiles and then moving to print. The program systematically brings into play a three-way sensory feedback system from the ear, eye, and mouth, with emphasis on verbal mediation and self correction.

The Lindamood materials do not include readers. In the ADD manual the Lindamoods advocate using either linguistic (e.g., see Chapter 6 for a description of the Merrill readers) or i.t.a.[1] readers in the beginning reading stages and they emphasize the importance of oral reading. For severely disabled readers, they suggest that the teacher first read the text aloud in order to model intonation, as well as to provide awareness of general content and vocabulary. Minimal coverage is given to reading comprehension in the ADD teacher manuals. Procedures that promote growth in reading comprehension through visual imagery have been developed by Nanci Bell (1991) for use in the Lindamood clinic, Lindamood-Bell Learning Processes (see Chapter 8).

The ADD techniques are designed for classroom use with small, homogeneous groups of students, and they can be applied in tutorial settings as well. The teacher uses a Socratic approach to instruction; questioning leads students to discover the alphabetic principle for themselves (Howard 1982).

The curriculum materials for the Lindamood ADD program are currently being distributed by PRO-ED. Patricia Lindamood is revising the Lindamood Auditory Conceptualization Test (1979) and the new edition will include more complex phoneme combinations than the earlier version. The present version of the LAC test includes segmentation of no more than four phonemes because many evaluators are unable to go beyond this level themselves (personal communication, August 1984). Lindamood plans to make both the revised LAC test and the ADD training program available in a computer-administered version which should help to standardize delivery.

---

[1] The Initial Teaching Alphabet uses altered spellings to regularize letter-sound relationships.

TEACHER TRAINING

Teacher training for the Lindamood ADD program is conducted in two five-day, nine-hour seminars. The first seminar teaches theory and demonstrates concepts and techniques. The second seminar usually follows immediately after the first and involves practical application of concepts and techniques.

Training is offered at Lindamood-Bell Learning Processes in San Luis Obispo, California. Alternatively, inservice training can be arranged in other geographic areas on request. As the duration of training is much shorter, inservice training costs are considerably less than those offered by Alphabetic Phonics and Slingerland.

EVALUATION AND IMPLEMENTATION

Analyses of data on the effectiveness of the ADD program have yielded generally positive results. Marilyn Howard (1982), conducting a ten-year longitudinal study in Arco, Idaho, found that average reading scores for children who had received ADD instruction as first graders rose by more than 30 percentile points over a five-year period. In a second report, Howard (1986) found that both boys and girls, and both kindergarten and first-graders trained in ADD made greater gains in word attack and reading skills than did controls.

A two-year study by the Institute for Training and Research in Auditory Conceptualization (INTRAC 1983) investigated the effects of incorporating the Lindamood program with the Ginn basal reader program in first- through fourth-grade classrooms in the Santa Monica public schools. INTRAC compared academic progress in these classrooms to progress in classrooms using only the Ginn program. At the end of the first year, superior gains were evidenced in the experimental classrooms as compared to the control classrooms, not only in auditory conceptualization but also on the spelling, reading, and word attack subtests of the Wide Range Achievement Test (WRAT) and Woodcock Reading Mastery Tests (WRMT). At the end of the second year of ADD training, students in the experimental classrooms increased their lead over the control subjects.

As a result of the favorable outcome for ADD instruction in the INTRAC study, the Santa Monica school board voted in the third year to provide inservice training for teachers and to include ADD curriculum in all kindergarten through second-grade classrooms in the school district.

One recent training study (Alexander et al. 1991) used ADD with ten children with dyslexia ranging in age from 7 through 12 who were attending an after-school remedial center. Treatment was sustained until all levels of ADD had been completed. Treatment time varied from 38 to 124 hours, with an average of 65 hours. Significant progress was made by the group in terms of standardized reading scores. While there was no control group in this study, an important experimental comparison was made: there was no difference at posttest between Word Identification and Word Attack subtests on the Woodcock Reading Mastery Tests. There was little in the research literature before this study to suggest that children with dyslexia could be taught to read nonsense words effectively along with gains in real word reading following remediation. As mentioned in Chapter 4, ADD is one component of a large scale, federally funded longitudinal intervention study being carried out by a research team directed by Joseph Torgesen at Florida State University in Tallahassee.

15

The Slingerland Approach

BACKGROUND AND RATIONALE

The Slingerland Approach was designed by Beth Slingerland as an Orton-Gillingham adaptation for use with whole classes of students. The program provides an alternative setting for at-risk beginning readers. As with other Orton-Gillingham programs, the Slingerland Approach is based on the premise that language depends on intersensory functioning. Multisensory activities are incorporated into all levels of the program to promote the development of automatic visual, auditory, and kinesthetic associations.

The first teacher education course was developed in 1960 in the Pacific northwest and the program has its headquarters at the Slingerland Institute in Bellevue, Washington. Hundreds of Slingerland classrooms now exist on the West Coast and more have sprung up in other parts of the United States.

The program was designed as preventive instruction for children who have been identified by the Slingerland Screening Tests as having *specific language disability* (SLD) and therefore are at risk for reading failure. The screening tests are usually administered at the end of kindergarten or the beginning of first grade. Children so identified receive Slingerland instruction in place of the traditional language arts curriculum; most remain in Slingerland classrooms for at least two years. The curriculum can also be used in the upper grades. Older children entering a school using the Slingerland Approach are tested using other versions of the screening tests, which are available up through the high school level, and then provided with the Slingerland curriculum where appropriate.

CURRICULUM AND INSTRUCTION

The Slingerland curriculum has three components: Learning to Write, the Auditory Approach, and the Visual Approach. Training begins

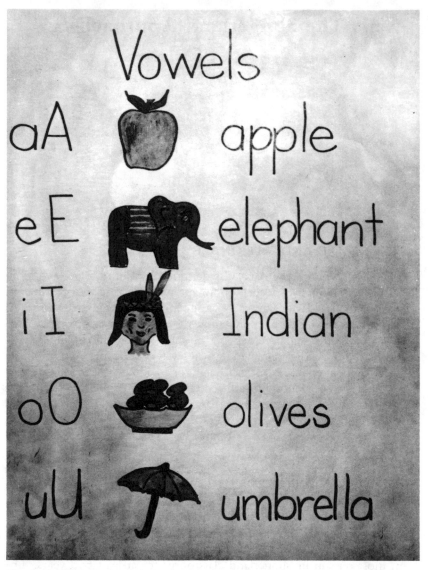

Slingerland Wall Card. Photograph from A Multi-Sensory Approach to Language Arts for Specific Language Disability Children *by Beth H. Slingerland. (Reproduced with permission from Educators Publishing Service, Cambridge, MA. Copyright 1971.)*

with handwriting. Ten consonants and a vowel are taught during the first several months of training. In each case, an individual letter is written on large paper in manuscript (or in cursive beginning in the third year of the program). The students trace the letter with two fingers and then with the blunt end of a pencil before using the sharpened end to trace the letter. The next step is to use paper folded in thirds for tracing, copying, and writing from memory after listening to the teacher say the sound of the letter. This *Visual-Auditory-Kinesthetic* (V-A-K) association is believed to lead toward automatic recall. After a formation has been mastered, students are given a key word (on a flash card or a wall chart) to go with the letter sound. As they form the letter with an arm swing, they must provide the letter name, the key word, and the letter sound. Both unison and individual responses are used in the Slingerland Approach. In answering individually, the child usually stands up in order that the rest of the class can observe, as well as hear, the response.

The second component, the Auditory Approach, leads to spelling. Here, too, the stimulus is presented orally and linked with a kinesthetic response. The teacher says each letter sound and asks individual children to name the letter while forming it in the air, then to name its key word and give its sound. The teacher then holds up an alphabet card and has the class repeat the procedure in unison, thus completing the V-A-K linkage for a particular letter.

A technique which Slingerland calls *blending*[1] is introduced with oral activities for beginning readers (students who are very young or severely dyslexic students). The teacher pronounces a c-v-c word, such as *hat*, and the class repeats the word. Then an individual child produces the initial sound /h/, says the name *h*, and places a card with the corresponding letter into a pocket chart. The child repeats the word, pronounces the /a/ sound before naming it, and places the letter *a* next to the *h*, and then repeats this procedure for the final /t/ sound. Eventually, most students are able to approach this task beginning with the vowel sound, as in the following oral response: "Hat - /a/ - *a* ; hat - /h/ - *h*; hat - /a/ - *a*; hat - /t/ - *t*.; hat - *h* - *a* - *t*." Once students are able to do this, and can form the letters correctly on lined paper, writing accompanies the pocket chart activity in *written blending* or spelling. The teacher dictates words, phrases, and sentences, and as the student's proficiency increases, she encourages creative writing.

The third component is the Visual Approach, which leads to reading. Here the stimulus is presented in written form. Decoding or *unlocking words* is not taught until the Auditory Approach *blending* skills are in place, usually in the second semester of first grade, as explained in a

---

[1] Note that the term *blending* is used in the Slingerland Approach to refer to what is more often called *segmenting* or the analysis of a spoken word into individual phonemes.

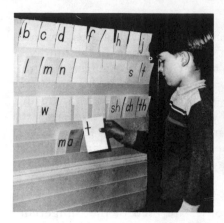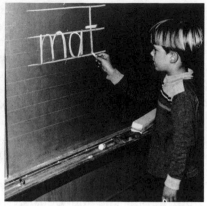

Spelling Activities in the Slingerland Program. Photographs from A Multi-Sensory Approach to language Arts for Specific Learning Disability Children *by Beth H. Slingerland. (Reproduced with permission from Educators Publishing Service. Copyright 1971.)*

1993 supplement provided by Educators Publishing Service with the original materials (Slingerland 1971). Decoding instruction begins with c-v-c words. Beginning readers are asked to pronounce the initial consonant sound, then the vowel sound, to blend the two, then to pronounce the final consonant sound, and to blend the entire word.

Once older or more competent students are able to *unlock words* letter by letter, from left to right, they are taught to look first for the vowel in each word and to say its name, its sound, and then the whole word. One recent change included in a 1993 supplement to the three 1971 curriculum manuals is that the key word is no longer used to unlock words as in the earlier version of the program.

Consonant clusters or blends, (e.g., *bl-*, *-lk*) are taught as two distinct letter sounds rather than as units. That is, the word *black* is conceptualized as being made up of four sounds: /b/-/l/-/a/-/ck/. Strings of letters that represent a single sound or *phonogram* (e.g., *th*, *ea*, *tch*) are taught as single units of sound, as are inflectional endings such as *-ed* and *-ing*.

Text reading is taught initially via a whole-word approach, usually with whichever basal reader program is used in the school. It can begin, according to Slingerland, at the same time as it is introduced in the other first grade classrooms and is conducted in small groups. A considerable amount of lesson time is spent on *preparation for reading* in which students practice recognizing and reading words and phrases from the text. The teacher writes a new list of words on the chalkboard and the students learn to recognize the words, pronounce the words, and identify their meanings. Toward the last end, the teacher might, for example, ask a student to find the word in the list that "tells the name of a girl" (Jill) or "tells what children do" (swim). Phrases are taught in the same way, and fluency and intonation are emphasized, with the teacher modeling by reading aloud.

The teacher structures a portion of each day's text reading by breaking several sentences into phrases (e.g., Teacher: "What three words tell where the pony ran?" Student: "to the barn"). The teacher guides comprehension using this technique.

Although the basic Slingerland curriculum is designed for the first two primary grades and is described in corresponding teacher guides (Books 1 and 2), a third year curriculum has been developed for Slingerland students who need further support after second grade, as well as older reading-disabled students who were not identified earlier (Book 3). Cursive writing is introduced in this curriculum (Slingerland 1971).

The curriculum continues to evolve as new techniques and materials are incorporated. For example, the key word for short *i* has been changed from *Indian* to *inch*. These changes are included in a short addendum available with the 1971 revision of Books 1-3. The addendum stresses the importance of ongoing change in response to program usage and states that the changes will be incorporated into the next revisions of the three books.

TEACHER TRAINING

Training as a Slingerland teacher involves participation in a four-week teacher-training course. This training usually takes place during the summer within summer school classrooms established for children identified in the Slingerland program as having a specific language disability and provides graduate credits at an affiliated college or university. Staff members from the Slingerland Institute or Slingerland teachers within the school district serve as teacher trainers. The program is coordinated by a certified Slingerland director, who has had two years of Slingerland instruction, plus a third year of classroom supervision, followed by experience as a Slingerland staff teacher.

Dolores Ballesteros and Nancy Royal (1981) describe the organization of a Slingerland summer school training program in a large school district. The program director is responsible for the overall management of the training program, which involves evaluating the training staff. He or she also gives lectures to the teacher-participants on language development, reading, and learning disabilities, phonics, and multisensory techniques. Staff teachers must be well versed in the Slingerland techniques and must be approved by the Slingerland Institute. Each staff teacher works with fifteen teacher-participants, demonstrating the teaching techniques within a classroom and meeting with teachers for discussion and daily lesson planning. In addition to attending lectures and classroom demonstrations, each teacher-participant works daily with an individual child, under the supervision of a staff teacher. A clerical staff member is hired when the number of teacher-participants exceeds forty-five.

School district expenses for a Slingerland summer school training program include staff salaries, minimal supply costs for children's materials and minimal printing costs, in addition to a teacher-participant service charge to the Slingerland Institute for in-service staff and Slingerland materials. Teacher participants usually pay for teacher's materials and university credit where it is available. All Slingerland training programs must be planned through the Slingerland Institute in Bellevue, Washington. Summer schools are held only in districts providing administrative support for teachers interested in Slingerland instruction.

EVALUATION AND IMPLEMENTATION

The Slingerland method has been enthusiastically received in a large number of school districts throughout the country, particularly in the Pacific Northwest, where it originated, and in California. In many cases, parents have been instrumental in starting Slingerland programs and in some cases have even threatened to file suit unless their children were provided with this instruction (Lovitt and DeMier 1984). Ballesteros and Royal (1981) describe how the program served as a voluntary magnet for racial integration in schools in southern California; Slingerland classes were established in high-minority schools in the San Diego area with two-thirds of the enrollment space reserved for nonminority children from the district that had requested Slingerland instruction. Moreover, through parental petition, Slingerland classes were established here through the twelfth grade.

Considerable research has addressed the question of program effectiveness. John Litcher and Leonard Roberge (1979) conducted a three-year study with first-grade children receiving Slingerland instruction, comparing their year-end achievement with matched control children in other schools. They reported significantly higher achievement for the Slingerland children. However, because they did not describe the instruction provided to the control subjects, the meaning of the comparison is difficult to interpret.

Beverly Wolf (1985) measured progress on the Metropolitan Achievement Test (MAT) for children in Slingerland classes, some of whom were considered to be language disabled as determined by the Slingerland Screening Tests, and some of whom were not. She conducted an ex post facto analysis of first-to-second-grade gain scores as compared to the scores of children in traditional classrooms. Instruction in the conventional classrooms, which served as the control treatment, was not described in detail, but appears to have been an eclectic basal reader approach. Thus two experimental groups received Slingerland instruction, those with SLD and those without SLD, and two control groups received conventional instruction, one with SLD and one without. The outcome of the analysis indicated that Slingerland instruction produced significantly greater gains than did conventional instruction on the language section of the MAT (listening comprehension; punctuation and capitalization; usage, grammar, and syntax; spelling; and study skills) for both SLD and non SLD students. On the reading section (word and sentence reading; vocabulary; literal, inferential, and evaluative comprehension) the advantage of Slingerland training over conventional instruction approached but did not achieve significance. However, scores of the Slingerland students were less variable than those of the conventionally instructed group. On the other hand, the superiority of Slingerland instruction over conventional instruction was not evidenced in the reading scores for the non-SLD students.

Another ex post facto investigation (McCulloch 1985) compared California Achievement Test (CAT) scores of 15 children with SLD who received three years of Slingerland training with 15 children with SLD who had been taught in conventional classrooms during the first three grades. Statistical analyses demonstrated significantly higher reading and language scores for the Slingerland trained children. Spelling scores, in contrast, did not reveal significant between-group differences. The study's author, Clara McCulloch (personal communication, May 9, 1994) explains that Slingerland students are taught to spell using an auditory approach consistent with Orton's assertion that a clear-cut auditory pattern of the spelling word must be present. The CAT spelling task is virtually a visual proofreading (orthographic) task, and may not tap phonology which McCulloch considers more related to spelling.

School-wide and district-wide evaluation studies of the Slingerland Approach have yielded generally positive results. For example, a study conducted in 1980 by the Bureau of Child Educational Services (BOCES) in South Huntington, New York, determined that by third grade, Slingerland students had achieved reading gains equal to children in regular classrooms, although they did not reach the same reading level. The Slingerland Institute has stated emphatically that the achievement levels of students with SLD should not be compared to those of normal students, but instead, expected year-to-year gains should be assessed, as in this study.

One observation that was disconcerting to Diana Clark as she visited schools and reviewed research for the earlier edition of this book (Clark 1988) is the finding that Slingerland instruction has not always been sufficient to meet the needs of all children at risk for reading failure. Clara McCulloch commented (personal communication, May 9, 1994) that the Slingerland Approach was designed for children with Specific Language Disability. Children who are severely dyslexic may require more individualized instruction than a group setting can provide. Children with reading problems because of other handicapping conditions (e.g., children who are mentally retarded or emotionally disturbed) may have their needs met more adequately in other special programs.

16

Recipe for Reading

BACKGROUND AND RATIONALE

Recipe for Reading is another adaption of the Orton-Gillingham approach (Gillingham and Stillman 1960) and, like the Orton-Gillingham, is designed for one-to-one tutorial use. It was developed in the 1950s by Nina Traub and first used in Ossining, New York, with parents serving as tutors for learning-disabled children in the community. Because of its success, funding was obtained in the early 1970s to place the program in five Ossining elementary schools (Traub 1982).

The Traub method applies a synthetic phonics approach, teaching individual letter sounds in isolation before introducing syllables or words. All teaching follows a part-to-whole progression. Although the term *multisensory* does not appear in the manual, the use of visual, auditory, and kinesthetic reinforcement techniques is encouraged throughout the program. Traub developed a sequence for introducing letter sounds based on their visual, auditory, and kinesthetic characteristics. In the instructor's manual, available from Educators Publishing Service (Traub and Bloom 1975), Traub states that students who appear to have learning disabilities should be individually diagnosed and receive carefully planned individualized instruction.

CURRICULUM AND INSTRUCTION

The Traub method is designed for first- through third-grade students to be delivered on a one-to-one basis outside the classroom in half-hour sessions five days a week. In developing Recipe for Reading, Traub has greatly simplified the Orton-Gillingham curriculum. The teacher's manual (Traub and Bloom 1975) is clearly written, easy to follow, and relatively short. A curriculum sequence chart is printed on the inside cover.

Instruction begins by introducing seven consonants (hard *c* and *g*, *d*, *m*, *l*, *h*, and *f*) and two vowels (*a* and *o*). Explaining the rationale for her selection of these letters, Traub states in the manual that some letters are learned and written more easily than others. As examples, she maintains that *c*, *o*, *a*, and *d* have the same basic kinesthetic formations (circle to the left), hard *c* and *g* "seem to be among the easiest sounds perceived by the ear," *d* and *m* are two of the first sounds made by infants (i.e., "da-da," "ma-ma"). The letters *d* and *b* "are introduced at a considerable distance from each other, because they are the pair that are most commonly reversed and confused."

Each letter to be learned is first presented on a large piece of oak tag, written in one-inch thick strokes. The teacher gives the letter sound and then writes the letter. The child traces the letter and then writes it independently. When the child has done this successfully, the teacher says the letter name.

Both manuscript and cursive letter formations are taught in the Traub method. Special lined paper is provided to designate orientation points in letter formation. Each writing line is divided into four parallel lines. Letters with no stems should fill the space between the two middle lines, called *the little red house*. Upward letter stems should touch the top line ("the attic") and downward stems the bottom line (*the basement*). Directional cues for letter formations are provided at the top of each page—a bat and a ball for letters such as *b*, that turn to the right, and a drum and drumstick for those turning to the left. Many multisensory techniques are suggested for the student who has difficulty with letter formations, for example, walking on a letter formed with masking tape on the floor, forming a letter with rolls of clay and then tracing it with the eyes open and eyes shut, and writing in the air (*sky writing*).

Spelling precedes reading in the Traub approach. After the student has learned the sound and name for each of the first nine letters and is able to write each of these letters, the student is taught to spell c-v-c words with these letters. The teacher dictates words without the student's having seen the words in print. The student repeats the word, spells it aloud, and then writes it while spelling it aloud (simultaneous oral spelling). If the student has difficulty, he or she is asked to listen for the first sound and give its letter name as the teacher says the word, separating each phoneme. This procedure is repeated with the middle vowel and final consonant. The manual tells the teacher to dictate more naturally "as the child's auditory discrimination improves" (Traub and Bloom 1975).

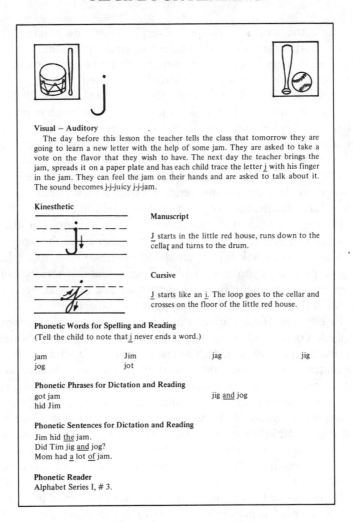

Visual – Auditory

The day before this lesson the teacher tells the class that tomorrow they are going to learn a new letter with the help of some jam. They are asked to take a vote on the flavor that they wish to have. The next day the teacher brings the jam, spreads it on a paper plate and has each child trace the letter j with his finger in the jam. They can feel the jam on their hands and are asked to talk about it. The sound becomes j-j-juicy j-j-jam.

Kinesthetic

Manuscript

J starts in the little red house, runs down to the cellar and turns to the drum.

Cursive

J starts like an i. The loop goes to the cellar and crosses on the floor of the little red house.

Phonetic Words for Spelling and Reading
(Tell the child to note that j never ends a word.)

jam	Jim	jag	jig
jog	jot		

Phonetic Phrases for Dictation and Reading

got jam   jig and jog
hid Jim

Phonetic Sentences for Dictation and Reading

Jim hid the jam.
Did Tim jig and jog?
Mom had a lot of jam.

Phonetic Reader
Alphabet Series I, # 3.

Lesson from Recipe for Reading *by Nina Traub with Frances Bloom. (Reproduced with permission from Educators Publishing Service, Cambridge, MA. Copyright 1975.)*

After the student spells the words, he is asked to read them as printed on *phonetic word cards* (flash cards), rather than in his own writing. If the student has trouble reading a word, the teacher places cards representing each letter (phonetic sound cards) under the word and has the student say each letter sound. Traub suggests many blending techniques but, like Gillingham and Stillman (1960), she emphasizes first blending the initial consonant and following vowel, for example, ba-t, rather than the vowel and final consonant, as in the phonic-linguistic approach (e.g., b-at). which she claims encourages the wrong directionality.

Once the student can spell several words, the teacher dictates phrases or short sentences for the student to write, providing the spelling for any nonphonetic word. After writing sentences, the student reads these sentences from *phonetic sentence cards* and when ready, graduates to reading *phonetic storybooks*, following the same procedures. In addition to these storybooks, Traub provides a list of phonetic readers from other publishers for supplementary reading. She suggests that teachers alternate oral reading with students to model fluency and expression and that they discuss the passage. Recognizing the low interest level of most phonetic readers, Traub recommends reading other materials aloud to the student to develop comprehension skills. She suggests asking the student to listen for the answer to a particular question as the text is read.

Having the student dictate his or her own stories is another suggested activity in Recipe for Reading. The teacher types the story, which is then made into a book for the child and others to read, much like the language experience approach. Traub maintains that this activity improves verbal expression and helps build a sight vocabulary. She also recommends using Dolch flash cards[1] for building sight vocabulary.

Briefly, the Traub curriculum moves from one-syllable words, to two-syllable compound words (e.g., *pigpen*) to two-syllable phonetically regular words (e.g., *dislike*). In the last instance, the student first reads the individual syllables on cards and then puts them together to make words. All letter sounds or groups of letter sounds are introduced one by one: initial consonant blends, three-letter word endings (e.g. *ing, ank*), long vowel words with *magic e*, vowel digraphs, vowel–consonant combinations, diphthongs, nonphonetic word parts, such as *igh*, and common suffix rules, such as when to double final consonants before adding vowel suffixes. A special section on affixes and word roots is provided for older students.

Daily lessons begin with drill on previously learned letter sounds. Then new material is presented and taught as previously described. Depending on the student's ability level, word reading, sentence reading, and story book reading follow in order. Lastly, phonetic word games are played to reinforce learning.

Each student's work is dated and retained in a folder, and his progress carefully recorded. A count is kept of all words learned. Traub emphasizes the importance of making students aware of their progress. For younger children, particularly, she recommends ending lessons with an activity at which they are sure to succeed and acknowledging their success with some sign of approval. By way of additional encouragement, a list of all the books a student has read is included in his folder.

---

[1] The Dolch Basic Sight Vocabulary Cards (Dolch 1952) contain 220 of the words most frequently encountered by beginning readers.

In addition to the teacher's manual, there are now Recipe for Reading workbooks, writing paper, sequence pads for keeping records for individual children, and a series of 21 storybooks called the *Alphabet Series* and coordinated with the Recipe for Reading sequence. A comprehension component should be available shortly.

TEACHER TRAINING

All training for Recipe for Reading teachers or tutors was conducted by Traub, the program's author, until her death. Since then, her colleague, Connie Russo, has carried on the program and conducted the teacher training. The following description of the teacher training program was provided by Russo via telephone.

Training is usually done within a public school in daily, five-hour sessions over a two week period. It is best arranged during the summer when children are attending classes for remedial instruction. The first two hours are devoted to lecture. In the next two hours each teacher trainee applies the knowledge acquired from the lecture by tutoring two public school students for one hour each under supervision. The last hour involves a sharing and pulling together of all that has been learned that day among the fifteen or so teacher trainees.

When training is conducted during the school year, it is usually condensed into six hours of lecture without the tutoring practicum because of problems with classroom pull-out time. However, supervised tutoring experience is arranged individually for each teacher trainee during the year.

EVALUATION AND IMPLEMENTATION

A federally funded validation study, reported by Traub (1982), was carried out in 1976 by the MAGI Educational Service on the initial school implementation of Recipe for Reading in five Ossining, New York elementary schools. Results of this study indicated that second-grade Ossining students who were tutored with Recipe for Reading made significantly greater improvement in reading and spelling, as measured by posttest, than a control group of second-grade students from another district tutored using a different remedial method that was not described. Unfortunately, since the tests administered yield only total reading grade equivalents, it is not possible to ascertain which subskills (decoding, vocabulary, or comprehension) are most influenced by the Traub method.

As a result of this validation study, Ossining received a federal IV-C grant to continue and expand the use of Recipe for Reading. Traub (1982) states that subsequent to the program's implementation in Ossining, twenty-six different school districts had received similar grants to replicate the Ossining program and that she had trained the staff in these schools. She reports positive effects of Recipe for Reading, as measured by year-to-year comparison studies on student achievement conducted in several of these districts. One district cited the program's cost effectiveness, maintaining that personnel was the highest expense and that expense for materials was low. Another district cited enhanced motivation and improved attitude toward reading among students receiving Recipe for Reading instruction.

Recipe for Reading is most often used in self-contained special education classrooms and in resource rooms, or for early intervention with children who are at-risk. Though designed for one-to-one instruction, Russo maintains that the method is ideal for groups of as many as five students. Recipe for Reading is also used for whole-class and small group lessons in regular education settings. Classroom teachers who like to design their own materials rather than using a basal reading series seem to find Recipe for Reading more valuable than other phonics programs because the structure and sequence are clear but not lockstep or scripted, and because many of the ideas seem creative (e.g., practicing writing *p* in peanut butter) as well as linguistically sound. Cisqua-Rippowam, an independent school for high-achieving children in Bedford, New York, uses Recipe for Reading as a beginning reading program with all students.

17

Project Read (Enfield and Greene)

BACKGROUND AND RATIONALE

Project Read was developed in 1969 by Mary Lee Enfield and Victoria Greene for the public school district in Bloomington, Minnesota, in response to the growing number of children who did not seem to benefit from the basal reading program used in the district. It began as a three year experimental program to deliver direct, systematic phonics instruction within regular classrooms to students performing below the 25th percentile in reading and spelling. The major goals of the program were to provide cost effective reading instruction to students who were not learning in the district's reading program, to increase coordination between regular classroom instruction and remedial instruction, and to avoid the stigma of removal from the mainstream (Enfield 1976). The authors consider the program an alternative as well as a remedial approach to reading instructions (Enfield and Greene 1981).

Project Read is now being used with students in grades one through six who are functioning at the lowest reading levels, as well as with students identified as learning disabled. Though designed for the classroom teacher, the program may be used effectively in a resource center (Arkes 1986). Extensions of the program, covering reading comprehension and written expression, as well as phonology, are appropriate for intermediate and secondary students who are weak in these areas.

CURRICULUM AND INSTRUCTION

Project Read curriculum comprises three phases. Phase I instruction focuses on phonics, Phase II on reading comprehension, and Phase III on written expression. Phase I is essentially a modification of the Orton-Gillingham model of systematic, multisensory phonics instruction. Originally designed for grades one through three, Phase I has since been extended through grade nine. Instruction in basic phonics knowledge for grades one through three is outlined in a teacher's guide (Greene and Enfield 1985a). The guide provides a systematic sequence of skills and concepts that are covered in a series of sixty lessons, each of which may span several days or even a week of instruction. Specific techniques, many of which are multisensory, are described for teaching these skills and concepts. These include tracing letters in a sand tray (called the *memory box*), in the air, on a shag rug, a table, or a chalkboard. Raised letters are provided for showing directionality of confusable letters. Mouth positions are stressed in teaching consonant sounds, for example, for *b*, a voiced explosion of air, for *t*, a tongue bounce, for *m*, mouth closed. Finger puppets and key words are mnemonics suggested for teaching vowels, and children are given practice in identifying the vowels from among the other letters in the alphabet sequence. Long and short vowel markings are taught in the first lesson.

Each lesson introduces a new phonic element, such as a letter sound, and a particular concept, for instance, the fact that vowels have a significant value for building words. A lesson begins with review of previously learned material that includes both decoding and encoding practice. Hand signals are used to direct unison response. The teacher flashes letter cards and the students say the letter symbols. Next, new sounds are introduced and reinforced with multisensory techniques. Students then build words or syllables with letter cards and decode them. Various techniques for sound blending are described in the teacher's guide. Spelling practice follows with students saying the letter sound as they write each letter.

Oral reading is the last activity of each lesson. The program has incorporated the *SRA Basic Reading* linguistic series (Rasmussen and Goldberg 1976) for this purpose, although alternative materials are suggested in some of the lessons. Students are taught to follow along with a finger or pencil while reading and, if they have difficulty decoding, to trace over the particular letter or letters *to unlock the sound* (Greene and Enfield 1985a). Oral reading involves both *reinforcement reading*, where the material is usually phonetically regular and students are expected to have little decoding difficulty, and *stretch reading* in which the material may include unfamiliar words. Irregular words contained in reinforcement reading material are taught separately. In stretch reading the teacher supplies any words that may be beyond the students skill level.

Three categories of words are distinguished in Project Read: "green words" which are phonetically regular for both decoding and encoding (e.g., *cat*); "yellow words" which are regular for decoding but follow spelling generalizations for encoding (e.g., *back*); and "red words" which are irregular for both decoding and encoding (e.g., *the*).

One teaching point that distinguishes Project Read from other Orton-Gillingham oriented programs involves the teaching of consonant clusters or blends. While other programs teach digraphs such as *-ch* as a single sound and consonant clusters or blends such as *bl* as two sounds for reading and spelling, Project Read teaches both digraphs and clusters as single units. That is, the cluster *bl* is taught as a single sound (i.e., /bl/) rather than as two sounds (i.e., /b/-/l/) as in other Orton-Gillingham programs such as Alphabetic Phonics and Slingerland.

A continuation of Phase I for students in fourth through ninth grades focuses on vocabulary development by teaching affixes and common word roots. The curriculum is outlined in a second Phase I teacher guide, referred to as the Affix Guide (Greene and Enfield 1981). The guide presents a unique approach to unlocking word meaning. Rather than drawing attention to word roots, which may be elements too obscure to bear apparent meaning (for example, the syllable *dict* in the word *unpredictable*) students are taught to look for known parts (in this case *predict*), which are referred to as *word foundations*. After identifying the known foundation, the attending affixes are isolated and identified.

Another creative aspect of Greene and Enfield's curriculum is their application of the concept of comprehension to the understanding of affixed words. Students learn that these words actually represent phrases, for example, *unpredictable* equals "cannot be predicted." The teacher's guide presents pairs of sentences, one containing such a phrase, the other the corresponding affixed word. It also provides sentences that can be used for demonstration and reinforcement in dictation exercises, using the affixed words in meaningful context. A spelling guide incorporating a structured phonics approach is also included in the Project Read materials (Greene and Enfield 1985). The guide provides the teacher with valuable information about English spelling patterns and rules. It takes into consideration three relevant aspects of English graphemes: their origin (e.g., Anglo Saxon, Latin), their frequency, and their placement in words. In terms of frequency, Enfield and Greene maintain that teaching the least frequently encountered spellings for a particular phoneme first — for example, *ue* before *ew* — helps students learn to sort and classify words according to spelling patterns.

The syllable is the unit of emphasis in this spelling guide. According to Greene and Enfield, all syllables in the English language fall into one of seven categories: closed, open, vowel team, vowel-consonant-final *e*, diphthong, final consonant *le*, and vowel controlled by *r*. They stress the fact that the type of syllable determines the sound of the vowel or vowels it contains.

Phase II of Project Read focuses on reading comprehension and vocabulary development and begins when a student has mastered basic decoding skills, usually toward the end of first grade. However, major emphasis on comprehension instruction takes place in grades four through six. The curriculum is outlined in a teacher's guide (Greene and Enfield 1985b) which has incorporated instructional materials from other publishers for teaching reading comprehension skills, for example, the McGraw Hill Reading for Concepts series and the Barnell Loft Specific Skills Series. Most of these materials are nonfiction.

The guide distinguishes two levels of text analysis and presents a sequence of comprehension skills within each level. At the literal level these skills include identifying the subject of the text, selecting and defining unfamiliar words, noting punctuation and understanding its purpose, and determining whether the text material is fiction, nonfiction, or procedural (telling how to do something). At the interpretive level, the skills include identifying and sequencing the information in the text (either key facts or key procedural steps), finding the supporting details, making inferences, and drawing conclusions. Students also are taught to outline the organizational form of a text.

Multisensory activities are suggested to reinforce the concepts being taught. For example, having students write key facts on paper-cutout keys and paste the keys in the margins, pointing to the facts as written in the text, or having students feel an object hidden in a paper bag and make assumptions about that object from touch.

The major focus in the inference unit of the curriculum is on teaching students to look for clues in the text that lead to or support assumptions about the context. Toward this end the teacher may make an inferential statement and ask students to find the clues in the text that lead to this inference or the teacher may ask an inferential question for the students to answer and indicate the clues that led to their answer.

Phase III of Project Read encompasses instruction in written expression, provided systematically and incorporating multisensory techniques. Handwriting instruction, however, is not included in the program. The focus in this phase is on teaching sentence structure and paragraph development. Instruction moves from basic sentence structure (simple sentences) to complex sentences. Students are taught to diagram sentences; they spend considerable time at this activity. Concepts are practiced in creative writing experiences. Phase III extends from the end of grade one through grade nine and may be used as an alternative to the regular English program in grades five through nine (Arkes 1986).

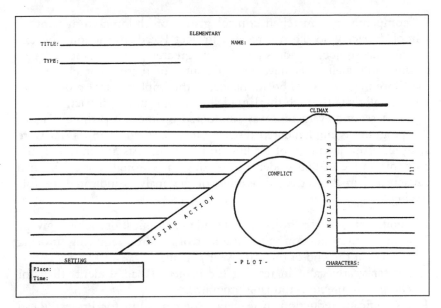

Diagram of Story Form from There's a Skeleton in Every Closet, Teacher Text *by Victoria E. Greene and Mary Lee Enfield. (Reproduced with permission from the authors. Copyright 1976.)*

TEACHER TRAINING

In the early stages of Project Read, training was carried out by ten former classroom teachers who had learned the program. Using demonstration and observational methods, they, in turn, taught the program in schools to elementary teachers as they worked with groups of low achieving students in their classrooms. At the end of two or three weeks, the classroom teacher took over full responsibility for the program, supported by periodic visits from the project staff for further observation, feedback, and demonstration as needed.

Since that time training has shifted to half-day workshops of five days each held during the summer in Bloomington at the Project Read Teacher Training Institute. Each workshop is devoted to one of three instructional areas: phonology, reading comprehension, or written expression. Training for workshop participants continues in the following school year with demonstration and observation of the program in their respective classrooms in the district.

EVALUATION AND IMPLEMENTATION

The first evaluation of Project Read was conducted by Mary Lee Enfield in 1976 as a pilot study. An experimental group of forty-five children in grades one through three, fifteen at each grade level, who were reading below the 25th percentile, received Project Read instruction.

As compared to a matched control group of children from another school district who did not receive Project Read instruction, the experimental subjects made significantly greater gains on measures of reading and spelling achievement. Because of these favorable results, the Bloomington school board mandated the implementation of Project Read in all first- through third-grade classrooms in the district.

A second evaluation was conducted on the initial three years of the program as implemented district wide (Enfield 1976). Data were analyzed from a battery of reading and spelling tests administered to a random sample of 665 students in grades one through three who had participated in Project Read. Results of the analyses indicated the following:

1. significant gains for Project Read students on most of the tests given;
2. a significant reduction in the number of children requiring tutoring services at the end of the three year period;
3. greater yearly gains in reading for Project Read students than for children in previous tutoring programs;
4. a significant reduction in teacher cost per pupil for Project Read students as compared to students in tutoring programs;
5. a district-wide reduction of students falling below grade level in reading after two years of Project Read implementation.

One of the major limitations of the study, as Enfield herself has pointed out, was the lack of a control group. She also acknowledges the possibility of a *Hawthorne effect* or performance enhancement due to the novelty of a program. More recently, Enfield and Greene evaluated the progress of students in grades two, four, and six of the Bloomington public schools who were receiving Project Read instruction (Enfield and Greene 1983). Separate evaluations were conducted on results of district-wide standardized testing in reading and spelling for non-learning disabled students in the Project Read program and students classified as learning disabled who received Project Read instruction. Both evaluations indicated that Project Read students were performing above 75 percent of their achievement potential (estimated on the basis of IQ). Enfield and Greene maintain that this performance level represents significant improvement for these students who were otherwise functioning in the bottom quartile of their class. Their claim, however, must be regarded as being based on subjective judgment.

Project Read is being used increasingly in public school districts around the country: Portland, Oregon; Irvine, California; Tampa, Florida, to name just a few. According to Enfield (personal communication), an enthusiastic leader is needed to convince the school administration to undertake a pilot study. In some instances leadership has come from a motivated teacher.

The town of Greenwich, Connecticut has implemented the program district-wide, without on-site supervision from Project Read staff, through the enthusiastic leadership of teachers and special education administrators. Initially, elementary classroom teachers from one elementary school attended the summer training session in Bloomington and implemented the phonics strand with the lowest achieving students in their classrooms. Subsequently, training has been provided routinely in all schools in the district and is an expectation for all teachers who teach reading either in the classroom or in special support situations. The Project Read phonics strand has been incorporated into the regular language arts curriculum, and is considered a bridge between the regular education classroom and special education settings. According to Nancy Eberhardt, who is the curriculum coordinator for Special Education in the district (personal communication, August 1, 1994), Project Read training is used as a vehicle "to help all teachers involved with beginning literacy instruction understand the profile of the learner who needs direct, concept-driven, multisensory education."

18

DISTAR

BACKGROUND AND RATIONALE

The Direct Instruction Model, which became known as DISTAR (Direct Instructional System of Teaching Arithmetic and Reading), was developed by Wesley Becker and Siegfried Engelmann at the University of Oregon. It was officially launched in 1968 as one of nine instructional models to be used in Project Follow-Through, a U.S. Government sponsored project to evaluate the effectiveness of promising educational programs for disadvantaged children in the first three grades.

Four basic assumptions form the theoretical rationale for the DISTAR model (Becker 1977). First, all children, regardless of background and developmental readiness, can be taught, and teachers must be held accountable for student failure. Second, basic skills acquisition underlies all successful learning; for children who are socioeconomically deprived, direct teaching of these skills is essential. Third, disadvantaged children generally lag behind advantaged students in basic skills acquisition due to the existing academic structure in most schools. The fourth assumption is that in order to close the achievement gap, disadvantaged youngsters must be taught more within the allotted instructional time than advantaged children.

Though originally designed for disadvantaged children, DISTAR has been used to teach children with a variety of constitutional handicaps, including learning disabilities. Writing in 1977, Norris Haring, Barbara Bateman, and Douglas Carnine stated:

> DISTAR's approach is representative of a growing trend in special education that shifts some attention from the child's strengths, weaknesses, or special etiology to an individualized remediation program for the tasks the child must learn (Haring, Bateman, and Carnine 1977).

Elsewhere in the same chapter, these strong advocates of Direct Instruction wrote:

> DISTAR's conceptualization encompasses all essential aspects of the teaching process—analyzing concepts, programming, teaching per se, classroom management, educational materials, and evaluation. It has developed a way of analyzing tasks that isolates the general concept or skill to be taught, and a way to program in which this general case is presented so impeccably that every child can learn it. It has techniques for teaching the general case and strategies for classroom management (Haring, Bateman, and Carnine 1977).

CURRICULUM AND INSTRUCTION

Becker (1977) outlined seven essential instructional components of the DISTAR model: 1) teaching general cases in order that learning can be generalized from selected examples to broader instances; 2) higher teacher-student ratio; 3) carefully structured daily curriculum; 4) rapid-paced, teacher-directed, small-group instruction with a high number of teacher/student interactions; 5) positive reinforcement; 6) carefully trained and supervised teaching staff; and 7) biweekly performance monitoring by means of criterion-referenced tests.

One special feature of DISTAR is that all instruction follows a script. The presentation books (flip-books) provide exact wording and precise directions for everything the teacher says and does in each lesson. Instruction is conducted in small groups with students seated in a semicircle close to the teacher in order to be able to see the one-inch printed letters and words in the teacher presentation books. The proximity additionally helps the teacher to monitor student response, much of which is done in unison. Teachers use hand signals, for example, a hand drop, a clap, a point, or other cue, to indicate the type and timing of the responses required. The presentation books ensure that all concepts deemed relevant by the program's developers are taught and practiced by the students. They include correction procedures and scripts for anticipated student errors.

DISTAR (Engelmann and Bruner 1983) is published by Science Research Associates, Inc. and is now formally referred to as SRA's Direct Instruction Programs. The programs provide instruction in reading, language, spelling, and arithmetic and cover grade levels one through six.

The language program has three levels. The first level is for preschool and primary students and focuses on teaching the language of instruction used in school, building vocabulary, developing oral language skills, and establishing the foundation for logical thinking. The second level builds a language foundation for reading comprehension, emphasizing reasoning skills, and teaches following directions and the meanings of words and sentences. The third level focuses on sentence analysis, both spoken and written, and deals with mechanics, as well as informational content.

The reading program (Reading Mastery) has six levels; only levels I and II, which extend from preschool through second grade, will be discussed here. Both decoding and comprehension are taught from the very beginning.

In Reading Mastery I, letters are referred to as sounds; in Reading Mastery II, letter names are taught. Prereading activities start with teaching the pronunciations of letter sounds. Diagrams are presented to teach the distinction between continuous sounds (e.g., /s/, /m/, /r/, certain digraphs, and all vowels) and stop sounds (e.g., /b/, /d/, /t/). Games are played to promote sequencing skills and to teach understanding of cue words, such as *first* and *next*. Oral blending activities begin in the first lesson and continue through the prereading lessons. Children are taught the difference between sounding out words (saying the letter sounds slowly) and pronouncing the words (saying them fast); the teacher uses hand signals in directing other activities. Rhyming activities are introduced to help children learn to blend initial sounds with word endings. Association between sounds and letter symbols is reinforced in take-home activities.

Letter sounds are introduced slowly in Reading Mastery I, about one every three to four lessons. Reading begins when six sounds have been learned. Each new sound to be taught is presented in a word; this word is used throughout the remainder of the program as a mnemonic device to cue the letter sound.

When new words are introduced, children are instructed first to sound out each word and then say it fast. Irregular words, for example, *is* and *was*, are also initially taught in this way, with the teacher providing the correct pronunciation. It is felt that treating irregular words in this manner, rather than teaching them as sight words, emphasizes their stable spellings. All words learned become part of the students' reading vocabulary and are incorporated first in simple sentences and later in stories.

A modified orthography is used in the early stages of the DISTAR reading program and phased out by the middle of Reading Mastery II. The modification is meant to compensate for the unbalanced ratio of sounds to symbols in the English language and to increase the number of words that can be read as regular words, as well as to highlight differences between visually similar letters. The major features of this orthography include printing silent letters (e.g., *e* in *made*, *i* in *maid*) in smaller type, placing a heavy macron over letters representing long vowel sounds, printing consonant blends as joined letters, slightly changing the configuration of *d* to distinguish it from *b*, and omitting upper case formations except for *I*.

Comprehension activities at the prereading level include interpreting pictures and ordering events in sequence. At the reading level, comprehension skills are taught first in simple sentences and then in stories. In the early stages, children are asked to predict something about the content of pictures by first reading words related to the picture but presented on a prereadng page. Once children are reading stories, oral comprehension questions, such as wh questions, are posed during the reading. In addition, the teacher summarizes the story and asks students to predict what will happen next.

In later stages, children answer written questions about the story. For explicit questions, the group is called upon to respond in unison, but for questions asking for divergent responses, such as giving opinions, individual response is requested. When students are able to read stories *the fast way* on first reading, each student's speed and accuracy are checked every fifth lesson. In addition, mastery tests are administered approximately every fifth lesson from the beginning of the program. Spelling instruction is optional in this program, though strongly encouraged. It is suggested that spelling be taught to the entire class if time does not

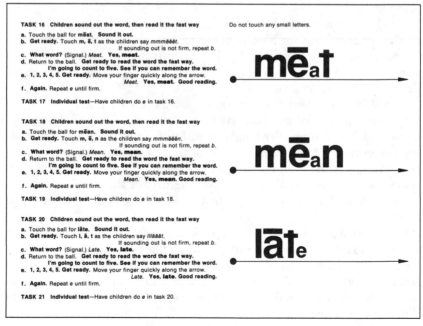

Teacher's Lesson Script from Reading Mastery I: Distar Reading *by Siegfried Engelmann and Elaine C. Bruner. (Reproduced with permission from Science Research Associates, Inc., Chicago, IL. Copyright 1983.)*

allow small-group practice. The spelling curriculum follows the sequence of the reading curriculum. Spelling activities begin with children writing letters for dictated letter sounds and move on to their writing words and sentences. The Spelling Mastery program begins in second grade and continues through sixth-grade level. It starts with teaching basic phonemic spelling strategies and memorization of high-frequency irregular spelling, and later teaches morphographs (word parts that have meaning, such as the ending *tion*) and spelling rules.

Handwriting instruction is included in the reading curriculum and begins in Lesson 7 when children are first asked to write letter sounds (letter names are not yet introduced). Students are taught manuscript letter formations through tracing exercises with faded prompts (the amount of the model letters shown is gradually diminished). Minimal emphasis is placed on handwriting or on written expression in the DISTAR curriculum.

The recommended time for reading lessons is twenty-five to thirty minutes of group instruction, followed by fifteen to twenty minutes of independent work, five minutes of work check for each group, and ten minutes of group spelling practice. Students are given take-home assignments from the first day of the program.

Scheduling for DISTAR may vary among schools. In one inner-city school, for example, approximately 60 percent of the school day is allocated to DISTAR reading, math, and language in the first three grades, with one hour per subject area (Meyer, Gersten, and Gutkin 1983).

TEACHER TRAINING

According to Becker (1977), a one-week preservice workshop, followed by one or two hours of inservice training a week is usually adequate for teachers to learn DISTAR. Manuals are provided for trainers, just as scripts are provided for teachers. The training procedure involves demonstration, guided practice, and feedback. In the case of the schools that participated in Project Follow-Through, a project manager (university staff member) trained teachers individually or in groups (Meyer, Gersten, and Gutkin 1983). After initial training, skilled teachers often supervised apprentice teachers within the classroom (Becker 1977).

EVALUATION AND IMPLEMENTATION

DISTAR gained prominence as the only one of the nine instructional models in Project Follow-Through to produce significant gains in basic skills as compared to a traditional instructional approach that was administered to a control group of disadvantaged children. Pre- and posttests on the Wide Range Achievement Test indicated that DISTAR students had moved, on average, from the 18th to the 84th percentile in reading (word decoding) on national norms and from the 8th to the 49th percentile in spelling (Becker 1977). DISTAR students did not show the same degree of advantage in reading comprehension on the Metropolitan Achievement Test (MAT), averaging 10 percentile points below the national average, but they still scored significantly higher than students in the other model programs in this area. In both spelling and language, DISTAR students met the national average on the MAT.

A later study, conducted as a follow-up of original DISTAR participants from one inner-city school in New York, looked at the progress of nine cohorts (classes) of those students who had completed three levels of the program (Meyer, Gersten, and Gutkin 1983). It was found that DISTAR students continued to score at or above grade level on standardized reading tests in grades four and five, and that they scored notably above a comparison group of disadvantaged students from the same school district who had not received DISTAR instruction

Tracing the progress of these same students into high school, Linda Meyer (1984) found that their advantage over the comparison group in reading persisted into ninth grade. Even more impressive was the finding that 34 percent of the DISTAR students had applied and been accepted to college, whereas only 1 percent of the non-DISTAR comparison students applied and 17 percent of these students were accepted. Furthermore, the dropout rate for DISTAR students was almost half that for comparison subjects.

DISTAR is not without its detractors, however. A common criticism is that the scripted lessons place too much restriction on teachers. Becker (1977) counters this complaint with the argument that scripts increase teacher accountability and help supervisors track teacher and student progress. Elsa Bartlett (1979), in comparing DISTAR with the Open Court basal program, finds that DISTAR's modified orthography is particularly detrimental to disadvantaged children who find it difficult to make the transition to traditional orthography. Bartlett also maintains that DISTAR does not provide enough literacy enrichment. However, Isabel Beck and Ellen McCaslin (1978), in comparing eight reading programs on several dimensions, conclude that DISTAR is the best program for compensatory education.

Although DISTAR has been used with young elementary school children classified as learning-disabled, some of whom may be dyslexic, research has not yet systematically investigated the effectiveness of the Reading Mastery program with this group of children. A recent study compared New Jersey children classified as perceptually impaired (learning disabled) in DISTAR classes with those in basal classes. No significant differences were found after a year of remediation and after two years, for the small number of remaining children, there were very small differences limited to word attack skills (Kuder 1990). The generalizability of these results is questionable; IQ scores were not available and the receptive vocabulary scores of these disadvantaged children were well below the normal range. Several studies have attempted to validate the success of Corrective Reading, the Direct Instruction remedial program for older learning disabled students (see Chapter 19).

The implementation of the DISTAR model, as part of the federally funded Project Follow-Through may be unique, and entailed several elements worth noting for school-change policy making. The first important implementation feature, after the provision of funds, was the sponsorship of each Follow-Through program by the program developer, in DISTAR's case, the University of Oregon, and the assignment of a project manger to train the teachers and install each program. According to Linda Meyer, Russell Gersten, and Joan Gutkin (1983) who studied the implementation of DISTAR at P.S. 137 in New York City, the project manager spends up to forty days a year at the school, conducting inservice training and acting as coordinator between students, parents, faculty, and administration. The project manager is actively involved in setting up classroom schedules, monitoring teacher and student performance, and assigning students and staff. It would be helpful to know if having an external change agent serve as principal administrator rather then a local school official is relevant to the program's success.

An extremely important factor in the P.S. 137 program has been strong parental involvement and support from the start (Meyer, Gersten, and Gutkin 1983). In fact, parents were largely responsible for the school's selection as a Follow-Through site, as well as for the choice of the Direct Instruction Model. Despite budget cuts and high teacher turnover, parents in this school apparently fought successfully to keep the DISTAR program in place for more than thirteen years.

Meyer, Gersten, and Gutkin (1983) assert that one of the major strengths of the DISTAR model that has promoted its longevity is the continuity and consistency from preservice to inservice training sessions to continuous classroom observation and demonstration. They cite the Rand Study (Berman and McLaughlin 1975) finding that hands-on technical assistance to teachers is crucial for bringing about educational change.

19

Corrective Reading

BACKGROUND AND RATIONAL

Corrective Reading (Englemann et al. 1980) is an extension of Wesley Becker and Siegfried Englemann's Direct Instruction Model (DISTAR), developed for students in fourth grade through twelfth grades who have failed to achieve in other reading programs. Corrective Reading instruction is intended to compensate for a wide range of constitutional and environmental deficiencies that contribute to reading failure; these include mild mental retardation, neurological impairment, emotional disturbance, socioeconomic deprivation, and language and cultural differences, as well as dyslexia or learning disabilities. Like DISTAR, the program is designed for group administration and is intended as a core rather than a supplementary reading program; it has been used in both special and regular education settings.

CURRICULUM AND INSTRUCTION

The Corrective Reading curriculum is divided into two strands, Decoding and Comprehension, each having three levels of skill development, levels A, B, and C. Lessons are carefully arranged in sequence so that the skills taught are cumulative. Students are given a test covering both decoding and comprehension, to determine their placement in the program. Special lessons at each curriculum level serve as entry points. Students may be placed in one or both of the curriculum strands; if in both, they must be in the same or a lower comprehension than decoding level, because the sequence of reading vocabulary in the comprehension strand corresponds to that in the decoding program.

The objective of the decoding program, according to the Series Guide (Englemann et al. 1980), is "to teach the skills required to accurately and fluently identify and pronounce words that appear in written passages." It should be pointed out, however, that the decoding strand also deals with reading comprehension; students are asked comprehension questions about passages they read orally.

Placement level in the decoding strand is determined by a student's speed and accuracy in reading a passage orally. Students not meeting baseline criteria are referred for DISTAR I instruction. Students with only minimal reading skills are placed in Level A: Word Attack Basics, which contains sixty lessons. The major instructional goal at this level is to teach the idea that most words are regularly spelled and can be read by blending the letter sounds. Individual letter sounds are taught, first in isolation and then in words. Words are read first in isolation and then in unrelated sentences to avoid predictable context and discourage guessing, the latter strategy being the one most of these students have relied on unsuccessfully to compensate for their lack of letter-sound knowledge.

Only the most commonly used sound for each letter symbol is introduced at this level. This is the stated rationale for teaching the short sound for the vowel *a* and the long sound for the vowel *e* in Lesson 1. Not until Lesson 23 is the short *e* sound introduced; long *a* is not presented until Level B. The digraph *ee* is presented at the same time as the open syllable for long *e* (as in "me"). This practice represents the principle of instructional economy whereby strategies and rules are kept as simple as possible (Gersten, Woodward, and Darch 1986). For this reason, too, terms such as *vowels, double consonants,* or *final e words* are avoided. Practice in discriminating vowel sounds is provided by having students identify medial sounds in one-syllable words, as in, "Which word has the middle sound /aaaa/: *bean, ban, ben?*"

As in DISTAR, pronunciation of letters and words is practiced by first sounding them out slowly and then saying them fast. When irregular words are first introduced in Lesson 46, the distinction is made between how they are spelled and how they are said. Students first sound out the words, pronouncing and blending the individual letter sounds, for example "wwwaaasss" for *was*. Then the teacher gives the correct pronunciation (i.e., "wuz").

According to the program's authors, 60 to 80 percent of Corrective Reading students enter at Level B: Decoding Strategies, which comprises 140 lessons. The focus of the curriculum at this level is on long and short vowels, vowel-consonant digraphs, vowel digraphs, diphthongs, and common word endings. Long-short vowel confusion errors are referred to as *same vowel mistakes*, and teachers are given specific instructions for correcting these errors. Students are asked to note the presence or absence of a final e in the word missed which indicates the pronunciation of the preceding vowel. After pronouncing the word correctly, the students repeat the word. The teacher then writes the word as the students mistakenly pronounced it and has them read it. She changes it back to its correct spelling and asks the students to read it again. This model-test-discriminate-retest approach is used as a correcting procedure throughout the program. For correcting vowel confusion errors in words with endings (e.g, saying "robe" for *robber*), the teacher underlines the word from the beginning to the second letter after the vowel (<u>robb</u>er), and students are told, "If the last letter of the underlined part is *e* or *i*, you hear a letter name in the word" (Englemann et al. 1978). Phonic rules are not taught as spelling rules in Corrective Reading as they are in most remedial approaches. Although Level A includes spelling dictation exercises, the Corrective Reading curriculum includes little direct spelling instruction. Two types of word reading exercises are provided at Level B: similar list presentation, which emphasizes orthographic differences between words that share features (e.g., *hat, hate, hated*) and random list presentation of unrelated words which requires remembering specific features of words.

In addition to word attack exercises, Level B involves group story reading which uses a round-robin format, each student reading a sentence or two. Stories contain words introduced in the lessons. Oral reading errors are corrected on the spot, and the student is asked to reread the sentence. The teacher asks comprehension questions during the story reading, calling on individual students to answer. The questions not only ensure that all students are following the text, but also provide a story grammar framework for comprehending its contents, for example: Who is the story about? What does he or she want to do? What happens when he or she tries to do it? What happens in the end? According to Russell Gersten, John Woodward, and Craig Darch (1986), who are strong proponents of Corrective Reading, students begin to "internalize these four questions and generalize this framework to other narrative material." From Lesson 81 on, students are asked to write answers to additional comprehension questions after the story has been read.

Oral reading checks are conducted at the end of each lesson in Level B. Students read aloud individually the same 100-word passage from the story read in that lesson, as well as a second 100-word passage from the previous lesson. Selected peers may act as checkers, according to the program's authors, but most studies of Corrective Reading application report the use of teacher aides for this purpose. Every fifth lesson requires a timed reading check, so that a record of speed as well as accuracy can be kept for each student.

Lesson 108

WORD-ATTACK SKILLS

Individual turns
After presenting each of the following exercises
to the group, call on individual students.
Each student should read one word or more.
Present words that were difficult for the group.

EXERCISE 1   Sound combination: **oi**
1. Print in a column on the board: **oil, voice,
   spoil, hoist, foiled, moist, joined.**
   Underline as indicated.
2. Point to **oi** in **oil.**
   What sound? Touch. *oy*
   Point to **oil.**
   What word? Signal. *Oil.*
3. Repeat step 2 for **voice, spoil.**
4. For each remaining word:
   Point to the word. Pause. **What word?** Signal.
5. Repeat the list until firm.

EXERCISE 2   Endings buildups
1. Print on the board: **heat, splash, boil, clamp.**
2. For each word:
   Point to the word. Pause. **What word?** Signal.
3. Change the words to **heater, splasher, boiler,
   clamper.** Repeat step 2.
4. Change the words to **heats, splashes, boils,
   clamps.** Repeat step 2.
5. Change the words to **heated, splashed, boiled,
   clamped.** Repeat step 2.
6. Repeat steps 1–5 until firm.
7. Change the words to **heater, splashes, boils,
   clamped.** Repeat step 2.
8. Repeat the exercise until firm.

EXERCISE 3   Word practice
1. Print on the board: **batch, scare, recall,
   invisible, upstairs, couch, watched, stinky,
   mirror, cracked, shelf, chairs, else, easy,
   spun, basement, quickly, Herman, slowly, Fern,
   women.**
2. For each word:
   Point to the word. Pause. **What word?** Signal.
3. Repeat the list until firm.

EXERCISE 4   Word conversions
1. Print on the board the words that are not in
   brackets:

fell [feel]	**call [carl]**	**poach [pouch]**
boiling [bailing]	**tool [toil]**	**coach [crouch]**
coach [couch]	**malt [melt]**	**pond [pound]**
beet [belt]	**want [went]**	**clod [cloud]**

2. For each word:
   Point to the word. Pause. **What word?** Signal.
3. Change each word to the word in brackets
   next to it. Then repeat step 2.
4. Convert each word back to its original form.
   Repeat steps until firm.

EXERCISE 5   Word practice on worksheet
1. Pass out the worksheet for lesson 108.
2. **Point to the underlined part of the first
   word.** Check.
   What sound? Signal. *ar.*
   What word? Signal. *Lark.*
3. For each word with an underlined part:
   Next word. Check.
   What sound? Signal.
   What word? Signal.
4. For each word that does not have an underlined
   part:
   Next word. Check.
   What word? Signal.
5. Repeat each row of words until firm.

GROUP READING

EXERCISE 6   Story reading
1. **Everybody, touch the story.** Check.
2. **The error limit for this story is twelve.**
   If the group reads the story with twelve errors
   or less, you can earn up to 10 points.
3. Call on a student to read the title.
   What do you think this story is about?
4. Call on individual students to each read one
   or two sentences.
5. Ask the comprehension questions below during
   the story reading. The numbers in the story
   indicate at what point each question should
   be asked. Call on individual students to
   answer each question.
   1. **In what ways was Irma going to have fun**
      with the paint?
   2. **Where did Irma rub the paint?**
   3. **Where didn't Irma rub the paint?**
      How would her eyes have spoiled the
      trick?
      How did Irma make her eyes look invisible?
   4. **What is the only part of Irma that is not**
      invisible?
      What kind of hand is Irma going to give
      her boarders?
   5. **What are the boarders doing?**
      What is the woman on TV doing?
   6. **Why is Irma talking in a loud voice?**
   7. **What did Irma's boarders do when they**
      saw the hand?
6. Award points quickly.
7. If the group makes more than twelve errors,
   tell them they earn no points for the story
   reading. Then do one of the following:
   a. If time allows, repeat the story reading
      immediately. If the group now succeeds,
      complete the lesson (individual checkouts)
      and do the next lesson the following day.
   b. If there isn't time to repeat the story
      reading, tell the group they will have to
      repeat the story the following day.
8. Point to the written comprehension questions.
   Remember: write the answers to the questions
   while the others are being checked out.

CHECKOUTS

EXERCISE 7   Individual reading checkouts
1. Each student reads to the checker:
   a. A 100-word passage from story 108 as the
      first reading of this lesson.
   b. A 100-word passage from story 107 as the
      second reading.
   Those who make no errors on the first reading
   automatically receive 5 points credit for the
   second reading. They do not do a second reading.
2. Each student records points in box C of the
   point chart.

EXERCISE 8   Written questions checkout
1. Call on individual students to answer each
   question. Remind the students to mark each
   incorrect answer.
2. **Answer key: 1.** He wanted Irma to help move the
   couch. **2.** She rubbed paint on a pair of sun
   glasses. **3.** Her right hand **4.** "Uh, buh,
   duh, buh, buh, uh."
3. Remind the students to record the points they
   earned on their charts.

END OF LESSON 108

Teacher's Lesson Script from Corrective Reading Series Guide *by Siegfried Engelmann, Wesley C.
Becker, Susan Hanner, and Gary Johnson. (Reproduced with permission from Science Research Associates,
Inc., Chicago, IL. Copyright 1978.)*

Level C: Skills Applications comprises 140 lessons. This top level of the decoding strand continues instruction in word attack skills, reviewing previously introduced digraphs, diphthongs, less common phonemes and syllables, and teaching new ones. It introduces some of the more common affixes. Exercises for teaching these elements follow the formats used in the lower curriculum levels.

Preparing students to read textbook material is a major objective of the Level C: Decoding curriculum. More than 600 new vocabulary words are introduced, defined, and presented in text. The basis for selecting these words, however, is not explained; the selections seem to vary widely in frequency rating (e.g., *prevented* as compared to *prestidigitator*). An effort is made to expose students to "sentence types and conventions that characterize text material" (Englemann et al. 1980), such as the passive voice. Group story reading at this level requires answering both literal and inferential comprehension questions in writing. In addition, students read nonfiction information passages during individual oral reading checks. After lesson 70 they also read together magazine and newspaper articles on topics of their choice.

The program's authors maintain that students who complete Level C are "fluent decoders who make only occasional decoding errors when reading materials that contain a fairly broad vocabulary and a variety of sentence types" (Englemann et al. 1980). The authors believe that although students may still have comprehension deficits that limit their overall reading ability, their decoding problems at this point are essentially remediated.

Although reading is involved, Corrective Reading's comprehension strand is devoted primarily to the development of cognitive skills and language skills that relate to academic work. Level A, called Thinking Basics, is geared to students who lack essential concepts underlying school curriculum content, who may have a limited store of background information for processing school material, and may also manifest difficulty repeating orally presented information. Each lesson has three segments. The first, Thinking Operations, teaches the following concepts, which are relevant to content area material: analogies and/or basic evidence, classification, deductions, definitions, description, inductions, opposites, same, statement inference, and true-false. These are taught directly by the teacher to the group, through example and repetition. In the second lesson segment, students apply these concepts in workbook exercises. In the third, the Information track, they are taught calendar facts (months, seasons, holidays) and biology facts (animals and their classifications); additionally, they learn to recite short poems.

While somewhat more advanced than Level A students, those entering Level B: Comprehension Skills may still lack basic information, such as calendar facts. The major thrust at this level is "to teach and reinforce a substantial amount of information and many operations" (Englemann et al. 1980). Areas covered in this curriculum include: Reasoning Skills (deductions, basic evidence, analogies, contradictions, and similes); Information Skills (classification, body systems, body rules, and economic rules); Vocabulary Skills (definition); Sentence Skills (parts of speech, subject/predicate, sentence combinations, and sentence analysis); Comprehension Skills (inference and following directions); and Writing Skills (writing directions, editing, writing paragraphs, and writing stories). Each lesson involves group oral work, oral workbook exercises, and independent workbook exercises. Students check each others' answers to these exercises.

At Level C: Concept Applications, the instructional emphasis is on teaching students to apply independently the skills they have learned. Five categories of application skills are taught in this curriculum: Organizing Information (main idea, outlining, specific-general, morals, and visual-spatial information); Operating On Information (deductions, basic evidence, argument rules, ought statements, and contradictions); Using Sources of Information (basic comprehension passages, words or deductions, maps, pictures and graphs, and supporting evidence); Communicating Information (definitions, combining sentences, editing, and getting meaning from context); and Using Information (writing directions, filling out forms, and identifying contradictory directions). The first two operational categories are classified as *higher-order skills* and the last three as *basic tools*. A major change in instructional procedure takes place at Level C—rather than the teacher's presenting scripted lessons, students read the lesson scripts in their workbooks. The teacher monitors their processing of the workbook exercises, asking questions to ensure understanding. Increasing demands are placed on writing performances at this level.

All Corrective Reading lessons are designed to be administered daily in 35-40 minute periods, although several effectiveness studies report somewhat longer periods and often more than one period per day. A lesson is designed to be covered within a single period but may be repeated if mastery is not attained by all students in the class. Individual mastery checks, as well as the monitoring of group responses, provide ongoing information on student performance and allow for repetition or acceleration of lessons if needed.

A point system serves as a behavior management device at all curriculum levels. Students are awarded points for successful performance in both group and individual activities throughout the Corrective Reading curriculum; a point schedule is provided for each lesson. In group activities, all students must meet performance criteria in order for any points to be awarded. Bonus points may be given for success or persistence on especially difficult activities or to encourage positive behaviors, such as being on time for lessons. Students keep records of points earned. Weekly summaries of accumulated points are intended to provide positive feedback to further reinforce student learning.

Behavior management also entails having each student who enters the program sign a contract indicating his or her willingness to cooperate and work hard. The teacher explains the point system, the need for daily class attendance, and the penalty for making negative comments about peers. The penalty for making fun of another student is paid by the group as a whole to further discourage this detrimental behavior.

As in DISTAR, the hallmark of Corrective Reading is its unique approach to direct group instruction. All lessons are scripted, teachers are told exactly what to say and do. All student exercises are presented in formats; similar activities follow the same formats, which simplifies the teacher's task and serves as a prompt for students to apply a learned skill to new examples. Correction procedures, both general and specific, are carefully spelled out for all activities. Hand signals are used by teachers to direct student response in unison. These allow for fast paced instruction, which is believed to help sustain student attention, increase student achievement, and reduce auditory memory demands on students. The signals include: the hand-drop, which indicates that students should respond in unison in naming items pointed to on the chalkboard or in their workbooks; the audible signal (clapping, finger snapping, foot tapping) to redirect student attention; the sound-out signal (the teacher runs her finger along a line under the letter or word to be pronounced), which controls the pace of blending letter sounds; and the sequential-response signal (the teacher holds up one finger to call for a first response and then two fingers to signal a second response), as when students are asked to name two important facts in a story.

The materials used in Corrective Reading Instruction include: the Series Guide which provides an overview of the entire program; a teacher's manual for each level of a curriculum strand, which provides a curriculum guide for that level and the presentation scripts for each lesson; a student workbook which contains stories to be read and/or exercises to be carried out; and, at Level C, a student textbook which contains the lesson scripts to be read by the students themselves.

TEACHER TRAINING

Teacher preparation for Corrective Reading has not been formalized as in some other remedial programs and may vary with schools and school districts, depending upon their requirements and their budgets. However, training can be arranged through The Association for Direct Instruction (see Resource and Teacher Training Guide in Appendix). On the East Coast it is provided by the Center for Direct Instruction which is based in New York City. This training is usually conducted in one six-hour session, most often in a school, though sometimes in university-sponsored workshops offering graduate credit. Follow-up on-site supervision in classrooms or further consultation to schools is available for an additional fee.

Reporting on the implementation of Corrective Reading with learning disabled and mildly retarded adolescents in a rural/suburban school district, Edward Polloway and Michael Epstein (1986) indicate that teacher preparation involved two full days of in-service training. The first session provided an overview of the program and the instructional methodology, as well as information about placement testing, grouping, and scheduling. The second session focused specifically on teaching techniques. However, even with two training sessions, considerable variability in teacher competence was noted during program implementation.

Epstein and Cullinan (1981) employed teacher aides in their implementation of Corrective Reading. The aides were trained directly in the classroom and received weekly follow-up supervision alongside the classroom teachers. Cynthia Herr (1984) has found teacher aides to be extremely useful for monitoring oral reading checks and supervising work with adult students in Corrective Reading.

EVALUATION AND IMPLEMENTATION

Studies have investigated the use of Corrective Reading with students having a range of mild handicapping conditions, as well as with students for whom English is a second language (Polloway and Epstein 1986). Several of these adults have examined the program's effectiveness with students classified as learning disabled. Polloway and Epstein (1986), for example, measured the effectiveness of Corrective Reading with a mixed group of students who were educable mentally retarded (EMR) and learning disabled (LD) in grades 6-12, by comparing reading gains achieved over a year of Corrective Reading instruction to gains made in the previous year of special education instruction. Using the Peabody Individual Achievement Test (PIAT), they found significantly greater gains after Corrective Reading instruction than in the previous year for subjects who were EMR as well as LD in both word recognition and reading comprehension. Although the subjects with LD had greater gains than the subjects with EMR on word recognition scores, no significant differences were found in reading comprehension gain scores between the two subject types. However, Polloway and Epstein suggest that the latter finding may be due to the failure of the PIAT to tap the comprehension skills taught in Corrective Reading. In support of this suggestion, they cite teachers' claims that the PIAT underestimates student achievement in this area.

Epstein and Cullinan (1981) investigated the effects of a federally funded model implementation of Corrective Reading with nine-year-old students classified as learning disabled. (It is worth noting that their Slosson IQ scores ranged only from 76 to 86.) Subjects were randomly assigned to self-contained classrooms, two of which used Corrective Reading. The other classroom used unspecified remedial procedures and served as the control condition. At the end of one school year, reading scores (posttest only) were higher for both groups receiving Corrective Reading than the comparison group. However, John Lloyd along with Epstein and Cullinan, in reporting on the same study, acknowledge that neither of the experimental groups reached normal reading achievement levels in that year and suggest that more instructional time is needed to reach such a goal (Lloyd, Epstein, and Cullinan 1981). It should also be mentioned that the number of subjects in each group was low (seven to eight), as was the case in the Polloway and Epstein study (four to eight). Though optimal for instructional purposes, such small samples weaken the validity of the outcome analyses.

In terms of program implementation, Epstein and Cullinan (1981) maintain that although the planning, training, and evaluation costs of Corrective Reading are considerably higher than the cost of most basal reading programs, the expense is on par with that of other learning disability programs. A greater challenge, but one worth meeting they believe, is convincing school personnel of the need for carefully supervised, highly structured, task-oriented direct instruction with learning disabled children.

20

Project READ (Calfee)

BACKGROUND AND RATIONALE

Project READ was developed by Robert Calfee and his associates at Stanford University, in collaboration with an elementary school in the Palo Alto area of California. It is a metacognitive approach to both decoding and comprehension and includes highly explicit instruction. While developed for regular classroom use rather than for children with reading problems, its explicit nature makes it an instructional possibility for children with dyslexia.

Project READ was initiated in 1981 with an assessment of curriculum needs carried out through teacher workshops. This led to the creation of a teacher's manual, THE BOOK: *Components of Reading Instruction* (Calfee and Associates 1981-1984) which serves as the curriculum guide for Project READ. The Program serves as the primary literacy component of Stanford's Accelerated Schools program and is used in more than thirty schools in California, as well as Project READ sites in other places (e.g., Chicago, New York, Pittsburgh, and Omaha).

In a 1989 description of READ distributed by Calfee Projects at Stanford, the central goal is stated as, "competence in applying language as a tool for thinking and for communication." Calfee and his colleague Marcia Henry maintain that the subject matter and materials in most schools are fragmented, and that the teachers are not provided with a conceptual framework for teaching. Project READ seeks to remedy these deficiencies by providing a "parsimonious and coherent theoretical framework for representing the various elements that comprise a reading program" (Calfee and Henry 1985).

Calfee and Henry (1985) distinguish two kinds of learning: *learning-by-doing* which is experiential and incremental, and the more formal, school-based *learning-by-knowing*. Stressing the need to teach children how to learn by knowing, the authors state:

> A major goal of schooling is to transmit to the student the most significant facets of our cultural heritage, knowing that it is most efficiently transferred through learning-by-knowing. In addition, the school teaches the student how to acquire knowledge in this fashion (learning to learn, if you will, of a special variety) (Calfee and Henry 1985, p. 145).

THE BOOK emphasizes four instructional propositions, the first being *simplicity*; complex tasks should be broken down into a "small number of relatively coherent subtasks." The second is that language skills (reading, writing, speaking, and even listening) are *interrelated* and should be taught as such. The third is that teaching the *formal use of language* is one of the most important goals of schooling. The fourth proposition is that *direct teaching*, combined with *small group discussion*, is an essential component of effective reading instruction.

Although READ was originally developed for children in regular elementary classrooms, its structures and strategies have been used successfully with a wide range of populations including those who are at risk for reading failure (Calfee, personal communication, May 5, 1994). See the discussion of Project READ with children who are dyslexic at the end of this chapter.

CURRICULUM AND INSTRUCTION

The basic curriculum components of Project READ are: 1) decoding, 2) vocabulary, 3) comprehension of narrative text, and 4) comprehension of expository text. Critical to the program's philosophy of coherence and parsimony is the fact that any lesson should focus on only one of these curriculum areas at a time. The program was designed to be adapted to any basal reading series, and recent use with literature-based curriculum is said to work equally well.

The original instructional format for lessons had four fairly conventional parts: 1) the *opening* with an introduction and stated lesson goal, 2) the *middle activity* which includes discussion, question asking, problem solving, summarizing, and recording results, 3) the *closing*, with a review of what was accomplished in the lesson, and 4) *follow-up activities* which incorporate practice and reinforcement of the new skills. This format was revised during the late 1980s. The new format is called CORE, which stands for Connect, Organize, Reflect, and Extend. The objective for this new format was to produce a constructivist learning environment. Calfee feels that the old format can also be useful. Teachers are urged to develop a script for each lesson that they teach.

Decoding skills are organized around a traditional sequence of letter sounds with short vowels first, followed by long vowels, vowel digraphs, and then polysyllabic words. Common sight words, called *weirdo words*, are taught early in the program. Spelling is taught together with reading.

One notable feature of the decoding curriculum is the attention given to etymology in instruction for children in the third grade and above. This portion of the program was developed by Marcia Henry and is called the *Words* program. In teaching word attack strategies, a major distinction is made between words of Anglo-Saxon and Romance origins. Anglo-Saxon words are taught first; these are short words, often with short vowels, but they tend to include many digraphs that are needed to code the Anglo-Saxon sounds, which are more numerous than our 26 letter alphabet. Words with a Romance origin are taught later; they tend to be longer and to have sounds such as the schwa that are in unaccented syllables and thus harder to read and spell. Words with Greek roots tend to be used in technical vocabulary and are taught to older children (Calfee and Henry in press; Henry 1988,). Henry's materials are available as a guide called *Words* and a series of tutoring books and student word lists based on word origins and structure (Henry 1990; Henry and Redding 1990).

A recent innovation is a downward extension of Henry's Words program for younger students. The new *Metaphonics* program was designed for use in kindergarten and first-grade classrooms but is currently being used in second- and third-grade classrooms as well. It includes eight blocks of instruction, beginning with teacher assessment of phonological awareness and phonics knowledge, and progressing through instruction in phonological awareness that stresses articulation and manipulation of phonemes, followed by letter sound associations for short *a* and five consonants, and on through a fairly conventional Gillingham-like sequence. The distinguishing characteristic of *Metaphonics*, as with much of Calfee's READ, is the emphasis on teacher-student discussion rather than rote learning (Henry, personal communication, September, 1994).

Metaphonics was developed in California where whole language instruction is prevalent. Henry notes the popularity of the *Metaphonics* cirriculum with teachers who use it in Salinas, California with Chapter 1 and inclusion students, as well as with regular education students. These teachers are provided with two days of training before school opens and then an additional three hours of inservice training each month during the school year. Research is being conducted but the results are not yet available.

Vocabulary, in Project READ, is always taught using a conceptual framework rather than through memorization. Calfee has incorporated two innovative instructional techniques that he refers to as *webbing* and *weaving*. Webbing involves teaching each new word within a set of words that are semantically related, as opposed to presenting them in unrelated word lists. In the webbing script the teacher selects a target word or concept and tells the students to generate related words. These words are then arranged by the class into categories, and a webbing diagram is drawn up. See the script provided here.

The weaving script begins with a group of words, selected by the teacher, that are discussed by the class and organized as conceptual

---

```
SCRIPT:   Webbing

                        AIM:  To make students aware of how words are related
    STUDENTS' PREREQUISITES:  Knowledge of basic meanings of target words
     TEACHER'S PREPARATION:   Select target word
                              Choose categories for web
```

OPENING

> Today we're going to study about how words are related so we can get a better understanding of what a word means.
>
> (Explain the concept of a web)
>
> Today we're going to work with the word _____

MODAL
MIDDLE ACTIVITY

    FREE GENERATION

> What are some of the things the word _____ (write on board) makes you think of?
>
> Let's go around the room, each of you tell me what you think of when you hear _____. Let's see if everyone can give a different answer.
>
> I'll write on the board what you say, and we'll try to organize your answers.
>
> (Write responses in a webbing plan as illustrated in Blackboard Examples . . . then:)

    Categorization

> Look how the words are arranged.
>
> Why do you think I put certain words together?
> Why are . . . (e.g., fur, black nose, pointed ears together?)
> Why are . . . (e.g., bark, bite, run together?)
>
> Can you think of any other words to add to the web?

CLOSING

> What have we learned about the word _____?
>
> What are some of the categories we used to organize our web?
>
> Why did we put certain words in the same category?
>
> How did webbing help us understand word meanings?

```
THE BOOK
Calfee/Stanford  81/83a                                      Vocabulary
```

Teacher's Lesson Script from THE BOOK *by Robert Calfee and Associates, 1981-1984, School of Education, Stanford University, Palo Alto, CA. (Reproduced with permission from the author.)*

structures, either hierarchical semantic networks or matrixes. Numerous activities can be used in the weaving script such as finding evidence, making comparisons, and hypothesizing relationships. Calfee suggests that a weaving lesson can provide preparation for writing.

Building morphological knowledge is an important aspect of effective vocabulary instruction, particularly at the secondary level, according to Calfee. He advocates teaching recognition and meaning of morphological elements by first presenting concrete examples and only later introducing the rules. This places responsibility on teachers to acquire more than the rudimentary linguistic knowledge provided in most teacher preparation programs.

Comprehension instruction begins at the text level; there is no mention in THE BOOK of syntax or grammar, and there are no directions for teaching comprehension at the sentence level. Calfee makes a major distinction between narrative and expository text. Narrative comprehension is taught first. Students are taught to recognize the elements of story structure (e.g., characters, setting, sequence of events, and main theme) through activities such as graphing the action or making outlines of the episodes.

Calfee points out that most children come to school with a basic knowledge of story structure and that beginning literacy materials almost always involve narrative structures. In contrast, they receive little exposure to exposition in these grades and they are rarely provided with knowledge of expository structure. THE BOOK provides a classification of expository styles, focusing on two basic categories — description and sequence. Suggested teaching activities include discussing the structure and purpose of the text, making outlines, locating and labeling topic sentences, and diagramming.

Project READ teaches test-taking strategies as well. Instruction in this area also involves the use of scripts and provides a conceptual framework by incorporating webbing activities into the scripts.

TEACHER TRAINING

Training for Project READ teachers involves a three-day summer institute. There are four major objectives: 1) to familiarize teachers with READ's theoretical foundations, 2) to enable teachers to evaluate reading instructional materials from the basal reader series or literature-based programs used in their schools in terms of this framework, 3) to demonstrate the use of instructional scripts, and 4) to demonstrate small group problem solving as an instructional approach. A recent innovation in the summer institute involves assigning teachers to work with a team to develop a thematic project. Calfee reports that this has been quite successful for helping these teachers integrate the components of the READ model in practical form.

In the fall, following the workshop, staff members visit the target schools to demonstrate sample scripts and to help teachers apply the project's principles. The newly trained teachers are observed as they try out scripts in their classrooms. For additional support, two or three day-long follow-up sessions are held in each school for progress evaluation and further instruction as needed. All Project READ teachers are interviewed at the end of the school year to determine their overall impressions of the program and their success in implementing the program's philosophy. Monthly newsletters are circulated to provide up-to-date information on program development.

EVALUATION AND IMPLEMENTATION

Early research on Project READ was carried out in 12 California schools. Scores in these schools increased by one half to one full grade level equivalent (Calfee, Henry, and Funderberg 1988). The authors claim that the quantity and quality of student writing was also enhanced.

Informal evaluation procedures, based on observation and interviews, indicate improvement in teacher attitudes, morale, and self confidence, as well as teacher competence. In addition, teachers report a closer professional relationship with other faculty members (Calfee and Henry 1985). Parents and students are generally enthusiastic about the program. The most difficult skill for teachers to learn, apparently, is the development of scripts. Additional preparation time and ongoing support were deemed necessary for developing scripts in the first year that a new Project READ teacher used the program.

From these initial evaluations, Calfee and his associates drew several conclusions concerning the implementation of educational change in schools. Their first tenet is that any change must be initiated and sustained at the local school level (Calfee, Henry, and Funderberg 1988). A second premise, which has extensive empirical backing, is that the school principal must assume a strong leadership role. Before working with a school, Calfee and his colleagues make sure that they can count on the principal's support and even insist that the principal participate in the training program. Another condition, which they consider essential for effective reading instruction, is the creation of a common conceptual framework for this instruction. Too often, they maintain, new programs focus on only a single aspect of reading, which further fragments the existing curriculum. Consistent with the idea of school-wide involvement in change, Calfee has recently begun to think in terms of READ acting as a catalyst for change within a professional community.

In the first edition of this book Diana Clark raised the question of whether or not the instruction provided in Project READ was either appropriate or adequate for students with dyslexia. She pointed out that although the program's conceptual framework might have value for teachers working with reading-disabled students, these students might require a greater degree of explicit instruction in decoding than was offered by the program at that time (Clark 1988). Since then Marcia Henry has carried out research suggesting that late elementary age children instructed in Project READ did better than controls taught in regular basal classrooms on measures of phonological and morphological knowledge as well as reading and spelling (Henry 1989). In addition, *Metaphonics*, the downward extension of the phonics component of Project READ, is a promising early intervention program providing a highly structured introduction to reading through phonological awareness and phonics instruction.

21

Writing to Read

Writing to Read, recently updated as Writing to Read 2000, was designed as a beginning reading program for children in the educational mainstream rather than as a remedial program for children with dyslexia. It is described in this book because it embodies many of the instructional principles important for remediation of dyslexia. These include an emphasis on teaching letter-sound correspondences and mastery of the alphabetic principle, the built-in promotion of phonological awareness, the incorporation of multisensory activities, and the opportunity for extensive practice and overlearning. Furthermore, two additional aspects of the program may have potential for children with dyslexia: 1) a systematic method for teaching beginning reading through writing, and 2) the innovative application of computer technology for teaching these skills.

BACKGROUND AND RATIONALE

Writing to Read was created by John Henry Martin, a retired school superintendent with thirty-five years of experience as an educator. The program was developed in cooperation with International Business Machines Corporation (IBM) and piloted over a five-year period with nearly 1000 children. It was subjected to nationwide evaluation from 1981 to 1984 with over 10,000 children in 105 schools within 22 school districts in metropolitan, suburban, and rural settings.

The rationale for Writing to Read was derived from the theories of Maria Montessori (1964), Carol Chomsky (1979), and other educators who have proposed that young children learn to read words that they themselves have composed more easily than words written by someone else (see Chapter 12, The Writing-Reading Relationship). In their book, *Writing to Read*, which describes the program, Martin and his co-author Ardy Friedberg, state that most normal children enter school knowing more than 2,000 words that they are able to combine in syntax "nearly as complex as that used by adults" (Martin and Friedberg 1986). It is assumed that these children can readily apply this knowledge to writing the letter sounds of English in words, sentences, and stories, which will lead them to grasp the alphabetic principle in a very short time. Writing to Read, according to Martin, teaches the alphabetic principle and phonemic spelling while utilizing the educational potential of the computer in combination with multisensory stimulation.

CURRICULUM AND INSTRUCTION

Writing to Read, and its recently updated version, Writing to Read 2000, were designed as a beginning reading program for children in grades K-1 and can be used with children who are nonreaders in grades 2-4. Originally intended to be set up in a center or special laboratory supervised by a specialist teacher and an assistant with classes visiting for an hour at a time, it can also be set up in the regular classroom and integrated into the school day in a less formal manner. The method uses cooperative learning, small group instruction, and classroom learning centers.

Despite the image of IBM's Writing to Read as a computer-based instructional program, the computer is only one of six *work stations* or centers: 1) the Computer center, 2) the Writing/Typing center, 3) the Activity center, 4) the Work Journal center, 5) the Make Words center, and 6) the Tape Library center. Instruction involves rotation through the different centers.

Pairs of students work at the Computer center where ten cycles or units of three words each are taught. Forty-two phonemes are introduced sound-by-sound within the context of these 30 words. Directions are presented to students via audio cassettes. A lesson begins with a picture (e.g., a cat) appearing on the screen. A voice on the cassette says the word aloud and asks the student to repeat it while the letters c-a-t flash on the screen. Then the voice introduces the sound of the initial phoneme /c/ and asks the student to say /c/ and then to type the correct letter with the original flashing model still present. As each letter is typed it is positioned in the student's version of the word that appears in the center of the screen. Errors are not accepted, thus encouraging self-correction. At the next step this procedure is repeated without the presence of the flashing model on the screen. Finally, the student is asked to say each letter sound in rhythm while clapping out the three phonemes in, for example, the word *cat*. This exercise is repeated for each of the three words in a cycle before the student takes a mastery test that involves spelling the three words. Depending on how successful these spellings are, the student either repeats this cycle of exercises or moves on to three new words in the next cycle.

Innovations introduced to the Computer center in Writing to Read 2000 include the use of stories in rhyming text so that the new cycle words can be seen in context. For example the nursery rhyme, "Hey Diddle Diddle" is used as part of the cycle including the words *cat, dog,* and *fish,* all of which occur in the rhyme. The cycle words are highlighted for emphasis in the rhyme. The rhymes provide both contextualized reading, and extra opportunities to view the cycle words, which helps students commit the new words to memory. During the introduction of the word *cat* in the initial exercise and its use in the rhyme, there are 31 iterations of this word.

Another innovation in Writing to Read 2000 is the option of skipping some of the exercise units in the computer programs. For example, a teacher can choose to skip over several *cat* exercises for a child who has learned this word before the end of the cycle. The content of the original Writing to Read remains the same so that some portions can be updated by a school while retaining the original computer center. System requirements for running Writing to Read and information about upgrades are available from IBM's EduQuest 800 number listed in the resource guide at the end of this book.

Most of the creative work done by students in the program is carried out at the Writing/Typing center. Martin determined that children are particularly enthusiastic about keyboarding because it renders perfect reproductions of the words they wish to write and obviates the labor of penmanship. Children use either an IBM Selectric typewriter, or in the newer Writing to Read 2000, the IBM Primary Editor Plus word processor. Children are encouraged to type words and then sentences and stories. At every stage they are encouraged to edit their work. Students using the Primary Editor Plus can use text-to-speech read back and a spell check to help in the editing process. Student files can be saved and teacher management features include controlled use of the spell check and an option for either enabling or disabling the voice on the text-to-speech read back.

At the Make Words center, materials such as plastic letters are available for assembling into words. Many of these materials are self-correcting so that a picture cue triggers the spelling of a word that cannot be assembled without the correct spelling. These activities and materials have been completely revised in the new Writing to Read 2000 version.

At the Activity center, hand-formed letters are practiced using tactile materials . For example, clay is available for shaping letters or letters can be traced in sand before they are written using soft lead pencils. Martin stresses the multisensory aspect of these activities.

At the Work Journal center, students again follow directions on an audiotape. Here a worksheet format is used to practice writing by hand the cycle words learned on the computer. There is also an opportunity to work with the rhyming text again at the Work Journal center. Conventional orthography is stressed on the worksheets as well as letter-sound relationships. For example, silent *e* is included in correctly spelled words on the worksheets, but in a *dimmed* or lightly printed form to indicate that silent *e* should be used in spelling but that it cannot be heard in a word. This center also includes opportunities to write stories by hand in journals.

In the Tapes Library center there are 23 trade books available for reading or for listening using ear phones and an audio cassette. Children are encouraged to follow along in the book as they listen to cassettes. Children's literature has been selected for this center based on the occurrence of the cycle words, providing another opportunity to read or listen to the words in context following the initial introduction through use of the computer exercises. For example, the story *Julius Pig* is used following the introduction of the cycle word *pig* on the computer.

Martin has also developed a readiness program for four year olds to prepare them for the Writing to Read curriculum. This program, called *Get Set for Writing to Read*, uses the computer to teach alphabet and basic segmentation skills. The alphabet is first introduced in an activity that involves listening to an audio cassette of the Alphabet Song while using an alphabet board to locate letters. Next children listen to nursery rhymes and folk songs focusing on specific letter sounds, and follow along in Verse and Rhyme Books. Target letters are emphasized in bold-face type. Children then move to the computer, first working on the Computer Alphabet Program which introduces both uppercase and lowercase letters along with animation and voice synthesizer. Later they use the Syllable and Segment program which illustrates the concept that many words share the same sounds and letter combinations. The program is intended to span an eighteen-week period, at the end of which, according to Martin, children have learned a significant number of basic skills and concepts. These include: visual discrimination, letter recognition, uppercase and lowercase letter names, fine motor skills, eye-hand coordination, keyboard familiarity, auditory memory, auditory sequencing, the concept that letters make words, and the concept that words contain segments or syllables that are repeated in other words.

TEACHER TRAINING

IBM initially offered a three-day leadership training workshop on Writing to Read after which newly trained teachers returned to their schools to conduct on-site in-service workshops for other school faculty desiring training. Currently, IBM provides an initial Writing to Read 2000 training session on-site, with a follow-up visit in 90 days. Training is provided by former teachers and is customized through contracts designed to fit the specific needs of individual schools. Unlike some of the remedial programs described in this book, training in Writing to Read is not strictly controlled; there is no certification requirement that must be met before using the curriculum.

EVALUATION AND IMPLEMENTATION

Writing to Read has been used by over 6 million students in more than 11,000 schools. The original nationwide evaluation study of Writing to Read was carried out by the Educational Testing Service (ETS) (Murphy and Appel 1984). In the second year of the program (1983-1984) a core sample of 3,210 children in randomly selected schools within the participating districts was compared with a control group of 2,379 children in schools not using Writing to Read. Pre- and posttest scores on standardized reading tests were compared across groups for both kindergarten and first-grade students. Schools were allowed to make their own test selections from among five widely accepted nationally normed instruments. Spelling achievement was measured using a list of ten dictated words. Writing samples on a specified topic were collected from kindergarten and first-grade children, and from first-grade children who had received Writing to Read instruction in kindergarten but not in first grade. These writing samples were scored qualitatively by trained teachers and compared with writing samples from control students.

Analysis of the data in the ETS study is complicated and the findings are difficult to interpret. In summarizing the major conclusions, however, Murphy and Appel (1984) affirm that the program functions well as a system, that children are able to handle the technology and had no difficulty adjusting to the rotational format of the work stations in the learning laboratory. The evaluators also maintain that Writing to Read students in kindergarten and first grade progressed faster than comparison students in reading, that they learned to write better, and that they spelled as well as comparison students despite the lack of direct instruction in spelling. Parents, as well as teachers, apparently responded favorably to Writing to Read.

Martin (1985) acknowledges that formative evaluation studies of his program revealed that 3 to 5 percent of the children did not respond to instruction. At the same time, he contends that no incidence of dyslexia or severe reading disability was found among Writing to Read students. This claim, however, may be founded less on fact than on Martin's understanding of dyslexia, which he defined as "the reversal or jumbling of letters and words in speech and writing which impairs the ability to read and to learn" (Martin and Friedberg 1986). Martin suggests that rather than dyslexia, "severe retardation in language development," as manifested by a vocabulary of less than 200 words, may have been the cause of failure in many of these children. Because children with dyslexia are so rarely diagnosed as early as kindergarten or early first grade, it remains to be established, therefore, whether or not Writing to Read is effective with children who are dyslexic.

Writing to Read is used in several New York City special education settings with poor urban children who are at risk for reading difficulty. In one of these Writing to Read laboratories, the teacher commented during an observation by Diana Clark that the program moved too quickly for most of these children. For example, all five short vowels are introduced in the first two cycles of the ten cycle program, whereas ordinarily all of the short vowels are not introduced this quickly or this early in kindergarten. This teacher also commented that the sequence of the program seemed arbitrary rather than linguistically based. This teacher was very enthusiastic about the program's introduction of the writing process early in kindergarten. She commented that this demanded a lot of teacher involvement and that she considered this to be a positive aspect of the program. Keep in mind that these poor urban children do not fit the current description of children specifically at risk for dyslexia (see Chapter 2), but these comments are included because they seem applicable to all children at risk for reading difficulty.

Based on serving 120 students a day, IBM's estimated cost in 1988 for installing Writing to Read in a school, starting with an empty room, ranged from $15,000 to $18,000, with the cost per student over a five year period estimated as $25 (Clark 1988). This kind of estimate per student is no longer possible because the range of choices in equipment is so wide. Most schools today already own some computers and the possible configurations available from IBM are almost endless, ranging from new software to be used with existing computers in classrooms to fully equipped Writing to Read laboratories.

22

Reading Recovery

BACKGROUND AND RATIONALE

Reading Recovery was first developed by Marie Clay in New Zealand during the mid 1970s. It was conceived as an early intervention program for the lowest achieving children at time of entry into what is called first grade in the United States, and was closely linked, both philosophically and systemically, with New Zealand's national reading scheme. After a year of a kindergarten program that focuses on early literacy skills, children are screened individually by their teachers and approximately the lowest 20 percent are selected for Reading Recovery intervention at the beginning of first grade. This involves reading in a one-to-one setting for half an hour a day with a master teacher who has received a year of additional training in Reading Recovery methods. The aim is to provide help before reading failure is established, and then to discontinue this special help and to return these children to their regular classroom reading groups as quickly as possible, with 12 weeks as the goal. Children who have not returned to their regular classroom after 20 weeks are usually referred for a more intensive kind of help and represent roughly one percent of all of the children in a particular grade.

During the 1984-1985 school year Marie Clay and her New Zealand colleague, Barbara Watson, together with a group headed by Gay Sue Pinnell at Ohio State University, brought Reading Recovery to the Columbus, Ohio public schools. Ohio schools have played a leadership role in the American whole language movement, which is philosophically linked to the New Zealand national reading scheme in some (but not all) characteristics, and thus Ohio provided a receptive site for this program. State funding was available for the project very early, and by 1987 it had been selected for federal funding as part of the U.S. Department of Education's National Diffusion Network. By 1993 there were Reading Recovery training sites in 44 states (Lyons, Pinnell, and DeFord 1993).

Reading Recovery views reading as the act of constructing meaning. While this is a sensible view, the emphasis on meaning can be provocative to some advocates of phonics instruction who see children with dyslexia as already over-relying on meaning and needing direct instruction in phonics. However, Reading Recovery is a highly complex early intervention system involving structural changes in a school as well as training in the particulars of the teaching method. It assumes a philosophical stance in which children are provided with strategies for self-monitoring with the thought that training will be discontinued once they have internalized these strategies and are reading at the level of their classroom's middle reading group. Marie Clay talks at length about inner controls; one of her books is titled *Becoming Literate: the Construction of Inner Control* (1991). The rhetoric will sound familiar to those of us who remember the late 1960s and its emphasis on the child as learner, except that there is great rigor to the Reading Recovery teacher training and to the expectations placed on the child as an independent learner.

CURRICULUM AND INSTRUCTION

Reading Recovery tutoring involves an entry phase for observing what the child already knows, prior to implementation of the teaching program. During this *roaming around the known* phase the teacher works daily to build the child's confidence in strategies that are already in place, and observes carefully in order to plan instruction based on the child's strengths.

After this two week period, instruction begins. Each half hour lesson is structured around four steps: 1) re-reading familiar books, 2) re-reading the most recent book with a *running record* of observed strategies and miscues jotted down by the teacher, 3) a letter-oriented lesson based on a pattern observed to be difficult for the student during the previous day's new book, 4) a writing lesson based on this book, and finally, 5) introduction of a new book.

There is no standard sequence of reading materials in Reading Recovery and this represents a radical difference between Reading Recovery and other programs described in this book. The reading materials are small readers called *little books*, each with a complete story, profusely illustrated in color, and with short, repetitive, predictable text.

The 700 books used by Reading Recovery are organized into a sequence of 20 increasingly more difficult beginning reading levels, but within each level books are read in different orders by different children. No child is expected to read every book or to reach a specific level before being discontinued from Reading Recovery lessons.

Ideally, similar books are used in the classroom as well. According to Trika Smith-Burke, of New York University, Reading Recovery has been used in schools using other classroom reading schemes. For example, the Ginn Readers were used in classrooms in the early days of Reading Recovery in Ohio, and phonetically based texts are used in classrooms in the Greenwich, Connecticut public schools, which use both Reading Recovery and Enfield and Green's Project Read. Smith-Burke feels that the optimal situation involves consistency between the classroom and Reading Recovery in regard to both books and teaching philosophy.

A new book is introduced at the end of a lesson and then reread during the next lesson. Before a child reads a new book, the tutor invites the child to make sense of the story from the title and pictures, and in this conversation the tutor uses words that the child will be reading. Once the child begins to read, the teacher steps back, encouraging the child to practice strategies for figuring out new words independently. Both letter cues and context cues are encouraged. When the teacher does help, he or she directs the child's attention in a way that encourages successful problem solving rather than simply providing the answer. The child is encouraged to *cross-check* to see that information from different sources is in agreement (e.g., "If the word is *meanies,* what letter would you expect to see at the beginning?").

During the two Reading Recovery tutoring lessons observed within a training session at New York University during the summer of 1994, the child, in each case, began by choosing two books that were old favorites to read aloud. Then the child was asked to read the new book from the last lesson. During this reading the tutor kept a running record of those strategies and letter patterns that were mastered as well as those that needed work. The scheme for observing a child's reading strategies is highly elaborated in both the Reading Recovery literature (Clay 1993a, 1993b) and during training. Observational records provide information to be used in making decisions about instruction. Unlike the traditional error analysis, running records involve observations of effective strategies as well as miscues. Help from the tutor during oral reading tended to involve encouraging the child to try a particular strategy, and this occurred only after the child had tried to solve the problem independently.

This running record was followed by a short lesson (less than two minutes) using plastic letters to teach a strategy for reading a letter pattern that had been misread in a previous lesson. In one case this involved the *all* word family. The tutor made a point of linking the unknown *all* words (e.g., *fall*, *call*) to those which were already known by the child (e.g., *all*, *ball*). During earlier phases in the development of Reading Recovery, these short *teaching points* were incorporated into reading sessions and presented spontaneously when the child seemed ready for new learning. They are now provided separately so as not to interrupt the focus on comprehension during book reading.

This lesson was followed by a short writing lesson that involved what is called *joint problem solving* (Lyons, Pinnell, and DeFord 1993). The child composed a sentence aloud based on interest in a recent book, and then wrote it down. Several words were spelled by having the child segment phonemes aloud. The tutor asked, "What letter would you expect to see?" and then wrote each letter in a series of Elkonin-type boxes she had prepared for this word (Elkonin 1963, 1973). Hard words were simply spelled out for the child. The completed sentence was cut up into words, scrambled, and then reassembled by the child as the tutor said the sentence aloud. Marie Clay (1992) built this writing activity into the program in order to capitalize on the reciprocal relationship between reading and writing, and to strengthen phonological awareness skills through the segmenting and spelling boxes. Clay calls this *invented spelling*, but note that the child does not actually misspell words as in many American classrooms using this technique. In Reading Recovery the child receives teacher support in building words correctly from patterns that have been internalized, and the teacher simply spells out others or parts of others that are, as yet, too difficult for the child.

The final activity in these observed lessons was the introduction of a new book. Prior to reading the new book, the child was engaged in conversation about the pictures and was encouraged to discuss background knowledge of the content and to make predictions about the story. At this point in the lesson some children in Reading Recovery tutoring have read as many as five short books during the half hour lesson. The ratio of time actually spent reading text to time engaged in reading-related activities is higher in Reading Recovery than in other programs described here. The efficiency of the lessons was striking. Almost all of the time was spent with the child actually engaged in reading. The books were so carefully chosen and the tutor so in touch with the child's reading that the direct instruction, while minimal, was highly focused and seemed to be quite effective.

TEACHER TRAINING

To enter a Reading Recovery training program in the United States, teachers must be certified and must have at least three years of classroom experience. They must be nominated by their school districts, with only about half of the nominated teachers accepted for training.

Teachers in training (and ultimately, Reading Recovery teachers) work with four children for half an hour each during the morning, and then return to their old jobs as classroom or resource room teachers in the afternoon.

During the year-long training period, teachers attend weekly sessions at a Reading Recovery training center. These centers are university-based, such as the ones at Ohio State University and New York University. Trainees take turns bringing a child for a demonstration lesson, which takes place *behind the glass* or one-way mirror. The other trainees watch and are guided in their observations by a teacher trainer who holds a doctoral degree, is affiliated with a university, and has been trained as a Reading Recovery teacher trainer. The emphasis during these observations is on decision making for a particular situation rather than simply learning standard techniques. Trainers focus on the reading process and on the impact of a particular teaching point. Careful observation of the child is a major focus.

EVALUATION AND IMPLEMENTATION

A number of large scale research studies have been carried out to evaluate Reading Recovery in the United States (see DeFord, Lyons, and Pinnell 1991). The consensus is that roughly 65-85 percent of Reading Recovery children are successfully returned to regular classroom reading groups (Center et al. 1995; DeFord, Lyons, and Pinnell 1991). Several recent studies seem particularly thorough and illuminating. The first teased apart the effective components of this highly complex teaching model. An evaluation team led by Ohio Reading Recovery trainer Gay Sue Pinnell (Pinnell et al. 1994) analyzed the effective characteristics of Reading Recovery through a comparison of other interventions with some but not all of its attributes. There were five groups in the experiment: 1) Reading Recovery, 2) Reading Recovery with a shorter teacher training period, 3) another one-to-one tutoring program using direct instruction, 4) Reading Recovery instructional techniques used by trained teachers with small groups rather than with individuals, and 5) controls in existing Chapter One pullout classes. This study used 324 of the lowest achieving first-grade children from 10 Ohio school districts. In addition to pre- and posttest measures of reading and writing, extensive analyses of videotaped lessons were carried out. Data from all of these sources suggested that Reading Recovery worked better than any of the other models, and that its effectiveness was the result of several key factors: 1) working one-to-one with students, 2) the framework of the lessons, and 3) the teacher training model with an expectation of ongoing learning in a supportive atmosphere. Tim-

othy Rasinski comments, in regard to this study, that the lengthy training of Reading Recovery's already skilled teachers and the intensity of
the one-to-one instruction may account for at least some of its effectiveness; the composition of the lesson itself may not be the crucial factor
in considering the program's effectiveness (Rasinski 1995).

A second study with similarly positive conclusions about Reading
Recovery was carried out by researchers who are not directly involved
with this program (Wasik and Slavin 1993). Note that Robert Slavin is
one of the developers of Success for All, a multi-faceted program for
urban at-risk children in the primary grades. Five programs are described
in Wasik and Slavin's report: 1) Reading Recovery, 2) Success for All,
3) Prevention of Learning Disabilities, 4) The Wallach Tutoring Program,
and 5) Programmed Tutorial Reading, all designed for at-risk children
in the primary grades. Wasik and Slavin compared effect sizes for the five
programs as reported by independent researchers. Effect sizes were largest
for Reading Recovery and Success for All, which the researchers attribute
to use of certified teachers, one-to-one delivery of the programs, and
well articulated models of the reading process. This last point is an
important one; understanding basic reading processes is an important
feature of Reading Recovery teacher-training; trainees are not taught
to teach from scripts but, rather, to observe for signs of processes and
strategies, and to use these observations in planning instruction.

Wasik and Slavin also address the issue of cost effectiveness; both
Success for All and Reading Recovery are often criticized as being expen-
sive. Wasik and Slavin make the point that using special education funds
for early prevention can save money over the long term (Dyer 1992;
Slavin et al. 1992).

A third study was carried out in Rhode Island by a Reading
Recovery trainer and a university researcher, both from New Zealand
(Iverson and Tunmer 1993). It attempted to answer questions about a
common criticism of Reading Recovery: what is perceived by many
special educators as a lack of direct instruction in phonetic knowledge
and phonological awareness. Two groups of Reading Recovery teachers
were trained, one in the usual Reading Recovery training program and
the other in the usual program with the addition of phonics and phonological awareness instruction. Both programs were found to be effective,
but children in the Reading-Recovery-plus-phonics program were discontinued from tutoring sooner than those in the regular Reading
Recovery program.

Unlike many of the other remedial programs described here,
there is systematic research to describe characteristics of those children
who have not been successfully discontinued from Reading Recovery
and to document what the eventual outcome was for them. Marie Clay
attempts to answer these questions with preliminary results from a New

Zealand study (Clay 1992). Most of the highest functioning of the unsuccessful children in this study did eventually read within the average range after about two years. About a third of the unsuccessful children had low intelligence and were provided with other forms of support. A small number had psychological problems believed to be interfering with learning to read.

One criticism of the Reading Recovery research that has been carried out by Clay and others directly associated with the program is that these researchers have failed to include the reading scores of children who have not been successfully discontinued in follow-up studies of ability to maintain gains (Center et al. 1995). Yola Center states that as many as 30 percent of children are removed from Reading Recovery programs because of failure to make progress. This would tend to skew the success-rate statistics. Center and her colleagues report data from a study carried out in Australia in which Reading Recovery children were compared to controls receiving group-based extra instruction. Reading Recovery children were significantly stronger than controls at the time that the Reading Recovery children were discontinued from one-to-one help, but this advantage faded over the subsequent weeks and months.

Because Reading Recovery is so widely used and is, thus, in the public eye to a greater degree than many of the other programs described here, the quality of the research has been more rigorously controlled. The research is characterized by larger studies and by studies with control groups. Even critics of Reading Recovery (e.g., Center et al. 1995; Rasinski 1995) agree that this individual instruction is effective. Overall, the research carried out on Reading Recovery appears to be both thorough and positive. To date, there is no research on the success rate of Reading Recovery instruction with children screened in kindergarten as being specifically at-risk for dyslexia.

23

The Wilson Reading System

BACKGROUND AND RATIONALE

The Wilson Reading System is one of the few remedial programs that was developed especially for adults and adolescents with dyslexia. It was developed by Barbara A. Wilson who was originally a special educator in the public schools in Massachusetts. When she became concerned about students who had reading difficulty despite average or better cognitive ability, she sought additional training in the Orton-Gillingham approach at the Language Disorders Unit of Massachusetts General Hospital. She remained there for five years once her training was completed, working with adults with dyslexia. The Wilson Reading System was based on this training and was developed through Wilson's private tutoring practice at the Wilson Learning Center. This center was established in 1985 in Hopedale, Massachusetts with her husband, Edward J. Wilson, as business manager. The Wilsons began publishing the Wilson Reading System materials in 1988 and began providing teacher training in 1989. By 1991 their focus had changed from tutoring in a private setting to disseminating information about the program to teachers in the public sector through establishment of the Wilson Language Training Corporation (WLT). In 1993 this new center for disseminating materials and training was moved to Millbury, Massachusetts.

The Wilson Reading System is based on Orton-Gillingham principles and is a multisensory, synthetic approach to teaching reading and writing to students with language-based difficulties in written language. It has many characteristics in common with other Orton-Gillingham based programs such as Alphabetic Phonics (e.g., sounds are taught to automaticity and then used to decode phonetically controlled text; language structure is taught in a systematic, cumulative way; there is constant review and repetition). It is an integrated system for teaching all aspects of decoding and encoding.

Wilson believes that many older poor readers have begun to think of English as so lacking in regularities that it is impossible to learn. Through the introduction of English as a system, students are taught to trust the system right from the beginning as they learn to be able to count on what they have been taught.

CURRICULUM AND INSTRUCTION

The Wilson Reading System is designed for adults and for students in grades 5-12, but can be used with younger children as well. Wilson believes that one-to-one tutoring presents an ideal setting because of myriad self esteem issues usually present for the older poor reader. However, her program has also been used successfully in school settings with small groups or even as the spelling curriculum for an entire class.

The program (Wilson 1988c) is sequenced in 12 steps that are based on 6 syllable types (i.e., closed syllables, syllables with vowels and silent *e*, open syllables, syllables ending in a consonant with *-le*, *r*–controlled syllables, and diphthong syllables). One innovation Wilson brings to the Orton-Gillingham approach is emphasis on these syllable types right from the beginning. Words are coded by the student, as is typical of other Orton-Gillingham programs (e.g., see Alphabetic Phonics, Chapter 13). However, complex diacritical marks are not used; only the short and long vowel codings and crossing-out of the silent e are used. Instead, a simplified syllable marking is used with a code for each of the syllable types. See the codings for the 6 syllable types. The traditional Orton-Gillingham *slashing* of syllables is not used (e.g., *con/trast*). Instead, words are *scooped* or underlined by syllables. Wilson points out that this emphasizes the left-to-right movement of reading; she does not "slash" words between syllables because she doesn't want students moving to the center of the word first as they view it. The underlining mimics the left–to-right movement used during reading.

Steps 1-3 introduce closed syllables with short vowels in single syllable words with 3 sounds (e.g., *bat*), with 4-6 sounds (e.g., *shrimp*) and in polysyllabic words (e.g., *consultant*). Step 1 instruction begins with phonemic segmentation in consonant-vowel-consonant (c-v-c) words. Steps 1 and 2 strongly emphasize phonological awareness with segmenting and blending of phonemes up to six sounds. Finger tapping is used for

SYLLABLE MARKING

Six Types of Syllables:

	code	vowel markings
1. Closed	(c)	cŭp c
2. V- E	(e)	bāke e
3. Open	(o)	hē o
4. R- Controlled	(r)	pork r
5. C- le	(c- le)	tle c- le
6. Diphthong	(d)	bait d

To mark syllables:

1. Underline the syllable(s):
    e.g.   <u>re</u> <u>port</u>

2. Identify type of syllable(s):
    Put the syllable code under the line for each syllable:
    e.g.   <u>re</u> <u>port</u>
             o   r

3. Mark the vowel(s):
    e.g.   r<u>ē</u> <u>port</u>
             o   r

analyzing spoken words into phonemes for spelling. This is similar to the technique called *finger spelling* in Project Read (Enfield and Greene) described in Chapter 17. Wilson also uses finger-to-thumb tapping of phonemes for helping children blend sounds at Steps 1 and 2.

Steps 4–5 introduce long vowels in syllables with silent *e* such as in *shine* and in open syllables such as in *program*. Step 6 introduces suffixes in unchanged base words such as *punished* and in consonant-*le* words such as *dribble*. During Steps 1–6 the word lists are controlled so that there are no possible alternative pronunciations. Through Step 6 the student reads only phonetically controlled text based on the 6 word-types that have been introduced and thus every word can be decoded using phonetic concepts.

Step 7 focuses on what Wilson calls *sound options* for *c* and *g* following *e, i,* and *y* (e.g., *decency, gigantic*). Step 8 introduces *r*-controlled syllables in words such as *market*. Step 9 introduces diphthong syllables in words such as *plain, thyroid,* and *light*. Step 10 introduces suffixes added to changing basewords such as *postponing* and *lagging*. Step 11 includes contractions and advanced suffixes. Step 12 introduces advanced concepts such as the *i* before *e* rule and silent letters. Both real and nonsense words are taught for reading and spelling at each of these steps.

Within each of the 12 steps there are additional substeps, providing 56 substeps in all. Instructors are urged to follow the carefully laid out sequence and to introduce concepts in the suggested order.

Lesson plans are consistent in structure and are outlined in the *Instructor Manual* (Wilson 1988b). Detailed directions are provided, with each lesson utilizing the following basic plan:

1. *Sound Cards.* A typical lesson begins with sound cards used to introduce a new sound and then to drill old sounds. After a quick drill, the teacher makes words using the phoneme cards to teach and practice the skill being taught. As students advance through the program, syllable and suffix cards are used here as well. Wilson believes that the manipulation of these sound cards at every lesson and with every concept is unique to her program. That is, the cards are used first thing in a lesson and then re-used at other points (e.g., in preparation for a writing lesson).

2. *Word Cards.* These cards, each with a printed word, are used to present and practice words using the sounds that were introduced and drilled on the sound cards above. The content from both the Sound Cards and Word Cards is tied to the 12 Steps and their 56 substeps. The 390 Word Cards are color coded to keep them organized into the correct sequence.

3. *Word List Reading.* Student readers include word lists that are read and then charted to keep ongoing records of a student's progress in

terms of accuracy. Lists of both real and nonsense words are provided for each substep. The Instructor Manual notes that this represents the third teaching of a concept within any particular lesson, the first two taking place at the Sound Card and Word Card levels of the lesson.

4. *Sentence Reading.* The student readers also contain sentences composed of the above words. As with stories in the Student Readers (see below) any words that cannot be decoded using patterns previously taught have been boxed at the top of a page and the instructor simply reads them aloud to the student.

5. *Preparation for Written Work.* Activities in this portion of the lesson prepare the student for the spelling dictations that follow. The student practices a particular concept by spelling with sound cards, syllable cards, and suffix cards.

6. *Written Work.* Materials include a Dictation Book with detailed directions for writing words with the different syllable types. This section of the lesson begins with a *What says* activity. For example, the instructor asks, "What says /b/?" and the student is expected to respond with both the correct letter name and the keyword. Once mastered, the keyword is used only as needed. In addition, the Dictation Book includes both word lists and sentences for spelling at every level. Dictated words are to be taken from prior lists, for review, as well as from current lists. This is followed by dictation of several sentences. A sequence of 12 workbooks is available and can be used to extend the learning of concepts for writing words.

7. *Reading/Listening.* The 12 phonetically controlled Student Readers are based on the 12 steps of the System. Words that have not yet been covered in the sequence appear in a small box at the top of the page and are read aloud to the student before a reading passage is undertaken. As with the sentences, the student reads the passage silently first before reading it aloud. If the student cannot read a word whose pattern has already been taught (and which thus does not appear in the box), the word is to be written on paper, underlined by syllable, and coded by syllable type. After the passage has been read silently, the student retells the story from the Student Reader in his or her own words. The final step in a lesson involves reading the story aloud to the student with the emphasis on comprehension.

All of the materials used in the program are available from WLT with the exception of the outside reading materials introduced after Step 6. The materials are color coded so that the Student Reader, the Student Workbook, and the Word Cards from a particular step of the system are the same color.

The Sound Cards are also color coded, but not by step. Consonants and consonant units are one color, vowels and vowel units another, and

and word families (e.g., *an*, *ung*) and complex suffixes (e.g., *tion*, *ture*) are yet another. Unlike the Initial Reading Deck cards in Alphabetic Phonics (see Chapter 13), but like that program's Advanced Reading Deck, the Wilson Sound Cards include no diacritical marks or key word pictures on the front. A letter or letters appear on the front for the student to see. The pronunciation, a key word, and the system step at which the sound option is introduced appear on the back for the instructor to see. Instructors are warned to take care not to introduce all sounds at once but to introduce them sequentially and with much review and repetition. Smaller color-coded versions of the Sound Cards, about the size of Scrabble tiles and called *Mini Sound Cards*, are also available for assembling into words. Consonant clusters are assembled from multiple cards, while the letters in a consonant digraph (e.g., *th*) occur on the same Mini Sound Card, as is the case with the larger Sound Cards. In this regard the system is like Alphabetic Phonics and unlike Project Read (Enfield and Greene); in the latter method consonant clusters are taught as single units.

When a new sound is introduced, the student copies information from the Rules Notebook into a personal notebook designed for keeping notes on new concepts. This notebook is used for concepts introduced in other portions of the lesson as well. The emphasis is on the learner's responsibility for taking over management of newly learned concepts. The notebook has sections for sounds, syllables, spelling rules, and sight words.

The content of the Student Readers is geared toward the interests of older readers in so far as possible. As with most phonetically controlled text based on c-v-c words the earliest stories include instances of the words *cat* and *hat*, but in the Wilson stories, content involves words based on more adult interests such as *prom, kiss, Red Sox,* and *job*. Many of the stories are about high school activities or about issues related to self suffi-ciency such as job hunting or finding a place to live away from home. See the sample text from Student Reader Six (Wilson 1988b), which focuses on suffix endings in unchanging basewords. Supplementary reading materials that follow the 12-step system are also available from WLT. These include student readers and a short novel about a young adult who leaves home to live on his own (Brown 1992, 1994).

It was a hot, spring day in Alabama. Cathy Jones suddenly had a call. The man on the line had a job for her singing in a local establishment! She had been recommended by a friend. She strongly wanted to be a big-time singer. She shyly responded, "Yes."

Text from "Cathy Gets a Job" in Student Reader Six in the Wilson Reading System *by Barbara A. Wilson. (Reproduced with permission from Wilson Language Training, Millbury, MA. Copyright 1988b.)*

Through Step 6 of the program, outside reading is discouraged. The Instructor Manual states that this is to discourage guessing and to encourage the reliable use of letter cues in decoding. After mastery of material from the first six steps, non–controlled text from other sources can be used in the lessons as well as the readers. Instructors are also urged to read aloud to students, with selections made from high interest materials.

Test Forms are available for initial placement in the series and for assessment of mastery of the concepts taught in each of the 12 steps. Instructors are urged to begin with Step 1; the program start-points suggested after initial testing range from Step 1:1 through Step 1:3. For students who can learn the concepts quickly, an accelerated version is available in the form of a Program Overview which is really designed for use in teacher training sessions. In other words, for relatively proficient readers, steps should be reviewed quickly, and never skipped. Progression through all of the steps can take anywhere from 6 months to 3 years.

TEACHER TRAINING

Training and certification in the Wilson Reading System are carried out by the Wilson Language Training Corporation (WLT) in Millbury, Massachusetts. On-site training is available to school systems and adult literacy centers nationwide. Publications from WLT list 12 teacher trainers, in addition to Barbara Wilson, all trained in the Wilson System up to trainer level, and many trained in the Orton-Gillingham method at Massachusetts General Hospital as well as in the Wilson System.

WLT offers an initial two-day introductory workshop, called an *overview*, which can include a number of topics depending on a school's needs. Topics include descriptive information, both about dyslexia and about the Wilson system. WLT also offers extended training that eventually results in what is called *Level One Certification* for individual participants. Certification training typically takes place over the course of a summer or in monthly seminars during the school year. There are six follow-up observations of instructors-in-training carried out while they work with their students, to insure that the system has been properly mastered.

EVALUATION AND IMPLEMENTATION

The Wilson Reading System is relatively new but initial research is encouraging. Pretest-posttest records from schools using the method indicate gains ranging from 1.6 to 2.4 years for Wilson System students over the course of one school year.

A well-controlled study (Guyer, Banks, and Guyer 1993) was carried out with 30 students with dyslexia enrolled in the Higher Education for Learning Problems (HELP) program at Marshall University in West Virginia. These students ranged in age from 18-32, had a mean IQ of 110, and earned reading achievement scores at least one standard deviation below IQ scores. Most had been diagnosed with dyslexia prior to entering college and all were enrolled in the HELP program in order to receive remedial assistance with a range of academic problems such as study skills and proofreading papers for course work. The experimental group received spelling instruction using the Wilson System and was compared with controls receiving instruction in a nonphonetic spelling method and with those receiving no instruction. Both trained groups were tutored by learning-disabilities specialists with prior training in both the Wilson System and in the nonphonetic spelling method. After two hour-long lessons a week for 16 weeks the group receiving tutoring in the Wilson System was significantly stronger than either control group on spelling skills as measured by the Spelling subtest of the Wide Range Achievement Test (WRAT-R). While not formally documented, the authors note that several professors commented that these students' con-textualized spellings improved over the course of the semester as evidenced in papers.

A recent report from WLT describes a second study carried out with 220 student-teacher pairs from Massachusetts, Maine, and New Jersey (Wilson 1995). Of the 220 students, 92 were in grades 3-4 and 128 in grades 5-12. Criteria for selecting students involved a special education evaluation indicating IQ in the low average to high average range, reading at least two years below grade level, and lack of outstanding emotional factors. In all cases there was a history of poor progress made with other reading programs in one-to-one or small group settings. About a third had been retained at least one grade. About half were in regular classrooms with at least a third of the day spent in pull-out settings. Most of the other students were in full time special education settings for the entire day. Tutors attended a two-day Wilson training session and monthly seminars from September through June. During this time they tutored the subjects, with the number of sessions ranging from 55-100. Different forms of the posttest presented different results, but with forms combined, the average growth from pre- to posttest was 4.5 grade levels on the Word Attack Test of the Woodcock Reading Mastery Tests and 1.5 grade levels on the Reading Comprehension Test. These results are impressive in light of the minimal progress made by these students in other programs. Wilson points out that the current practice of placing special education students into remedial work without specially designed reading programs needs to be examined.

The Wilson Reading System has been implemented in a number of educational settings nationwide such as public school special education classes, private schools geared toward students with dyslexia, clinics offering reading remediation, adult literacy programs, and prisons.

24

Curriculum Planning: A Case Study

The issue of determining the appropriate instructional treatment for a particular student is crucial. As educators, this should be our principal concern, whether we are school administrators responsible for implementing and funding remedial or preventive curricula, or teachers working directly with students.

This book concludes with an illustration of this process, using the case history of KM. Her end-of-first-grade evaluation was outlined in Chapter 3, and is used here as the starting point in planning an instructional program for her.

KM'S REMEDIAL PLAN

SETTING

Having come to the conclusion that KM was dyslexic because her reading was so poor in relationship to her superior IQ and because of her unusually slow serial naming rate, our first consideration in formulating an educational plan involved choosing an appropriate setting. We wondered if KM should stay in her present school or if she should move to a school with a more traditionally structured phonics program. Would she do well in a special education setting? In looking at a plan for KM we wanted to keep in mind that while she appeared to need direct instruction in both reading and spelling, she did extremely well in school in math and in activities involving oral language.

KM attended a school with a whole-language curriculum and without any direct instruction in phonics. This did not present an ideal situation. On the other hand, we didn't think KM belonged in a special education setting. There are many wonderful schools in New York City that provide specialized environments, tailored to children with dyslexia and other learning disabilities, and we often recommend them to families of children with dyslexia. However, we thought that KM ought to remain in a regular classroom setting because she functioned very well in areas other than reading and writing. We wanted to keep her with other children who functioned at a high level intellectually because she thrived on the cognitive stimulation.

We would have preferred to see KM receive an hour a day of language arts instruction that included direct instruction in letter-sound associations, and guided practice using this knowledge in reading. Three of the programs reviewed here offer this in regular classrooms for children KM's age. The Slingerland program, and both Calfee's Project READ and Enfield and Greene's Project Read involve direct instruction in phonics in regular classrooms. Recipe for Reading is also used by some regular classroom teachers to supplement the curriculum. These programs were not available in KM's school.

Another possibility that occurred to us involved resource room. In cases where a phonics-based classroom program is not available, a resource room is often an appropriate option for children needing direct instruction in phonics but not in need of a full-day special education classroom. This was not available in KM's school. Even in public schools where the option is mandated, the educational approach is not always appropriate. Few resource room teachers have specialized training in the programs reviewed here.

After-school tutoring appeared to be the most workable plan. Even if specialized help had been available in her school, few schools offer this help on a one-to-one basis. Reading Recovery is a notable exception but KM was too old for this program. One-to-one help appears to be crucial for successful remediation. For a discussion of this see Wasik and Slavin's (1993) comparison of several reading programs.

KM'S INITIAL CURRICULUM PLAN

KM was tutored by graduate students under our supervision in the Child Study Center for two years. We initially designed her tutoring plan by reviewing remedial programs believed to work well with children with word-reading problems, and by looking at KM's particular profile.

Letter Knowledge

We wanted a program in which KM's difficulty responding automatically and rapidly to stimuli would be minimized. A sight word approach would have involved learning thousands of words to the automatic level. In a synthetic phonics approach there are only 98 letter-sound correspondences to be learned. We knew that KM was relatively strong in blending sounds and we reasoned that automatizing 98 sounds seemed less daunting than memorizing thousands of sight words to the point at which they could be retrieved quickly. Learning these 98 sounds would allow her to use letter cues to sound out new words.

For this letter-sound training, we chose the Initial Reading Deck (IRD; Cox 1971) from Alphabetic Phonics and began each session over the two years of tutoring by asking KM to respond to each letter or unit of letters with its sound. We began with just a few consonants she knew already and worked on speed of response. We added a new card roughly once a week. We also worked on response time for encoding; we said a sound and asked KM to say the letter name as quickly as she could. For KM, only about 5 minutes per tutoring session were spent on these two activities combined.

Segmenting/Spelling

We knew that KM was able to segment to some degree, but that she struggled with spelling when she needed to retrieve letter names for these segments and to think at the same time while composing. We did some phonological awareness training with KM in the form of segmentation/spelling (see Chapter 5). It is a principle of Orton-Gillingham training to provide practice in isolation before asking a child to juggle several skills or strategies at once. For each new letter-sound pattern KM was taught using the IRD, she was asked to segment words into component phonemes, and then to represent each phoneme with a letter or letters, either with tiles or through handwritten spellings. That is, when the digraph *th* was taught, KM was asked to segment the spoken word with into the sounds /w/-/i/-/th/, and then to spell it with lettered tiles. Spelling was often extended to written sentences. The spelling dictation portion of this technique can be found in a number of Orton-Gillingham programs such as Alphabetic Phonics and Recipe for Reading.

Phonetically Controlled Text for Oral Reading

It is fairly common practice with children with dyslexia to use text that provides practice in newly learned phonetic patterns, and that is limited to patterns that have been introduced already. With KM, we began with *Mac and Tab* from the Primary Phonics series (Makar 1985) available from Educators Publishing Service, but we could have used any number of books limited to short vowels introduced one at a time in a synthetic phonics format. KM read these little books with good accuracy but continued to sound out each word, letter-by-letter. Practice with the IRD helped her sound out each letter with increasing speed, but she failed to increase her retrieval rate for whole words.

Formative assessment at that point indicated rapid growth in non-sense word reading. KM's score on the Word Attack Test of the WRMT jumped from 61 to 94 in about 6 months, while her Word Identification score remained at 78. Because of her poor growth rate in reading real words as sight words, we switched her to the Merrill Linguistic Readers, Books B and C (1986) toward the end of her first year of tutoring. We thought that the emphasis on rimes (rather than the phonemic units used in synthetic phonics) would help her retrieve units of letters (e.g., *an*, *itch*) more quickly, and would encourage a switch from letter-by-letter reading to more automatic reading of units of letters in words. By the fall of her second year of tutoring KM began to read whole words more automatically but her reading rate remained slow. Should we have started with the Merrill Readers earlier, rather than with a synthetic program? Linnea Ehri's research indicates not. Her work suggests that phonics knowledge and the letter-by-letter strategy facilitate both the sort of analogy reading that the Merrill readers encourage (Ehri and Robbins 1992) and the acquisition of a sight word vocabulary (Ehri 1992).

Narratively Controlled Text: Trade Books

While many of the Orton-Gillingham programs limit early reading to phonetically controlled text (e.g., Alphabetic Phonics, Wilson Reading System) we saw KM's inability to integrate various cue systems as a problem that we wanted to remediate from the beginning. We tried to choose text that was interesting and that included (but was not limited to) exemplars of phonetic patterns she was practicing in other activities. This provided additional exposure to the pattern introduced with the IRD during a particular lesson and to words using that pattern introduced in the segmenting/spelling activity and read in the phonetic text. For example, during the end of KM's second grade year (her first year of tutoring) when we worked on consonant digraphs and blends with short vowels, we used the Harper I-Can-Read book, *The Grandma Mix-Up* (McCully 1988). The text is rich in this word type, but it also has a strong and compelling story line and lively illustrations. For many children with dyslexia, this sort of text might be inappropriate, but keep in mind that from the start KM had at least a marginally developed sense of phonological awareness and of the alphabetic principle. She simply lost this strategy in any sort of applied situation. Focus during the reading of narrative text was similar to that found in Reading Recovery lessons; KM was encouraged to develop strategies for using letter cues as well as context cues, and for checking her own reading by being sure that there was consistency between these cue systems. Roberta, her tutor, took notes during that period indicating that while KM easily read words with blends (e.g., *sled*, *slip*) in isolated situations such as games, she still over-relied on context and simply guessed when she read them in text. KM's reading during this period was characterized by poor motivation, and doggedness about holding on to inefficient and incomplete strategies. She had trouble focusing and was quite resistant to reading. She loved to have Roberta read aloud to her.

Note that this lesson outline, with a balance between phonics practice and trade book reading, is similar to one developed by Benita Blachman (Blachman 1987; Blachman et al. 1994).

ONGOING ASSESSMENT

Most preventive and remedial programs include a series of curriculum-based measures designed to tell us if a child has mastered a set of concepts and is ready to move on to new learning. For example, see Chapter 13, Alphabetic Phonics. Because KM tended to read more accurately given words out of context, we wanted to keep track of her application of a concept in contextualized reading rather than in isolation. For this reason we used the Reading Recovery (see Chapter 22) *running record* system of on-going assessment of reading in trade books to be sure KM had mastered a principle before we introduced new material. Keeping a log of observations allows immediate modifications to even the best-laid plan.

KM'S SECOND YEAR OF TUTORING

Tutoring sessions continued to be based on the instructional elements outlined above, beginning with a review of consonant blends and digraphs before moving into long vowels. Her second-year tutor, Sally, proceeded slowly with any new material, knowing that KM was apt to revert to inefficient strategies when overwhelmed. KM began this year reading from simple I-Can-Read trade books at the late first-grade level and read from Merrill readers D, E, and F throughout the year. Miscues collected while reading trade books continued to indicate problems in using all available letter cues (e.g., She read *tale* as "talk," *dirt* as "dry," and *calls* as "cries"). We continued to use lettered tiles for segmenting/spelling activities (e.g., "Spell *hid*. Change it to *hide*. Change it to *side*") in order to reinforce letter order and a sequence of particular letter-sound patterns. To encourage more rapid retrieval, some of these words were put on cards for timed reading. KM enjoyed trying to beat her own record, so we kept charts of her time from session to session and this was a successful activity in terms of motivation.

By the end of this year, her third-grade year in school, KM was reading short chapter books (e.g., *Something Queer at the Lemonade Stand*, *The One in the Middle is a Green Kangaroo*), and Random House Step-up Classics at roughly the third grade level (e.g., a retelling of *Peter Pan*). Trade book activities focused on meaning. In her final tutoring report, her tutor Sally noted, "KM's confidence in herself as a reader has risen dramatically. She will go back and re-read the text or sound out words to make meaning." KM still read quite slowly, but she was beginning to read whole phrases more smoothly.

Writing had become an issue in school; KM became reluctant to invent spellings and became a perfectionist about getting spellings right. Her story content became limited to words she knew how to spell. Her tutor provided structured writing experiences consistent with Orton-Gillingham methods, in which sentences were built up from previously practiced words. Cursive handwriting was undertaken and KM enjoyed this. She was less resistant to writing when dictations were approached as practice in cursive writing. Letter formations were taught in groups using terminology and formations from Alphabetic Phonics (e.g., *swing up letters*).

KM'S FINAL EVALUATION

At the end of her second year of tutoring KM moved to another state. We administered a second formal evaluation to accompany her to her new school where she would enter the fourth grade. Her scores were no longer discrepant from age peers but continued to be lower than predictions based on her superior range IQ. Note that KM's oral language scores, after remediation, continued to be higher than reading comprehension which, in turn, was stronger than word reading and spelling.

KM's Standard Scores over the Course of 2 Years of Tutoring

	1992	1993	1994
PIAT General Information (oral questions)	—	—	138
PPVT (oral vocabulary)	124	—	—
WIAT Listening Comprehension	—	—	120
WIAT Reading Comprehension	—	—	103
WIAT Basic Reading (word lists)	81	87	94
WRMT Word Identification (word lists)	78	78	95
WRMT Word Attack (nonsense words)	61	94	99
WIAT Spelling (dictated words)	84	88	94

KM's time on serial naming on the RAN continued to be several standard deviations slower than age norms. She demonstrated a significant discrepancy between reading accuracy and reading speed when we administered oral passages from the Gray Oral Reading Test (GORT-3). This is consistent with results from Wood and Felton (1994) indicating that rapid naming problems persist into adulthood and inhibit the development of reading rate.

KM's final piece of writing for us described her new home. Note that she over-relied on phonological spelling rather than using conventional orthography. Even in regard to phonics, not all vowel patterns or basic spelling rules for adding suffixes were in place. Her writing was spare in comparison with her gregarious oral style.

> My house is verry cold! But cossy. My room is verry small.
> I have a farm. there are lots of play gouns in the park. There are 5 Maces. There are 2 J.C. penes. Good by.
> P.S. I mess my friends.

Writing is often the last skill to fall into place once children with dyslexia have had successful remedial training. KM's final tutoring report listed the following areas for further work: 1) letter-sound training in the remaining vowel digraphs, and in hard and soft *c* and *g*; 2) practice of accuracy and fluency in phonetically controlled text such as Merrill Reader G; 3) practice of accuracy and fluency as well as higher level thinking in interesting trade books; and 4) encouragement of self-initiation of written expression.

No single reading program meets all of the instructional requirements of students with dyslexia. We chose to construct a program for KM from the components of a number of different programs. Had any of the age-appropriate programs described in Part III of this book been available in KM's school from the beginning of first grade, we are confident that she would have learned to read more easily than she did. However, any of these programs would have needed some adjustments to best fit KM's needs.

SUMMARY

The lessons to be learned from watching KM and other children with dyslexia learn to read and write can be summarized as follows:

1) Be sure that all children are screened in kindergarten for early signs of dyslexia.
2) Begin treatment as early as possible if there is any question of dyslexia. This is especially crucial for children in families with other affected members.
3) Provide direct instruction in phonological awareness and synthetic phonics and teach these children how to integrate these strategies with meaning-based strategies.
4) Read aloud to these children in order to provide intellectual stimulation and a knowledge base ordinarily acquired through reading.
5) Provide on-going assessment in order to modify and adjust the curriculum.

Tutors and teachers involved with these children need to continue their own professional development through conferences, additional training, and readings from the research. Those of us who work with children and adolescents with dyslexia should take a greater role than we have in the past in planning their language arts curriculums. In addition to using the research results of others to plan curriculum, we should also be documenting and sharing what we ourselves are doing, thereby adding to the research base.

References

Aaron, P. G., and Phillips, S. 1986. A decade of research with dyslexic college students. *Annals of Dyslexia* 36:44-68.

Adams, M. J. 1990. *Beginning to Read: Thinking and Learning about Print.* Cambridge, MA: The MIT Press.

Aho, M. S. 1967. Teaching spelling to children with specific language disability. *Academic Therapy* 3:45-50.

Alexander, A. W., Andersen, H. G., Heilman, P. C., Voeller, K. K. S., and Torgesen, J. K. 1991. Phonological awareness training and remediation of analytic decoding deficits in a group of severe dyslexics. *Annals of Dyslexia* 41:193-206.

Anderson, R. C., Hiebert, E. H., Scott, J. A., and Wilkinson, I. A. G. 1984. *Becoming a Nation of Readers.* Washington, D.C.: National Institute of Education.

Arkes, J. 1986. The ABCs of Project Read. Bloomington, MN: Bloomington Public Schools.

Arter, J. A., and Jenkins, J. R. 1979. Differential diagnosis-prescriptive teaching: A critical appraisal. *Review of Educational Research* 49:517-55.

Askov, E., and Greff, N. 1975. Handwriting: Copying versus tracing as the most effective type of practice. *Journal of Educational Research* 69:96-98.

Badian, N. A. 1988. Predicting dyslexia in a preschool population. In *Preschool Prevention of Reading Failure*, eds. R. L. Masland and M. W. Masland. Parkton, MD: York Press.

Baker, L., and Brown, A. L. 1984. Metacognitive skills in reading. In *Handbook of Reading Research*, ed. P. D. Pearson. New York: Longman.

Ball, E. W., and Blachman, B. A. 1991. Does phoneme segmentation training in kindergarten make a difference in early word recognition and developmental spelling? *Reading Research Quarterly* 26:49-66.

Ballesteros, D. A., and Royal, N. L. 1981. Slingerland-SLD instruction as a winning voluntary magnet program. *Bulletin of The Orton Society* 31:199-211.

Bandura, A. 1982. Self-efficiency mechanism in human agency. *American Psychologist* 37(2): 122–47.

Bannatyne, A. 1971. *Language, Reading, and Learning Disabilities*. Springfield, Il.: Charles C Thomas.

Barenbaum, E. M. 1983. Writing in the special class. *Topics in Learning and Learning Disabilities* 3:12–20.

Barger, E. J. 1982. The effect of the Glass Analysis technique for decoding words on the reading and spelling achievement of 7 to 10-year-old remedial readers. Ph.D. diss., George Washington University, Washington, D. C.

Barron, R. W. 1980. Visual and phonological strategies in reading and spelling. In *Cognitive Processes in Spelling*, ed. U. Frith. New York: Academic Press.

Bartlett, E. J. 1979. Curriculum, concepts of literacy, and social class. In *Theory and Practice of Early Reading, Vol 2*, eds. L. B. Resnick and P. A.Weaver. Hillsdale, NJ: Lawrence Erlbaum Associates.

Bateman, B. 1979. Teaching reading to learning disabled and other hard-to-teach children. In *Theory and Practice of Early Reading, Vol. 1*, eds. L. B. Resnick and P. A. Weaver. Hillsdale, NJ: Lawrence Erlbaum Associates.

Beck, I. L., and McCaslin, E. S. 1978. An analysis of dimensions that affect the development of code-breaking ability in eight beginning reading programs. Pittsburgh, PA: Learning Research and Development Center, University of Pittsburgh. (ERIC Document Reproduction Service No. ED 155 585).

Beck, I. L., Omanson, R. C., and McKeown, M. G. 1982. An instructional redesign of reading lessons: Effects on comprehension. *Reading Research Quarterly* 17:462–81.

Becker, W. C. 1977. Teaching reading and language to the disadvantaged – What we have learned from field research. *Harvard Educational Review* 47:518–43.

Bell, N. 1986. *Visualizing and Verbalizing for Language Comprehension and Thinking*. Paso Robles, CA: Academy of Reading Publications.

Bell, N. 1991. Gestalt imagery: A critical factor in language comprehension. *Annals of Dyslexia* 41:246–60.

Benton, A. L. 1985. Visual factors in dyslexia: An unresolved issue. In *Understanding Learning Disabilities: International and Multidisciplinary Views*, eds. D. Duane and C. K. Leong. New York: Oxford University Press.

Berlin, D. 1887. *Eine Besondere Art der Wrotblindheit (Dyslexie)*. Wiesbaden: J. F. Bergman.

Berliner, D. 1981. Academic learning time and reading achievement. In *Comprehension and Teaching*, ed. J. T. Guthrie. Newark, DE: International Reading Association.

Berman, P., and McLaughlin, M. 1975. Federal programs supporting educational change, Vol. 4: The findings in review (Report No. R–1589/4). Santa Monica, CA: Rand Corp. (ERIC Document Reproduction Service No. ED 108 330).

Berninger, V. W., and Abbott, R. D. 1994. Redefining learning disabilities: Moving beyond aptitude-achievement discrepancies to failure to respond to validated treatment protocols. In *Frames of Reference for the Assessment of Learning Disabilities*, ed. G. R. Lyon. Baltimore, MD: Paul H. Brookes Publishing Co.

Bertin, P., and Perlman, E. 1991. *Preventing Academic Failure*. Cambridge, MA: Educators Publishing Service.

Biemiller, A. 1970. The development of the use of graphic and contextual information as children learn to read. *Reading Research Quarterly* 6:75–96.

Birch, H. G. 1962. Dyslexia and maturation of visual function. In *Reading Disability: Progress and Research Needs in Dyslexia*, ed. J. Money. Baltimore, MD: The Johns Hopkins University Press.

Birch, H. G., and Belmont, L. 1964. Auditory-visual integration in normal and retarded readers. *American Journal of Orthopsychiatry* 34:852–61.

Birsh, J. 1988. Multisensory teaching and discovery learning in Alphabetic Phonics. Paper presented at the Fifteenth Annual Conference of the New York Branch of the Orton Dyslexia Society, March 5, 1988.

Bissex, G. L. 1980. GNYS at WRK: A Child Begins to Write and Read. Cambridge, MA: Harvard University Press.

Blachman, B. A. 1987. An alternative classroom reading program for learning disabled and other low-achieving children. In Intimacy with Language: A Forgotten Basic in Teacher Education, ed. R. Bowler. Baltimore: The Orton Dyslexia Society.

Blachman, B. A., Ball, E. W., Black, R. S., and Tangel, D. M. 1994. Kindergarten teachers develop phoneme awareness in low-income, inner-city classrooms: Does it make a difference? Reading and Writing: An Interdisciplinary Journal 6:1-18.

Black, J. L., Oakland, T., Stanford, G., Nussbaum, N., and Balise, R. R. 1994. An Evaluation of the Texas Scottish Rite Hospital Dyslexia Program. Unpublished report from the Texas Scottish Rite Hospital.

Blaskey, P., Scheiman, M., Parisi, M., Ciner, E. B., Gallaway, M., and Selznick, R. 1990. The effectiveness of Irlen filters for improving reading performance: A pilot study. Journal of Learning Disabilities 23:604-12.

Bloomfield, L., Barnhart, C. L., and Barnhart, R. K. 1965. Let's Read. Cambridge, MA: Educators Publishing Service.

BOCES Regional Office of Planning and Evaluation. 1980. A study of the South Huntington School District Slingerland Program. Suffolk County, NY: Author.

Boder, E. 1971. Developmental dyslexia: A diagnostic screening procedure based on three characteristic patterns of reading and spelling. In Learning Disorders: Vol. 4, ed. B. D. Bateman. Seattle, WA: Special Child Publications.

Boder, E., and Jarrico, S. 1982. The Boder Test of Reading-Spelling Patterns. New York: Grune and Stratton.

Boettcher, J. V. 1983. Computer-based education: Classroom application and benefits for the learning disabled. Annals of Dyslexia 33: 203-19.

Bonig, R. A. 1982. Specific Skill Series. Baldwin, NY: Barnell Loft Ltd.

Bradley, L. 1981. The organization of motor patterns for spelling: An effective remedial strategy for backward readers. Developmental Medicine and Child Neurology 23:83-91.

Bradley, L. 1985. Dissociation of reading and spelling behavior. In Understanding Learning Disabilities: International and Multidisciplinary Views, eds. D. Duane and C. K. Leong. New York: Plenum Press.

Bradley, L., and Bryant, P. E. 1979. Independence of reading and spelling in backward and normal readers. Developmental Medical Child Neurology 21: 504-14.

Bradley, L., and Bryant, P. E. 1983. Categorizing sounds and learning to read - a causal connection. Nature 301:419-21.

Bradley, L., and Bryant, P. E. 1985. Rhyme and Reason in Reading and Spelling. Ann Arbor, MI: University of Michigan Press.

Brady, S., and Fowler, A. E. 1988. Phonological precursors to reading acquisition. In Preschool Prevention of Reading Failure, eds. R. L. Masland and M. W. Masland. Parkton, MD: York Press.

Brady, S., Poggie, E., and Rapala, M. 1989. Speech repetition abilities in children who differ in reading skill. Language and Speech 32:109-22.

Brady, S., Shankweiler, D., and Mann, V. 1983. Speech perception and memory coding in relation to reading ability. Journal of Experimental Child Psychology 35:345-67.

Breitmeyer, B. G. 1993. Sustained (P) and transient (M) channels in vision: A review and implications for reading. In Visual Processes in Reading and Reading Disabilities, eds. D. M. Willows, R. S. Kruk, and E. Corcos. Hillsdale, NJ: Lawrence Erlbaum Associates.

Brigance, A. H. 1977. Brigance Diagnostic Inventory of Basic Skills. North Billerica, MA: Curriculum Associates.

Brigance, A. H. 1991. *Brigance Diagnostic Inventory of Early Development*. North Billerica, MA: Curriculum Associates.

Brightman, M. F. 1986. An evaluation of the Impact of the Alphabetic Phonics Program in the Kinkaid School from 1983-1985. Houston, TX: Neuhaus Foundation.

Brown, A. L., Palincsar, A. S., and Armbruster, B. B. 1984. Instructing comprehension-fostering activities in interactive learning situations. In *Learning and Comprehension of Text*, eds. M. Mandl, N. L. Stein, and T. Trebasso. Hillsdale, NJ: Lawrence Erlbaum Associates.

Brown, J. 1992. *Stories for Older Students*. Millbury, MA: Wilson Language Training.

Brown, J. 1994. *Travels with Ted*. Millbury, MA: Wilson Language Training.

Bruck, M. 1990. Word recognition skills of adults with childhood diagnoses of dyslexia. *Developmental Psychology* 26:439-54.

Bruck, M., and Treiman, R. 1990. Phonological awareness and spelling in normal children and dyslexics: The case of initial consonant clusters. *Journal of Experimental Child Psychology* 50:156-78.

Bryant, N. D. and others. 1980. The effects of some instructional variables on the learning of handicapped and nonhandicapped populations: A review. *Integrative Reviews of Research: Vol. I*, 1-70. New York: Teachers College, Institute for the study of Learning Disabilities.

Bryant, P. E. 1968. Comments on the design of developmental studies of cross-modal matching and cross-modal transfer. *Cortex* 4:127-28.

Bryant, P., and Bradley, L. (1985). *Children's Reading Problems*. New York, Basil Blackwell

Bryant, S. 1979. Relative effectiveness of visual-auditory versus visual-auditory-kinesthetic-tactile procedures for teaching sight words and letter sounds to young disabled readers. Ed.D. diss., Teachers College, New York.

Byrne, B. 1981. Deficient syntactic control in poor readers: Is a weak phonetic memory code responsible? *Applied Psycholinguistics* 2:201-12.

Byrne, B., and Fielding-Barnsley, R. 1991. Evaluation of a program to teach phonemic awareness to young children. *Journal of Educational Psychology* 83:451-5.

Byrne, B., and Fielding-Barnsley, R. 1993. Evaluation of a program to teach phonemic awareness to young children: A 1-year follow-up. *Journal of Educational Psychology* 83:104-11.

Calfee, R. and Associates. 1981-1984. *The Book: Components of Reading Instruction*. Unpublished manuscript.

Calfee, R., and Henry, M. K., 1985. Project READ: An inservice model for training classroom teachers in effective reading instruction. In *The Effective Teaching of Reading: Theory and Practice*, ed. J. Hoffman. Newark, DE: International Reading Association.

Calfee, R., and Henry, M. In press. Strategy and skill in early reading acquisition. In *Essays in Memory of Dina Feitelson*, ed. J. Shimron.

Calfee, R., Henry, M. K., and Funderberg, J. 1988. A model for school change. In *Changing School Reading Programs*, eds. J. Samuels and D. Pearson. Newark, DE: International Reading Association.

Calfee, R., Lindamood, P., and Lindamood, C. 1973. Acoustic-phonetic skills and reading; Kindergarten through twelfth grade. *Journal of Educational Psychology* 64:293-98.

Calkins, L. M. 1983. *Lessons from a Child*. Portsmouth, NH: Heineman.

Cardon, L. R., Smith, S. D., Fulker, D. W., Kimberling, W. J., Pennington, B. F., and DeFries, J. C. 1994. Quantitative trait locus for reading disability on chromosome 6. *Science* 266:276-79.

Carlisle, J. F. 1993. Selecting approaches to vocabulary instruction for the reading disabled. *Learning Disabilities Research and Practice* 8:97-105.

Carpenter, D. 1983. Spelling error profiles of able and disabled readers. *Journal of Learning Disabilities* 16:102-4.

Carroll, J. B. 1963. A model of school learning. *Teachers College Record* 64:723-33.

Catts, H. W. 1986. Speech production/phonological deficits in reading disordered children. *Journal of Learning Disabilities* 19:504-8.

Catts, H. W. 1989. Defining dyslexia as a developmental language disorder. *Annals of Dyslexia* 39:50-64.

Center, Y., Wheldall, K., Freeman, L., Outhred, L., and McNaught, M. 1995. An evaluation of Reading Recovery. *Reading Research Quarterly* 30:240-63.

Chall, J. S. 1978. A decade of research on reading and learning disabilities. In *What Research Has to Say about Reading*, ed. J. Samuels. Newark, DE: International Reading Association.

Chall, J. S. 1983a. *Learning to Read: The Great Debate.* New York: McGraw-Hill.

Chall, J. S. 1983b. *Stages of Reading Development.* New York: McGraw-Hill.

Chall, J., Roswell, F. G., and Blumenthal, S. H. 1963. Auditory blending ability: A factor in success in beginning reading. *The Reading Teacher,* 17:113-18.

Childs, S. B., and Childs, R. S. 1971. *Sound Spelling.* Cambridge, MA: Educators Publishing Service.

Childs, S. B., and Childs, R. S. 1973. *The Childs Spelling System: The Rules.* Cambridge, MA: Educators Publishing Service.

Chomsky, C. 1971. Write first, read later. *Childhood Education* 47:296-99.

Chomsky, C. 1979. Approaching reading through invented spelling. *Theory and Practice of Early Reading*, eds. L. B. Resnick and P. A. Weaver. Hillsdale, NJ: Lawrence Erlbaum Associates.

Cicci, R. 1983. Disorders of written language. In *Progress in Learning Disabilities: Vol. 5*, ed. H. Myklebust. New York: Grune and Stratton.

Clark, D. B. 1988. *Dyslexia: Theory and Practice of Remedial Instruction.* Parkton, MD: York Press.

Clarke, L. K. 1988. Invented versus traditional spelling in first graders' writings: Effects on learning to spell and read. *Research in the Teaching of English* 22:281-309.

Clay, M. M. 1991. *Becoming Literate: The Construction of Inner Control.* Portsmouth, NH: Heineman.

Clay, M. M. 1992. A second chance to learn literacy. In *The Assessment of Special Education Needs: International Perspectives*, ed. T. Cline. London: Routledge.

Clay, M. M. 1993a. *Observation Survey.* Portsmouth, NH: Heineman.

Clay, M. M. 1993b. *Reading Recovery: A Guidebook for Teachers in Training.* Portsmouth, NH: Heineman.

Cone, T. E., Wilson, L. R., Bradley, C. M., and Reese, J. H. 1985. Characteristics of LD students in Iowa: An empirical investigation. *Learning Disability Quarterly* 3(3):211-20.

Connors, C. K. 1978. Critical review of Electroencephalographic and neuropsychological studies in dyslexia. In *Dyslexia: An Appraisal of Current Knowledge*, eds. A. L. Benton and D. Pearl. New York: Oxford University Press.

Cox, A. R. 1971. *Initial Reading Deck.* Cambridge, MA: Educators Publishing Service.

Cox, A. R. 1977. *Situation Spelling.* Cambridge, MA: Educators Publishing Service.

Cox, A. R. 1984. *Structures and Techniques.* Cambridge, MA: Educators Publishing Service.

Cox, A. R. 1985. Alphabetic phonics: An organization and expansion of Orton-Gillingham. *Annals of Dyslexia* 35:187-98.

Cox, A. R. 1989 *Situation Reading.* Cambridge, MA: Educators Publishing Service.

Cox, A. R. 1992. *Foundations for Literacy: Structures and Techniques.* Cambridge, MA: Educators Publishing Service.

Critchley, M. 1970. *The Dyslexic Child.* Springfield, IL: Thomas Publishing Company.

Cronbach, L. J., and Snow, R. B. 1976. *Aptitude and Instructional Methods.* New York: Irvington.

Cunningham, A., and Stanovich, K. 1990. Early spelling acquisition: Writing beats the computer. *Journal of Educational Psychology* 82:159-62.

Cunningham, P., and Cunningham, J. 1992. Making words: Enhancing the invented spelling-decoding connection. *The Reading Teacher* 46:106-15.

DeCecco, J. P. 1968. *The Psychology of Learning and Instruction.* Englewood Cliffs, NJ: Prentice-Hall.

DeFord, D. E., Lyans, C. A., and Pinnell, G. S. 1991. *Bridges to Literacy: Learning from Reading Recovery.* Portsmouth, NH: Heineman.

DeFries, J. C., Olson, R. K., Pennington, B. F., and Smith, S. D. 1991. Colorado reading project: An update. In *The Reading Brain: The Biological Basis of Dyslexia,* eds. D. Duane and D. Gray. Parkton, MD: York Press.

Denckla, M. B. 1977. Minimal brain dysfunction and dyslexia: Beyond diagnosis by exclusion. In *Topics in Child Neurology,* eds. M. E. Blau, I. Rapin, and M. Kinsbourne. New York: Spectrum Publishers.

Denckla, M. B. 1978. Critical review of Encephalographic and neuropsychological studies in dyslexia. In *Dyslexia: An Appraisal of Current Knowledge,* eds. A. L. Benton and D. Pearl. New York: Oxford University Press.

Denckla, M. B. 1979. Childhood learning disabilities. In *Clinical Neuropsychology,* eds. K. M. Heilman and E. Valenstein. New York: Oxford University Press.

Denckla, M. B. 1986. Issues of overlap and heterogeneity in dyslexia. In *Biobehavioral Measures of Dyslexia,* eds. D. B. Gray and J. F. Kavanagh. Parkton, MD: York Press.

Denckla, M. B. 1987. Applications of disconnection concepts to developmental dyslexia. *Annals of Dyslexia* 27:51-63.

Denckla, M. B., LeMay, M., and Chapman, C. A. 1985. Few CT scan abnormalities found even in neurologically impaired learning disabled children. *Journal of Learning Disabilities* 18:132-6.

Denckla, M. B., and Rudel, R. 1974. Rapid "automatized" naming of pictured objects. colors, letters, and numbers by normal children. *Cortex* 10:186-202.

Denckla, M. B., and Rudel, R. G. 1976a. Naming of object-drawings by dyslexic and other learning disabled children. *Brain and Language* 3:1-15.

Denckla, M. B., and Rudel, R. G. 1976b. Rapid automatized naming (R.A.N.): Dyslexia differentiated from other learning disabilities. *Neuropsychologia* 14:471-79.

Dobson, L. 1985. Learn to read by writing: A practical program for reluctant readers. *Teaching Exceptional Children* 18:30-36.

Dolch, E. W. 1952. *Basic Sight Vocabulary Cards.* Champaign, IL: Garrard Publishing Co.

Dole, J. A., Duffy, G. G., Roehler, L. R., and Pearson, P. D. 1991. Moving from the old to the new: Research on reading comprehension instruction. *Review of Educational Research* 61:239-64.

Duane, D. D. 1983a. Underachievement in written language: Auditory aspects. *Progress in Learning Disabilities: Vol. 5,* ed. H. H. Myklebust. New York: Grune and Stratton.

Duane, D. D. 1983b. Neurobiological correlates of reading disorders. *Journal of Educational Research* 77:5-15.

Duane, D. 1992. Responses to Yale study on the nature of dyslexia. *Perspectives on Dyslexia* 18 (2):14.

Durkin, D. 1978-1979. What classroom observations reveal about reading comprehension instruction. *Reading Research Quarterly* 14:481-533.

Dyer, P. 1992. Reading Recovery: A cost-effectiveness and educational-outcomes analysis. *Educational Services Research Spectrum* 10:10-19.

Dykman, R. A., and Ackerman, P. T. 1991. Attention deficit disorder and specific reading disability: Separate but often overlapping disorders. *Journal of Learning Disabilities* 24:96-103.

Eden, G. F., Stein, J. F., Wood, M. H., and Wood, F. B. 1995. Verbal and visual problems in reading disability. *Journal of Learning Disabilities* 28:272-90.

Ehri, L. C. 1989. Movement into word reading and spelling: How spelling contributes to reading. In *Reading and Writing Connections*, ed. J. M. Mason. Boston: Allyn and Bacon.

Ehri, L. C. 1992. Reconceptualizing the development of sight word reading and its relationship to recoding. In *Reading Acquisition*, eds. P. B. Gough, L. C. Ehri, and R. Treiman. Hillsdale, NJ: Lawrence Erlbaum Associates.

Ehri, L. C. 1995. Teachers need to know how word reading processes develop to teach reading effectively to beginners. In *Thinking and Literacy: The Mind at Work*, eds. C. N. Hedley, P. Antonacci, M. Rabinowitz. Hillsdale, NJ: Lawrence Erlbaum Associates.

Ehri, L. C., and Robbins, C. 1992. Beginners need some decoding skill to read words by analogy. *Reading Research Quarterly* 27:12-26.

Ehri, L. C., and Sweet, J. 1991. Fingerpoint-reading of memorized text: What enables beginners to process the print? *Reading Research Quarterly* 26:442-62.

Ehri, L. C., and Wilce, L. S. 1985. Movement into reading: Is the first stage of printed word learning visual or phonetic? *Reading Research Quarterly:* 163-79.

Ehri, L. C., and Wilce, L. S. 1987a. Cipher versus cue reading: An experiment in decoding acquisition. *Journal of Educational Psychology* 79:3-13.

Ehri, L. C., and Wilce, L. C. 1987b. Does learning to spell help beginners learn to read words? *Reading Research Quarterly* 18:47-65.

Elkind, J., Cohen, K., and Murray, C. 1993. Using computer-based readers to improve reading comprehension of students with dyslexia. *Annals of Dyslexia* 43:238-59.

Elkonin, D. B. 1963. The psychology of mastering the elements of reading. In *Educational Psychology in the U.S.S.R*, eds. B. Simon and J. Simon. London: Routledge and Kegan Paul.

Elkonin, D. B. 1973. U.S.S.R. In *Comparative Reading*, ed. J. Downing. New York: MacMillan.

Enfield, M. L. 1976. An alternate classroom approach to meeting special learning needs of children with reading problems. Ph.D. diss., University of Minnesota, Minneapolis, MN.

Enfield, M. L., and Greene, V. E. 1981. There is a skeleton in every closet. *Bulletin of The Orton Society* 31:189-98.

Enfield, M. L., and Greene, V. E. 1983. An evaluation of the results of standardized testing of elementary Project Read and SLD students based on district wide tests administered in October, 1983. Bloomington, MN: Bloomington Public Schools.

Enfield, M. L., and Greene, V. E. 1985. *Project Read Practical Spelling Guide*. Bloomington, MN: Bloomington Public Schools.

Engelmann, S., and Bruner, E. C. 1983. *Reading Mastery I and II: DISTAR Reading*. Chicago: Science Research Associates.

Engelmann, S., Becker, W. C., Hanner, S., and Johnson, G. 1978. *Corrective Reading: Decoding B*. Chicago: Science Research Associates.

Engelmann, S., Becker, W. C., Hanner, S., and Johnson, G. 1980. *Corrective Reading Series Guide*. Chicago: Science Research Associates.

Englert, C. S. 1990. Unraveling the mysteries of writing through strategy intervention. In *Intervention Research in Learning Disabilities*. eds. T. E. Scruggs and B. Y. L. Wong. New York: Springer-Verlag.

Englert, C. S., Raphael, T. E., and Anderson, L. M. 1992. Socially mediated instruction: Improving students' knowledge and talk about writing. *Elementary School Journal*, 92: 411-449.

Englert, C. S., Raphael, T. E., Anderson, L. M., Gregg, S. L., and Anthony, H. M. 1989. Exposition: Reading, writing, and the metacognitive knowledge of learning disabled students. *Learning Disabilities Research* 5:5-24.

Englert, C. S., and Thomas, C. C. 1987. Sensitivity to text structure in reading and writing: A comparison of learning disabled and nonhandicapped students. *Learning Disability Quarterly* 10:93-105.

Epstein, M. H. , and Cullinan, D. 1981. Project EXCEL: A behaviorally-oriented educational program for learning disabled pupils. *Education and Treatment of Children* 4:357-73.

Farnham-Diggory, S. 1986a. Commentary: Time, now, for a little serious complexity. In *Handbook of Cognitive, Social, and Neurological Aspects of Learning Disabilities: Vol. 1*, ed. S. P. Cecci. Hillsdale, NJ: Lawrence Erlbaum Associates.

Farnham-Diggory, S. 1986b. Introduction to the third revised edition. In *The Writing Road to Reading*, eds. R. B. Spalding and W. T. Spalding. New York: Quill/William Morrow.

Farnham-Diggory, S. 1990. *Schooling*. Cambridge, MA: Harvard University Press.

Farnham-Diggory, S. 1992. *The Learning Disabled Child*. Cambridge, MA: Harvard University Press.

Felton, R., Naylor, and Wood, F. 1990. Neuropsychological profile of adult dyslexics. *Brain and Language* 39:485-97.

Felton, R., and Wood, F. 1989. Cognitive deficits in reading disability and attention deficit disorder. *Journal of Learning Disabilities* 22:2-13.

Fernald, G. M. 1943. *Remedial Techniques in Basic School Subjects*. New York: McGraw-Hill.

Fernald, G. M., and Keller, H. 1921. The effect of kinesthetic factors in development of word recognition in the case of non-readers. *Journal of Educational Research* 4:355-77.

Feuerstein, R. 1979. *The Dynamic Assessment of Retarded Performers: The Learning-Potential Assessment Device, Theory, Instruments, and Techniques*. Baltimore: University Park Press.

Filipek, P., and Kennedy, D. 1991. Magnetic resonance imaging: Its role in the developmental disorders. In *The Reading Brain: The Biological Basis of Dyslexia*, eds. D. D. Duane and D. B. Gray. Parkton, MD: York Press.

Fleisher, L. S., Jenkins, J. R., and Pany, D. 1979. Effects on poor readers comprehension of training in rapid decoding. *Reading Research Quarterly* 15:30-48.

Flowers, D. L. 1993. Brain basis for dyslexia: A summary of work in progress. *Journal of Learning Disabilities* 26:575-82.

Foorman, B., Francis, D. J., and Fletcher, J. M. April 1995. Early interventions for children with reading disabilities and at risk for developing reading disabilities. Paper presented at the annual meeting of the American Educational Research Association in San Francisco.

Frankiewicz, R. G. 1984. An evaluation of the impact of the Alphabetic Phonics Program in Cypress Fairbanks Independent School District from 1981 through 1984. Houston, TX: Neuhaus Foundation.

Frankiewicz, R. G. 1985. An evaluation of the Alphabetic Phonics Program offered in the on-to-one mode. Houston, TX: Neuhaus Education Center.

Frederiksen, J. R., and others. 1983. A componential approach to training reading skills. Final Report. Cambridge, MA: Bolt, Beranek, and Newman.

French, J., Ellsworth, N. J., and Amoruso, M. Z. 1995. *Reading and Learning Disabilities: Theory and Practice*. New York: Garland.

Frith, U. 1985. Beneath the surface of developmental dyslexia. In *Surface Dyslexia: Neuropsychological and Cognitive Studies of Phonological Reading*, eds. K. E. Patterson, J. C. Marshall, and M. Coltheart. London: Lawrence Erlbaum Associates, Ltd.

Frith, U. 1986. A developmental framework for developmental dyslexia. *Annals of Dyslexia* 36:69-81.

Frostig, M. 1967. Testing as a basis for educational therapy. *Journal of Special Education* 2:15-34.

Frostig, M., Lefever, D. W., and Whittlesey, J. R. B. 1964. *The Marianne Frostig Developmental Test of Visual Perception*. Palo Alto, CA: Consulting Psychologists Press.

Furner, B. A. 1983. Developing handwriting ability: A perceptual learning process. *Topics in Learning and Learning Disabilities* 3:41-54.

Galaburda, A. M. 1983. Developmental dyslexia: Current anatomical research. *Annals of Dyslexia* 33: 41-54.

Galaburda, A. M. 1985. Developmental dyslexia: A review of biological interactions. *Annals of Dyslexia* 35:21-34.

Galaburda, A. M., and Kemper, T. L. 1979. Cytoarchitectonic abnormalities in developmental dyslexia: A case study. *Annals of Neurology* 6:94-100.

Galaburda, A. M., Rosen, G. F., and Sherman, G. D. 1989. The neural origin of developmental dyslexia: Implications for medicine, neurology and cognition. In *From Reading to Neurons*, ed. A. M. Galaburda. Cambridge, MA: The MIT Press.

Ganschow, L. 1984. Analysis of written language of a language learning disabled (dyslexic) college student and instructional implications. *Annals of Dyslexia* 34:271-84.

Gardner, H. 1983. *Frames of Mind: The Theory of Multiple Intelligences*. New York: Basic Books.

Gates, A. I. 1927. *The Improvement of Reading: A Program of Diagnostic and Remedial Methods*. New York: MacMillan.

Gersten, R., Woodward, J., and Darch, C. 1986. Direct Instruction: A research-based approach to curriculum design and teaching. *Exceptional Children* 53:17-31.

Geschwind, N. 1982. Why Orton was right. *Annals of Dyslexia* 32:13-30.

Geschwind, N. 1983. Biological associations of left-handedness. *Annals of Dyslexia* 33:29-40.

Geschwind, N. 1986. The biology of dyslexia: The unfinished manuscript. In *Biobehavioral Measures of Dyslexia*, eds. D. B. Gray and J. F. Kavanagh. Parkton, MD: York Press.

Geschwind, N., and Behan, P. 1982. Left-handedness: Association with immune disease, migraine, and developmental learning disorder. *Proceedings of the National Academy of Science* 79:5097-5100.

Gillingham, A., and Stillman, B. 1960. *Remedial Training for Children with Specific Disability in Reading, Writing, and Penmanship*. Cambridge, MA: Educators Publishing Service.

Gillon, G., and Dodd, B. 1994. A prospective study of the relationship between phonological, semantic and syntactic skills and specific reading disability. *Reading and Writing: An Interdisciplinary Journal* 6:321-45.

Ginsburg, H. P., and Baroody, A. J. 1990. *Test of Early Mathematics Ability*. Austin, TX: PRO-ED.

Gittelman, R. 1983. Treatment of reading disorders. In *Developmental Neuropsychiatry*, ed. M. Rutter. New York: Guilford Press.

Glass, G. G., and Glass, E. W. 1976. *Glass Analysis for Decoding Only: Teachers Guide*. Garden City, NY: Easier to Learn.

Glass, G. G., and Glass, E. W. 1978a. *Glass Analysis for Decoding Only: Easy Starts Kit*. Garden City, NY: Easier to Learn.

Glass, G. G., and Glass, E. W. 1978b. *Glass Analysis for Decoding Only: Quick and Easy Alphabet Program*. Garden City, NY: Easier to Learn.

Godfrey, J. J., Syrdal-Lasky, A. K., Millaj, K. K., and Knox, C. M. 1981. Performance of dyslexic children on speech perception tests. *Journal of Experimental Child Psychology* 32:401-24.

Goodman, K. 1967. Reading: A psycholinguistic guessing game. *Journal of the Reading Specialist* 6:126-35.

Goodman, K. 1993. *Phonics Phacts*. Portsmouth, NH: Heineman.

Gordon, J., Vaughn, S., and Schumm, J. S. 1993. Spelling interventions: A review of literature and implications for instruction for students with learning disabilities. *Learning Disabilities Research and Practice* 8:175-81.

Goswami, U. 1986. Children's use of analogy in learning to read: A developmental study. *Journal of Experimental Child Psychology* 42:73-83.

Goswami, U. 1988. Orthographic analogies and reading development. *Quarterly Journal of Experimental Psychology* 40A:239-68.

Goswami, U., and Mead, F. 1992. Onset and rime awareness and analogies in reading. *Reading Research Quarterly* 27:152-62.

Gough, P., and Hillinger, M. L. 1980. Learning to read: An unnatural act. *Bulletin of The Orton Society* 30:179-96.

Gough, P. B. and Tunmer, W. E. 1986. Decoding, reading and reading disability. *Remedial and Special Education* 7:6-10.

Goulandris, N. K., and Snowling, M. J. 1991. Visual memory deficits: A plausible cause of developmental dyslexia? Evidence from a single case study. *Cognitive Neuropsychology* 8:127-54.

Grant, S. M. 1985. The kinesthetic approach to teaching: Building a foundation. *Journal of Learning Disabilities* 18:455-62.

Graves, D. H. 1978. *Balance the Basics: Let Them Write*. New York: Ford Foundation.

Graves, D. H. 1983. *Writing: Teachers and Children at Work*. Portsmouth, NH: Heineman.

Graves, D. H., and Stuart, V. 1985. *Write From the Start*. New York: New American Library.

Greenbaum, C. R. 1987. *The Spellmaster Assessment and Teaching System*. Austin, TX: PRO-ED.

Greene, V. E., and Enfield, M. L. 1981. *Project Read Affix Guide*. Bloomington, MN: Bloomington Public Schools.

Greene, V. E., and Enfield, M. L. 1985a. *Project Read Reading Guide: Phase I*. Bloomington, MN: Bloomington Public Schools.

Greene, V. E., and Enfield, M. L. 1985b. *Project Read Reading Guide: Phase II*. Bloomington, MN: Bloomington Public Schools.

Guyer, B. P., Banks, S. R., and Guyer, K. E. 1993. Spelling improvement by college students who are dyslexic. *Annals of Dyslexia* 43:186-93.

Hammill, D. 1985. Detroit Tests of Learning Aptitude -2. Austin, TX: PRO-ED.

Hammill, D. D., and Larsen, S. C. 1978. *The Test of Written Language*. Austin, TX: PRO-ED.

Hanna, P. R., Hodges, R. E., Hanna, J. L., and Rudolph, E. H. 1966. Phoneme-Grapheme Correspondence as Cues to Spelling Improvement. Washington, D.C.: Department of Health, Education, and Welfare, Office of Education.

Hansen, J. 1987. *When Writers Read*. Portsmouth, NH: Heineman.

Hardyck, C., and Petrinovich, L. F. 1977. Left-handedness. *Psychological Bulletin* 84-385-404.

Haring, N. G., and Bateman, B. 1977. *Teaching the Learning Disabled Child*. Englewood Cliffs, NJ: Prentice-Hall.

Haring, N. G., Bateman, B., and Carnine, D. 1977. Direct Instruction—DISTAR. In *Teaching the Learning Disabled Child*, eds. N. G. Haring and B. Bateman. Englewood Cliffs, NJ: Prentice-Hall.

Harste, J. C. 1985. Becoming a nation of language learners: Beyond risk. In *Toward Practical Theory: A State of Practice Assessment of Reading Comprehension Instruction. Final Report*, eds. J. C. Harste and D. Stevens. Bloomington, IN: Indiana University.

Henk, W. A., Helfeldt, J. P., and Platt, J. M. 1986. Developing reading fluency in learning disabled students. *Teaching Exceptional Children* 12:202-6.

Henry, M. 1988. Beyond phonics: Integrated decoding and spelling instruction based on word origin and structure. *Annals of Dyslexia* 38:259-77.

Henry, M. 1989. Children's word structure knowledge: Implications for decoding and spelling instruction. *Reading and Writing: An Interdisciplinary Journal* 2:135-52.

Henry, M. 1990. *Words: Integrated Decoding and Spelling Instruction Based on Word Origin and Word Structure*. Los Gatos, CA: Lex Press.

Henry, M. and Redding, N. C. 1990. *Tutor 1, Tutor 2, Tutor 3*. Los Gatos, CA: Lex Press.

Herr, C. M. 1984. Using Corrective Reading with adults. *Direct Instruction News*, Spring: 3-4.

Hill, J. R. 1981. *Measurement and Evaluation in the Classroom*. Columbus, OH: Merrill.

Hillocks, G. 1984. What works in teaching composition: A meta-analysis of treatment studies. *American Journal of Education* 93:133-70.

Hinshelwood, J. 1896. A case of dyslexia: A peculiar form of word blindness. *Lancet* 2:1451-54.

Hinshelwood, J. 1917. *Congenital Word Blindness*. London: H. K. Lewis.

Hirsch, E., and Niedermeyer, F. C. 1973. The effects of tracing prompts and discrimination training on kindergarten handwriting performance. *Journal of Educational Research* 67:81-83.

Hiscock, M., and Kinsbourne, M. 1982. Laterality and dyslexia: A critical view. *Annals of Dyslexia* 32:177-228.

Hohn, W. E., and Ehri, L. C. 1983. Do alphabet letters help prereaders acquire phonemic segmentation skill? *Journal of Educational Psychology* 75:752-62.

Hooper, S. R., Montgomery, J., Swartz, C., Reed, M. S., Sandler, A.D., Levine, M. D., Watson, T. E., and Wasileski, T. 1994. Measurement of written language expression. In *Frames of Reference for the Assessment of Learning Disabilities*, ed. G. R. Lyon. Baltimore, MD: Paul H. Brookes Publishing Co.

Hoover, W. A. October 1994. The simple view of reading: Analyses based on a monolingual sample. Paper presented at NATO Advanced Study Institute: Cognitive and Linguistic Bases of Reading, Writing, and Spelling, in Alvor-Algarve, Portugal.

Horn, E. 1960. Spelling. In *Encyclopedia for Educational Research*, ed. W. S. Monroe . New York: Macmillan.

Howard, M. 1982. Utilizing oral-motor feedback in auditory conceptualization. *Journal of Educational Neuropsychology* 2:24-35.

Howard, M. 1986. Effects of pre-reading training in auditory conceptualization on subsequent reading achievement. Ph.D. diss., Brigham Young University.

Hulme, C. 1981. *Reading Retardation and Multi-Sensory Teaching*. London: Routledge and Kegan Paul.

Hulme, C. 1988. The implausibility of low-level visual deficits as a cause of children's reading difficulties. *Cognitive Neuropsychology* 5:369-74.

Hulme, C., and Bradley, L. 1984. An experimental study of multisensory teaching with normal and retarded readers. In *Dyslexia: A Global Issue*, eds. R. Malatesha and H. Whitaker. The Hague: Martinus Nijhoff.

Hunt-Berg, M., Rankin, J. L., and Beukelman, D. R. 1994. Ponder the possibilities: Computer-supported writing for struggling writers. *Learning Disabilities Research and Practice* 9:169-78.

Hutchinson, L., Selig, H., and Young, N. 1990. A success story: A large urban district offers a working model for implementing multisensory teaching into the resource and regular classroom. *Annals of Dyslexia* 40:79-96.

Inhelder, B., and Piaget, J. 1958. *The Growth of Logical Thinking from Childhood to Adolescence*. New York: Basic Books.

Institute for Training and Research in Auditory Conceptualization (INTRAC). 1983. *Santa Monica Preventive Study*. San Luis Obispo, CA.

Iverson, S., and Tunmer, W. E. 1993. Phonological processing skills and the reading recovery program. *Journal of Educational Psychology* 85:112-26.

Jensen, A. R. 1980. *Bias in Mental Testing*. New York: Macmillan.

Johnson, D. J., and Grant, J. O. 1989. Written narratives of normal and learning disabled children. *Annals of Dyslexia* 39: 140-57.

Johnson, D. J., and Myklebust, H. R. 1967. *Learning Disabilities.* New York: Grune and Stratton.

Johnson, W. T. 1977. *The Johnson Handwriting Program.* Cambridge, MA: Educators Publishing Service.

Jorm, A. F. 1983. Specific reading retardation and working memory: A review. *British Journal of Psychology* 74:311-42.

Juel, C., Griffeth, P. L., and Gough, P. B. 1985. A longitudinal study of the changing relationships of word recognition, spelling, reading comprehension, and writing from first to second grade. Paper presented at the Annual Meeting of the American Educational Research Association, Chicago, April, 1985.

Just, M. A., and Carpenter, P. A. 1980. Theory of reading: From eye fixations to comprehension. *Psychological Review* 87:3329-54.

Kaplan, E., Goodglass, H., and Weintraub, S. 1983. *Boston Naming Test.* Philadelphia: Lea and Febiger.

Karweit, N. 1985. Time spent, time needed, and adaptive instruction. In *Adapting Instruction to Individual Differences,* eds. M. C. Wang and H. I. Walberg. Berkeley, CA: McCutchan.

Kaufman, A., and Kaufman, N. 1983. *Kaufman Assessment Battery for Children.* Circle Pines, MN: American Guidance.

Kaufman, A., and Kaufman, N. 1985. *Kaufman Test of Educational Achievement.* Circle Pines, MN: American Guidance.

Kavanagh, J. F., and Truss, T. J. eds. 1988. *Learning Disabilities: Proceedings of the National Conference.* Parkton, MD: York Press.

Keogh, B. D., and Pelland, M. 1985. Vision training revisited. *Journal of Learning Disabilities* 18:228-36.

Kibel, M. and Miles, T. R. 1994. Phonological errors in spelling of taught dyslexic children. In *Reading Development and Dyslexia,* eds. C. Hulme and M. Snowling. San Diego: Singular Publishing Group.

King, D. H. 1985. *Writing Skills for the Adolescent.* Cambridge, MA: Educators Publishing Service.

King, D. H. 1986. *Keyboarding Skills.* Cambridge, MA: Educators Publishing Service.

Kinsbourne, M., and Hiscock, M. 1981. Cerebral lateralization and cognitive development: Conceptual and methodological issues. In *Neuropsychological Assessment of the School-Age Child,* eds. G. W. Hynd and J. E. Obrzut. New York: Grune and Stratton.

Kinsbourne, M., and Warrington, E. K. 1963. Developmental factors in reading and reading backwardness. *British Journal of Psychology* 54:145-56.

Kintsch, W., and van Dijk, T. A. 1978. Toward a model of text and comprehension production. *Psychological Review* 85:363-94.

Kirk, S., McCarthy, J., and Kirk, W. 1968. *Illinois Test of Psycholinguistic Abilities.* Champaign, IL: University of Illinois Press.

Kirk, U. 1981. The development and use of rules in the acquisition of perceptual motor skills. *Child Development* 52:299-305.

Kuder, S. J. 1990. Effectiveness of the DISTAR reading program for children with learning disabilities. *Journal of Learning Disabilities* 23:69-71.

LaBerge, D., and Samuels. S. J. 1974. Toward a theory of automatic information processing in reading. *Cognitive Psychology* 6:293-323.

Leinhardt, G., Zigmond, N., and Cooley, W. W. 1980. Reading instruction and its effects. Paper presented at the Annual Meeting of the American Educational Research Association, April, 1980, Boston, MA.

Lesgold, A. M., and Resnick, L. B. 1982. How reading difficulties develop: Perspectives from a longitudinal study. In *Theory and Research in Learning Disabilities*, eds. R. F. Mulcahy and A. E. Wall. New York: Plenum Press.

Liberman, I. Y. 1973. Segmentation of the spoken word and reading acquisition. *Bulletin of The Orton Society* 23:65-77.

Liberman, I. Y. 1984. A language-directed view of reading and its disabilities. *Thalamus* 4:1-41.

Liberman, I. Y., Liberman, A. M., Mattingly, I., and Shankweiler, D. 1983. Orthography and the beginning reader. In *Orthography, Reading, and Dyslexia*, eds. J. P. Kavanagh and R. L. Venezky. Baltimore: University Park Press.

Liberman, I. Y., and Shankweiler, D. 1979. Speech, the alphabet, and teaching to read. In *Theory and Practice of Early Reading: Vol 2.*, eds. L. B. Resnick and P. A. Weaver. Hillsdale, NJ: Lawrence Erlbaum Associates.

Liberman, I. Y., and Shankweiler, D. 1985. Phonology and the problems of learning to read and write. *Remedial and Special Education* 6:8-17.

Liberman, I. Y., Shankweiler, D., Fischer, F. W., and Carter, B. 1974. Explicit syllable and phoneme segmentation in the young child. *Journal of Experimental Child Psychology* 18:201-12.

Liberman, I. Y., Shankweiler, D., Liberman, A. M., Fowler, C., and Fischer, F. W. 1977. Phonetic segmentation and recoding in the beginning reader. In *Toward a Psychology of Reading*, eds. A. S. Rober and D. L. Scarborough. Hillsdale, NJ: Lawrence Erlbaum Associates.

Lichter, J. H., and Roberge, L. P. 1979. First grade intervention for reading achievement of high risk children. *Bulletin of The Orton Society* 29:238-44.

Lindamood, P. C. 1994. Issues in researching the link between phonological awareness, learning disabilities, and spelling. In *Frames of Reference for the Assessment of Learning Disabilities*, ed. G. R. Lyon. Baltimore, MD: Paul H. Brookes Publishing Co.

Lindamood, P. C., Bell, N., and Lindamood, P. 1992. Issues in phonological awareness assessment. *Annals of Dyslexia* 42:242-59.

Lindamood, C. H., and Lindamood, P. C. 1975. *The A.D.D. Program, Auditory Discrimination in Depth: Books 1 and 2*. Austin, TX: PRO-ED..

Lindamood, C. H., and Lindamood, P. C. 1979. *The LAC Test: Lindamood Auditory Conceptualization Test*. Chicago: Riverside.

Lindamood, P. C., and Lindamood, C. H. 1980. Diagnosing and remediating auditory conceptual dysfunction. *Proceedings of the 18th Congress of the International Association of Logopedics and Phoniatrics* 2:148-77.

Lipa, S. B. 1984. Reading disabilities: A new look at an old issue. *Annual Review of Learning Disabilities* 2:51-55.

Lipson, M. Y., and Wixson, K. K. 1986. Reading disability research: A new look at an old issue. *Review of Educational Research* 56:111-36.

Livingstone, M. 1993. Parallel processing in the visual system and the brain: Is one subsystem selectively affected in dyslexia? In *Dyslexia and Development: Neurobiological Aspects of Extra-Ordinary Brains*, ed. A. M. Galaburda. Cambridge, MA: Harvard University Press.

Lloyd, J., Epstein, M., and Cullinan, D. 1981. Direct teaching for learning disabilities. In *Developmental Theory and Research in Learning Disabilities*, eds. J. Gottlieb and S. S. Strichart. Baltimore: University Park Press.

Lovegrove, W. 1992. The visual deficit hypothesis. In *Learning Disabilities: Nature, Theory, and Treatment*, eds. N. Singh and I. Beale. New York: Springer-Verlag.

Lovegrove, W. J., and Williams, M. J. 1993. Visual temporal processing deficits in specific reading disability. In *Visual Processes in Reading and Reading Disabilities*, eds. D. M. Willows, R. S. Kruk, and E. Corcos. Hillsdale, NJ: Lawrence Erlbaum Associates.

Lovitt, T. C., and DeMier, D. M. 1984. An evaluation of the Slingerland method with LD youngsters. *Journal of Learning Disabilities* 17:267-72.

Lubs, H., Duara, R., Levin, B., Jallad, B., Lubs, M., Rabin, M., Kushch, A., and Gross-Glenn, K. 1991. Dyslexia subtypes: Genetics, behavior, and brain imaging. In *The Reading Brain: The Biological Basis of Dyslexia*, eds. D. D. Drake and D. B. Gray. Parkton, MD: York Press.

Lubs, H., Rabin, M., Feldman, E., Jallud, B. J., Kushch, and Gross-Glenn, K. 1993. Familial dyslexia and medical findings in eleven three-generation families. *Annals of Dyslexia* 43:44-60.

Lundberg, I. 1985. Longitudinal studies of reading and reading difficulties in Sweden. In *Reading Research: Advances in Theory and Practice: Vol. 4*, eds. G. E. MacKinnon and T. G. Waller. New York: Academic Press.

Lundberg, I., Frost, J., and Petersen, O. P. 1988. Effects of an extensive program for stimulating phonological awareness in preschool children. *Reading Research Quarterly* 23:263-84.

Lyon, G. R. 1985. Identification and remediation of learning disability subtypes: Preliminary findings. *Learning Disabilities Focus* 1:21-35.

Lyon, G. R. ed. 1994. *Frames of Reference for the Assessment of Learning Disabilities*. Baltimore, MD: Paul H. Brookes Publishing Co.

Lyons, C. A., Pinnell, G. S., and DeFord, D. E. 1993. *Partners in Learning: Teachers and Children in Reading Recovery*. New York: Teachers College Press.

MacArthur, C. A., and Graham, S. 1988. Learning disabled students composing under three methods of text production: Handwriting, word processing, and dictation. *The Journal of Special Education* 21:22-42.

MacArthur, C. A., and Schneiderman, B. 1986. Learning disabled students difficulties in learning to use a word processor: Implications for instruction and software evaluation. *Journal of Learning Disabilities* 19:248-53.

MacArthur, C. A., Schwartz, and Graham, S. 1991. A model for writing instruction: Integrating word processing and strategy instruction into a process approach to writing. *Learning Disabilities Research and Practice* 6:230-6.

Makar, B. W. 1985. *Mac and Tab* (Primary Phonics series). Cambridge, MA: Educators Publishing Service.

Mann, V. A. 1986. Why some children encounter reading problems: The contribution of difficulties with language processing and phonological sophistication to early reading disability. In *Psychological and Educational Perspectives on Learning Disabilities*, eds. J. K. Torgeson and B. Y. L. Wong. New York: Academic Press.

Mann, V. A., and Liberman, I. Y. 1984. Phonological awareness and verbal short-term memory. *Journal of Learning Disabilities* 17:592-99.

Mann, V. A., Liberman, I. Y., and Shankweiler, D. 1980. Children's memory for sentences and word strings in relation to reading ability. *Memory and Cognition* 8:329-35.

Mann, V. A., Shankweiler, D., and Smith, S. 1984. The association between comprehension of spoken sentences and early reading ability: The role of phonetic representation. *Journal of Child Language* 11:627-43.

Mann, V. A., Tobin, P., and Wilson, R. 1987. Measuring phonological awareness through the invented spellings of kindergarten children. *Merrill-Palmer Quarterly* 33:365-91.

Maria, K. 1987. A new look at comprehension instruction for disabled readers. *Annals of Dyslexia* 37:264-78.

Maria, K. 1990. *Reading Comprehension Instruction: Issues and Strategies*. Parkton, MD: York Press.

Markwardt, F. C. 1989. *Peabody Individualized Achievement Test - Revised*. Circle Pines, MN: American Guidance.

Marsh, G., Freidman, M., Welch, V., and Desberg, P. 1981. A cognitive-developmental theory of reading acquisition. In *Reading Research: Advances in Theory and Practice: Vol. 3*, eds. G. Mackinnon and T. G. Waller. New York: Academic Press.

Martin, J. H. 1985. The Writing to Read system and reading difficulties: Some preliminary observations. In *Understanding Learning Disabilities*, eds. D. D. Duane and C. K. Leong. New York: Plenum Press.

Martin, J. H., and Friedberg, A. 1986. *Writing to Read*. New York: Warner Books.

Masonheimer, P. E., Drum, P. A., and Ehri, L. C. 1984. Does environmental print identification lead children into word reading? *Journal of Reading Behavior* 16:257-72.

McCulloch, C. 1985. The Slingerland approach: Is it effective in a specific language disability classroom? M.A. thesis, Seattle Pacific University, Seattle, WA.

McCully, E. A. 1988. *The Grandma Mix-up*. New York: Harper.

Menynuk, P., and Flood, J. 1981. Linguistic competence, reading, writing problems, and remediation. *Bulletin of The Orton Society* 31:13-28.

Metzger, R. L., and Werner, D. B. 1984. Use of visual training for reading disabilities: A review. *Pediatrics* 73:824-29.

Meyer, L. A. 1984. Long-term academic effects of the direct instruction project Follow-Through. *Elementary School Journal* 84:380-94.

Meyer, L. A., Gersten, R. M., and Gutkin, J. 1983. Direct Instruction: A Project Follow-Through success story in an inner-city school. *Elementary School Journal* 84:241-52.

Moats, L. C. 1983. A comparison of the spelling errors of older dyslexic and second grade normal children. *Annals of Dyslexia* 33:121-39.

Moats, L. C. 1993. Spelling error interpretation: Beyond the phonetic/dysphonetic dichotomy. *Annals of Dyslexia* 43:174-85.

Moats, L. C. 1994a. Assessment of spelling. In *Frames of Reference for the Assessment of Learning Disabilities*, ed. G. R. Lyon. Baltimore, MD: Paul H. Brookes Publishing Co.

Moats, L. C. 1994b. The missing foundation in teacher education: Knowledge of the structure of spoken and written language. *Annals of Dyslexia* 44:81-102.

Mokros, J. R., and Russell, S. J. 1986. Learner-centered software: A survey of micro-computer use with special needs students. *Journal of Learning Disabilities* 19:185-90.

Montessori, M. 1964. *The Montessori Method*. New York: Shocken Books.

Morais, J. Cary, L., Alegria, J., and Bertelson, P. 1979. Does awareness of speech as a sequence of phones arise spontaneously? *Cognition* 7:323-31.

Morocco, C. C., and Neuman, S. B. 1986. Word processors and the acquisition of writing strategies. *Journal of Learning Disabilities* 19:243-47.

Morris, D. 1981. Concept of word: A developmental phenomenon in the beginning reading and writing processes. *Language Arts* 58:659-68.

Morris, D. 1992. *Case Studies in Teaching Beginning Readers: The Howard Street Tutoring Manual*. Boone, NC: Fieldstream Publications.

Morris, D., and Perney, J. 1984. Developmental spelling as a predictor of first-grade reading achievement. *The Elementary School Journal* 84:441-57.

Murphy, R. T., and Appel, L. R. 1984. *Evaluation of the Writing to Read Instructional System*. Princeton, NJ: Educational Testing Service.

Myklebust, H. R. 1965. *Development and Disorders of Written Language: Vol. 1. Picture Story Language Test*. New York: Grune and Stratton.

Myklebust, H. R., and Johnson, D. J. 1962. Dyslexia in children. *Exceptional Children* 29:14-25.

Nockleby, D. M., and Galbraith, G. G. 1984. Developmental dyslexia subtypes and the Boder Test of Reading-Spelling Patterns. *Journal of Psychoeducational Assessment* 2:91-100.

O'Connor, P. D., Sofo, F., Kendall, L., and Olsen, G. 1990. Reading disabilities and the effects of colored filters. *Journal of Learning Disabilities* 23:597-603.

Oakhill, J., and Garnham, A. 1988. *Becoming a Skilled Reader*. Oxford: Basil Blackwell.

Obrzut, J. E., and Boliek, C. A. 1986. Lateralization characteristics in learning disabled children. *Journal of Learning Disabilities* 19:308-14.

Olson, R. K., Conners, F. A., and Rack, J. P. 1991. Eye movements in normal and dyslexic readers. In *Vision and Visual Dyslexia*, ed. J. F. Stein. London: Macmillan.

Olson, R. K., Forsberg, H., Wise, B., and Rack, J. 1994. Measurement of Word recognition, orthographic, and phonological skills. In *Frames of Reference for the Assessment of Learning Disabilities*, ed. G. R. Lyon. Baltimore, MD: Paul H. Brookes Publishing Co.

Olson, R. K., Kliegl, R., Davidson, B. J., and Folz, G. 1985. Individual and developmental differences in reading disability. In *Reading Research: Advances in Theory and Practice: Vol 4*, eds. C. E. MacKinnon and T. G. Waller. New York: Academic Press.

Olson, R. K., Wise, B. Conners, F., Rack, J. P., and Fulker, D. 1989. Specific deficits in component reading and language skills: Genetic and environmental influences. *Journal of Learning Disabilities* 22:339-48.

Olson, R. K., Wise, B., Conners, and Rack, J. P. 1990. Organization, heritability, and remediation of component word recognition and language skills in disabled readers. In *Reading and its Development: Component Skills Approaches*, eds. T. H. Carr and B. A. Levy. New York: Academic Press.

Orton, J. 1964. *A Guide to Teaching Phonics*. Cambridge, MA: Educators Publishing Service.

Orton, J. 1966. The Orton-Gillingham approach. In *The Disabled Reader*, ed. J. Money. Baltimore: The Johns Hopkins University Press.

Orton, S. T. 1928. Specific reading disability - strephosymbolia. *The Journal of the American Medical Association*, 90:1095-9.

Orton, S. T. 1937. *Reading, Writing, and Speech Problems in Children*. New York: Norton.

Orton Dyslexia Society. November 1994. Definition of the committee of members. In *Dyslexia: Newsletter of the New York Branch of the Orton Dyslexia Society*, ed. A. Bailin. Winter 1994.

Otto, W., Wolf, A., and Eldridge, R. G. 1984. Managing instruction. In *Handbook of Reading Research*, ed. P. D. Pearson. New York: Longman.

Palincsar, A. S. 1986. The role of dialogue in providing scaffolded instruction. *Educational Psychologist* 21:73-98.

Palincsar, A., and Brown, A. 1983. Reciprocal teaching of comprehension-monitoring activities (Technical Report No. 269). Urbana, IL: The University of Illinois, Center for the Study of Reading.

Palincsar, A., and Brown, A. 1985. Reciprocal teaching: A means to a meaningful end. In *Reading Education: Foundations for a Literate America*, eds. J. Osborn, P. T. Wilson, and R. C. Anderson. Lexington, MA: D. C. Heath.

Patterson, K. E., Marshall, J. C., and Coltheart, M. 1985. eds. *Surface Dyslexia: Neuropsychological and Cognitive Studies of Phonological Reading*. Hillsdale, NJ: Lawrence Erlbaum Associates.

Pavlidis, G. T. 1985. Eye movements in dyslexia: Their diagnostic significance. *Journal of Learning Disabilities* 18:42-50.

Pearson, P. D., and Fielding, L. 1991. Comprehension instruction. In *Handbook of Reading Research, Volume II*, eds. R. Barr, M. L. Kamil, P. B. Mosenthal, and P. D. Pearson. New York: Longman.

Peister, P., Fadiman, S., Pierce, K., and Fayne, H. 1978-1980. Integrative review of basic reading skills. *Integrative Reviews of Research: Vol. 1*. New York: Teachers College, Institute for the Study of Learning Disabilities.

Pennington, B. F. 1991. *Diagnosing Learning Disorders: A Neuropsychological Framework*. New York: Guilford Press.

Perfetti, C. A. 1984. Reading acquisition and beyond: Decoding includes cognition. *American Journal of Education* 93:40-60.

Perfetti, C. A. 1985a. Continuities in reading acquisition, reading skills, and reading disability. *Remedial and Special Education* 7:11-21.

Perfetti, C. A. 1985b. *Reading Ability*. New York: Oxford University Press.

Perfetti, C. A., Finger, E., and Hogaboam, T. 1978. Sources of vocalization latency differences between skilled and less skilled young readers. *Journal of Educational Psychology* 70:730-9.

Perfetti, C. A., and Hogaboam, T. 1975. Relationship between single word decoding and reading comprehension skill. *Journal of Educational Psychology* 67:461-69.

Perfetti, C. A., and Lesgold, A. M. 1979. Coding and comprehension in skilled reading and implications for reading instruction. In *Theory and Practice of Early Reading: Vol. 1*, eds. L.B. Resnick and P. A. Weaver. Hillsdale , NJ: Lawrence Erlbaum Associates.

Perfetti, C. A., and Roth, S. 1981. Some of the interactive processes in reading and their role in reading skill. In *Interactive Processes in Reading*, eds. A. M. Lesgold and C. A. Perfetti. Hillsdale, NJ: Lawrence Erlbaum Associates.

Pflaum, S. W., Walberg, H. J., Karegianes, M. L., and Rasher, P. 1980. Reading instruction: A quantitative analysis. *Educational Researcher* 9:12-18.

Piaget, J. 1970. *Structuralism*. New York: Basic Books.

Pinnell, G. S., Lyons, C. A., DeFord, D. E., Bryk, A. S., and Seltzer, M. 1994. Comparing instructional models for the literacy education of high-risk first graders. *Reading Research Quarterly* 29:8-39.

Poe, L. B. 1983. The effects of a supplemental intervention training program on first graders who lack segmentation ability. Ed.D. diss., University of Southern Mississippi, Hattiesburg, MS.

Pollatsek, A. 1993. Eye movements in reading. In *Visual Processes in Reading and Reading Disabilities*, eds. D. M. Willows, R. S. Kruk, and E. Corcos. Hillsdale, NJ: Lawrence Erlbaum Associates.

Polloway, E. A., and Epstein, M. H. 1986. The use of Corrective Reading (SRA) with mildly handicapped students. *Direct Instruction News*. 2-3.

Poplin, M. 1983. Assessing developmental writing abilities. *Topics in Learning and Learning Disabilities* 3:63-75.

Poplin, M., Gray, R., Larsen, S., Banikowski, A., and Mehring, T. 1980. A comparison of components of written expression abilities in learning disabled and non-disabled students at three grade levels. *Learning Disability Quarterly* 3:46-59.

Pressley, M., El-Dinary, P. B., Gaskins, I., Schuder, T., Bergman, J. L., Almasi, J., and Brown, R. 1992. Beyond direct explanation: Transactional Instruction of reading comprehension strategies. *The Elementary School Journal* 92:513-55.

Pressley, M., Gaskins, I. W., Cunicelli, E. A., Burdick, N. J., Schaub-Matt, M., Lee, D. S., and Powell, N. 1991. Strategy instruction at Benchmark School: A faculty interview study. *Learning Disability Quarterly* 14:19-48.

Pressley, M., Goodchild, F., Fleet, J., Zajchowski, R., and Evans, E. D. 1989. The challenges of classroom reading instruction. *Elementary School Journal* 89:301-42.

Pressley, M., Johnson, C. J., Symons, S., McGoldrick, J. A., and Kurita, J. A. 1989. Strategies that improve children's memory and of text. *Elementary School Journal* 89:3-32.

Punnet, A. F., and Steinhauer, G. D. 1984. Relationship between reinforcement and eye-movements during ocular motor training with learning disabled children. *Journal of Learning Disabilities* 17:16-20.

Rack, J. P., Snowling, M. J., and Olson, R. K. 1992. The nonword reading deficit in developmental dyslexia: A review. *Reading Research Quarterly* 27:28-53.

Raphael, T. E., and Englert, C. S. 1990. Reading and Writing: Partners in constructing meaning. *The Reading Teacher* 43:388-400.

Rashotte, C. A. 1983. Repeated reading and reading fluency in learning disabled children. Ph.D. diss., The Florida State University, Tallahassee, Fl.

Rashotte, C. A., and Torgesen, J. K. 1985. Repeated reading and reading fluency in learning disabled children. *Reading Research Quarterly* 20:180-88.

Rasinski, T. V. 1995. Commentary on the effects of Reading Recovery: A response to Pinnell, Lyons, DeFord, Bryk, and Seltzer. *Reading Research Quarterly* 30:264-70.

Rasmussen, D. E., and Goldberg, L. 1976. *SRA Basic Reading*. Chicago, Il: Science Research Associates.

Raynor, K. 1985. The role of eye movements in learning to read and reading disability. *Remedial and Special Education* 6:53-60.

Raynor, K. 1993. Directions for research and theory. In *Visual Processes in Reading and Reading Disabilities*, eds. D. M. Willows, R. S. Kruk, and E. Corcos. Hillsdale, NJ: Lawrence Erlbaum Associates.

Raynor, K., and Pollatsek, A. 1987. Eye movements in reading: A tutorial review. In *Attention and Performance XII: The Psychology of Reading*, ed. M. Coltheart. London: Lawrence Erlbaum Associates Ltd.

Read, C. 1970. Children's perceptions of the sounds of English phonology from three to six. Ph.D. diss., Harvard Graduate School of Education, Cambridge, MA.

Read, C. 1971. Preschool children's knowledge of English phonology. *Harvard Educational Review* 41:1-34.

Read, C. 1975. Lessons to be learned from the preschool orthographer. In *Foundations of Language Development: Vol. 2*, eds. E. H. Lennenberg and E. Lennenberg. New York: Academic Press.

Read, C. 1986. *Children's Creative Spellings*. London: Routledge and Kegan Paul.

Read, C., and Ruyter, L. 1985. Reading and spelling skills in adults of low literacy. *Remedial and Special Education* 6:43-52.

Reid, E. 1986. Practicing effective instruction: The Exemplary Center for Reading Instruction approach. *Exceptional Children* 52:510-519.

Resnick, L. B. 1979. Theories and prescriptions for early reading. In *Theory and Practice of Early Reading: Vol.2*, eds. L. G. Resnick and P. A. Weaver. Hillsdale, NJ: Lawrence Erlbaum Associates.

Richardson, E., and DiBenedetto, B. 1985. *Decoding Skills* Test. Los Angeles, CA: Western Psychological Services.

Richardson, E., DiBenedetto, B., and Adler, A. 1982. Use of the Decoding Skills Test to study the differences between good and poor readers. In *Advances in Learning and Behavioral Disabilities*, eds. K. D. Gadow and I. Bialer. Greenwich, CT:JAI Press.

Robinson, G. L. W., and Conway, R. N. F. 1990. The effects of Irlen colored lenses on students' specific reading skills and their perception of ability: A 12-month validity study. *Journal of Learning Disabilities* 23:588-96.

Robinson, H. 1972. Visual and auditory modalities related to methods for beginning reading. *Reading Research Quarterly* 8:7-39.

Robinson, H., and Schwartz, L. B. 1973. Visuo-motor skills and reading ability: A longitudinal study. *Developmental Medicine and Child Neurology* 15:281-86.

Rosenshine, B. 1983. Teaching functions in instructional programs. *Elementary School Journal* 83:335-40.

Rosenshine, B., and Stevens, R. 1984. Classroom instruction in reading. In *Handbook of Reading Research*, ed. P. D. Pearson. New York: Longman.

Rosner, J. 1974. Auditory analysis training with prereaders. *The Reading Teacher* 27:379-81.

Rosner, J. 1975a. *Helping Children Overcome Learning Disabilities*. New York: Walker and Company.

Rosner, J. 1975b. Test of auditory analysis skills. In *Helping Children Overcome Learning Difficulties*, New York: Walker and Co.

Rosner, J., and Simon, D. P. 1971. The auditory analysis test: An initial report. *Journal of Learning Disabilities* 4:384-92.

Roswell, F. G., and Chall, J. S. 1963. *Roswell-Chall Auditory Blending Test*. San Diego, CA: Essay Press.

Roswell, F. G., and Chall, J. S. 1992. *Diagnostic Assessment of Reading*. Chicago, Riverside Publishing Co.

Roth, S., and Beck, I. 1984. Research and instructional issues related to the enhancement of children's decoding skills through two microcomputer programs. Paper presented at the Annual Meeting of the American Educational Research Association, April, 1984, New Orleans.

Roy, B. J. 1986. A cooperative teacher education and language retraining program for dyslexics in West Texas. Paper presented at the Action in Research V, Conference, Jan., 1986. Lubbock, TX.

Rubin, H. and Eberhardt, N. C. In press. Facilitating invented spelling through language analysis instruction: An integrated model. *Reading and Writing: An Interdisciplinary Journal*.

Rumelhart, D. E. 1977. Toward an interactive model of reading. In *Attention and Performance VI*, ed. S. Dornic. Hillsdale, NJ: Lawrence Erlbaum Associates.

Rumelhart, D. E. 1980. Schemata: The building blocks of cognition. In *Theoretical Issues in Reading Comprehension*, eds. R. J. Spiro, B. C. Bruce, and W. F. Brewer. Hillsdale, NJ: Lawrence Erlbaum Associates.

Rutter, M. 1978. The prevalence and types of dyslexia. In *Dyslexia: An Appraisal of Current Knowledge*, eds. A. L. Benton and D. Pearl. New York: Oxford University Press.

Rutter, M. and Yule, W. 1975. The concept of specific reading retardation. *Journal of Psychology and Psychiatry* 16:181-97.

Ryan, M. C., Miller, C. E., and Witt, J. C. 1984. A comparison of the use of orthographic structure in word discrimination by learning disabled and normal children. *Journal of Learning Disabilities* 17:38-40.

Samuels, S. J. 1979. The method of repeated readings. *The Reading Teacher* 32:402-8.

Samuels, S. J. 1986. Automaticity and repeated readings. In *Reading Education: Foundations for a Literate America*, eds. J Osborn, P. T. Wilson, and R. C. Anderson. Lexington, MA: D. C. Heath.

Satz, P., Saslow, E., and Henry, R. 1985. The pathological left-handedness syndrome. *Brain and Cognition* 4:27-46.

Sawyer, D. J. 1987. *Test of Awareness of Language Segments*. Austin, TX: PRO-ED.

Schreiber, P. A. 1980. On the acquisition of reading fluency. *Journal of Reading Behavior* 12:177-86.

Seidenberg, M. S., and McClelland, J. L. 1989. A distributed, developmental model of word recognition and naming. *Psychological Review* 96:523-68.

Shanahan, T. 1984. The nature of the reading-writing relationship: An exploratory multivariate analysis. *Journal of Educational Psychology* 76:466-77.

Shanahan, T., and Lomax, R. 1985. An analysis and comparison of theoretical models of the reading-writing relationship. Paper presented at the Annual Meeting of the American Educational Research Association, April, 1985, Chicago.

Shaywitz, B. A. April 1993. Medical symposium of the New York Orton Dyslexia Society Annual Meeting.

Shaywitz, S. E., Escobar, M. D., Shaywitz, B. A., Fletcher, J. M., and Makuch, R. 1992. Evidence that dyslexia may represent the lower tail of a normal distribution of reading disability. *The New England Journal of Medicine* 326:145-50.

Shaywitz, S. E., and Shaywitz, B. A., eds. 1991. Introduction to the special issue on attention deficit disorder. *Journal of Learning Disabilities* 24:68-71.

Shaywitz, S. E., and Shaywitz, B. A., eds. 1992. *Attention Deficit Disorder Comes of Age: Towards the Twenty-First Century*. Austin, TX: PRO-ED.

Shaywitz, S. E., Shaywitz, B. A., Fletcher, J. M., and Escobar, M. D. 1990. Prevalence of reading disability in boys and girls. *Journal of the American Medical Association* 264:998-1002.

Shaywitz, S. E., Shaywitz, B. A., Schnell, C., and Towle, V. R. 1988. Concurrent and predictive validity of the Yale Children's Inventory: An instrument to assess children with attentional deficits and learning disabilities. *Pediatrics* 81:562-71.

Shepherd, M. J. and Uhry, J. K. April, 1993. Phonological awareness training: Case studies of children at-risk for dyslexia. Paper presented at the annual meeting of the American Educational Research Association in Atlanta.

Siegal, L. 1985. Psycholinguistic aspects of reading disabilities. In *Cognitive Development of Atypical Children*, eds. L. S. Siegal and F. J. Morrison. New York: Springer Verlag.

Siegel, L. S. 1989 IQ is irrelevant to the definition of learning disabilities. *Journal of Learning Disabilities* 22:469-78.

Silver, L. A. 1987. The "magic cure": A review of the current controversial approaches for treating learning disabilities. *Journal of Learning Disabilities* 20:498-512.

Silverman, R., Zigmond, N., Zimmerman, J.M., and Vallescorsa, B. 1981. Improving written expression in learning disabled adolescents. *Journal of Learning Disabilities* 16:478-82.

Slavin, R. E., Madden, N. A., Karweit, N. L., Dolan, L., and Wasik, B. A. 1992. *Success for All: A Relentless Approach to Prevention and Early Intervention in Elementary Schools.* Arlington, VA: Educational Research Service.

Slingerland, B. H. 1971. *A Multi-Sensory Approach to Language Arts for Specific Language Disability Children: A Guide for Primary Teachers, Books 1-3.* Cambridge, MA: Educators Publishing Service.

Slingerland, B. H. 1976. *Basics in Scope and Sequence of a Multi-Sensory Approach to Language Arts for SLD Children.* Cambridge, MA: Educators Publishing Service.

Slingerland, B. H. 1993. Supplement to *A Multi-Sensory Approach to Language Arts for Specific Language Disability Children: A Guide for Primary Teachers, Books 1-3.* Cambridge, MA: Educators Publishing Service.

Smiley, S., Oakley, D., Worthern, D., Campione, J., and Brown, A. 1977. Recall of thematically relevant material by adolescent good and poor readers as a function of written versus oral presentation. *Journal of Educational Psychology* 69:381-87.

Smith, F. 1978. *Understanding Reading: A Psycholinguistic Analysis of Reading and Learning to Read.* New York: Holt, Rinehart, and Winston.

Smith, F. 1979. Conflicting approaches to reading research and instruction. In *Theory and Practice of Early Reading: Vol. 2*, eds. L B. Resnick and P. A. Weaver. Hillsdale, NJ.: Lawrence Erlbaum Associates.

Smith, S. D., Kimberling, W. J., and Pennington, B. F. 1991. Screening for multiple genes influencing dyslexia. In *Neuropsychology and Cognition, Vol. 4, Reading Disabilities: Genetic and Neurological Influences*, ed. B. F. Pennington. Dordrecht, Netherlands: Kluwer Academic Publishing.

Snowling, M. J. 1980. The development of grapheme-phoneme correspondences in normal and dyslexic readers. *Journal of Experimental Child Psychology* 29:294-305.

Snowling, M. J. October, 1994. Phonology, dyslexia, and learning to read. Paper presented at NATO Advanced Study Institute in Alvor, Portugal.

Snowling, M., Goulandris, N., and Stackhouse, J. 1994. Phonological constraints on learning to read: Evidence from single case studies of reading difficulty. In *Reading Development and Dyslexia*, eds. C. Hulme and M. Snowling. San Diego: Singular Publishing Group.

Snowling, M. J., and Hulme, C. 1989. A longitudinal case study of developmental phonological dyslexia. *Cognitive Neuropsychology* 6:379-401.

Solan, H. 1990. An appraisal of the Irlen technique of correcting reading disorders using tinted overlays and tinted lenses. *Journal of Learning Disabilities* 23:621-3.

Spache, G. D. 1981. *Diagnostic Reading Scales*. Monterey, CA: CTB/McGraw-Hill.

Spalding, R. B., and Spalding, W.T. 1986. *The Writing Road to Reading*. New York: Quill/William Morrow.

Stanback, M., and Hansen, M. 1980. Integrative review of spelling. In *Integrative Reviews of Research: Vol. 1*. New York: Teachers College, Institute for the Study of Learning Disabilities.

Stanovich, K. E. 1980. Toward an interactive-compensatory model of individual differences in the development of reading fluency. *Reading Research Quarterly* 16:32-71.

Stanovich, K. E. 1981. Relationships between word decoding speed, general name-retrieval ability, and reading progress in first-grade children. *Journal of Educational Psychology* 73:809-15.

Stanovich, K. E. 1984. The interactive-compensatory model of reading: A confluence of developmental, experimental, and educational psychology. *Remedial and Special Education* 5:11-19.

Stanovich, K. E. 1986a. Cognitive processes and the reading problems of learning disabled children: Evaluating the assumption of specificity. In *Psychological and Educational Perspectives on Learning Disabilities*, eds. J.K. Torgesen and B. Y. L. Wong. New York: Academic Press.

Stanovich, K. E. 1986b. Matthew effects in reading: Some consequences of individual differences in the acquisition of literacy. *Reading Research Quarterly* 21:360-407.

Stanovich, K. E. 1988a. The right and wrong places to look for the cognitive locus of reading disability. *Annals of Dyslexia* 38:154-77.

Stanovich, K. E. 1988b. Explaining the differences between the dyslexic and the garden-variety poor reader: The phonological-core variable-difference model. *Journal of Learning Disabilities* 21:590-604.

Stanovich, K. E. 1991. Discrepancy definitions of reading disability: Has intelligence led us astray? *Reading Research Quarterly* 26:7-29.

Stanovich, K. E., Cunningham, A. E., and Cramer, B. 1984. Assessing phonological awareness in kindergarten children: Issues of task comparability. *Journal of Experimental Child Psychology* 38:175-90.

Stanovich, K. E., Cunningham, A. E., and Feeman, D. J., 1984. Intelligence, cognitive skills, and early reading progress. *Reading Research Quarterly* 19:278-303.

Stark, R. E., Bernstein, L. E., Condino, R., Bender, M., Tallal, P., and Catts, H. 1984. Four-year follow-up study of language impaired children. *Annals of Dyslexia* 34: 49-68.

Steeves, K. J. 1987. The use of computers in the education of the dyslexic child. Paper presented at the Fourteenth Annual Conference of the New York Branch of The Orton Dyslexia Society, March, 1987, New York.

Stein, J. F. 1993. Visuospatial perception in disabled readers. In *Visual Processes in Reading and Reading Disabilities*, eds. D. M. Willows, R. S. Kruk, and E. Corcos. Hillsdale, NJ: Lawrence Erlbaum Associates.

Stern, C., and Gould, T. 1965. *Children Discover Reading*. New York: Random House.

Stevenson, J. 1991. Which aspects of processing text mediate genetic effects? In *Neuropsychology and Cognition, Vol. 4, Reading Disabilities: Genetic and Neurological Influences*, ed. B. F. Pennington. Dordrecht, Netherlands: Kluwer Academic Publishing.

Stothard, S. 1994. The nature and treatment of reading comprehension difficulties in children. In *Reading Development and Dyslexia*, eds. C. Hulme and M. Snowling. San Diego, CA: Singular Publishing Group.

Strominger, A. Z., and Bashir, A. S. 1977. Longitudinal study of language-delayed children. Paper presented at the Annual Convention of the American Speech and Hearing Association.

Strother, M. E. 1984. Effects of automaticity training strategies on word recognition. Ph.D. diss., Arizona State University, Tempe, AZ.

Tallal, P. 1980. Language and reading: Some perceptual prerequisites. *Bulletin of The Orton Society* 30:170-78.

Tallal, P., and Stark, R. E. 1982. Perceptual/motor profiles of reading impaired children with or without concomitant oral language deficits. *Annals of Dyslexia* 32:163-76.

Tierney, R. J., and Cunningham, J. W. 1984. Research on teaching reading comprehension. In *Handbook of Reading Research*, ed. P. D. Pearson. New York: Longman.

Torgesen, J. K. 1985. Memory processes in reading disabled children. *Journal of Learning Disabilities* 18:350-57.

Torgesen, J. K. April 1995. Modeling growth in early reading skills: Individual and group differences. Paper presented at the annual meeting of the American Educational Research Association in San Francisco.

Torgesen, J. K., and Bryant, B. R. 1994. *Test of Phonological Awareness*. Austin,TX: PRO-ED

Torgesen, J. K., and Young, K. A. 1984. Priorities for the use of microcomputer with learning disabled children. *Annual Review of Learning Disabilities* 2:143-46.

Traub, N. 1982. Reading, spelling, handwriting: Traub Systematic Holistic Method. *Annals of Dyslexia* 32:135-45.

Traub, N., and Bloom, F. 1975. *Recipe for Reading*. Cambridge, MA: Educators Publishing Service.

Treiman, R. 1985. Onsets and rimes as units of spoken syllables: Evidence from children. *Journal of Experimental Child Psychiatry* 39:161-81.

Treiman, R. 1993. *Beginning to Spell*. Oxford: Oxford University Press.

Treiman, R., and Baron, J. 1983. Individual differences in spelling: The Phoenician-Chinese distinction. *Topics in Learning Disabilities* 3:33-40.

Turner, S., and Dawson, M. 1978. The teaching of reading: A review. *Journal of Learning Disabilities* 11:17-27.

Uhry, J. K. 1989. The effect of spelling instruction on the acquisition of beginning reading strategies. Ed.D. diss., Teachers College, Columbia University, New York. *University Microfilms International* 89:9033917.

Uhry, J. K. 1993a. Predicting reading from print awareness and phonological awareness skills: An early reading screening. *Educational Assessment* 1:349-68.

Uhry, J. K. 1993b. The spelling/reading connection and dyslexia: Can spelling be used to teach the alphabetic strategy? In *Reading Disabilities: Diagnosis and Component Processes*, eds. R. M. Joshi and C. K. Leong. Netherlands: Kluwer Publishers.

Uhry, J. K. October, 1994. Case studies of beginning readers at-risk for dyslexia: A follow-up study. Paper presented at the NATO Advanced Study Institute Cognitive and Linguistic Bases of Reading, Writing, and Spelling, Alvor, Portugal.

Uhry, J. K., and Shepherd, M. J. 1993a. Segmentation/spelling instruction as part of a first grade reading program: Effects on several measures of reading. *Reading Research Quarterly* 28:218-33.

Uhry, J. K. and Shepherd, M. J. 1993b. Writing disorder. In *Child and Adolescent Psychiatry Clinics of North America*, ed. L. B. Silver. 2:209-19.

Vaughn, S., Schumm, J. S., and Gordon, J. 1993. Which motoric condition is most effective for teaching spelling to students with and without learning disabilities? *Journal of Learning Disabilities* 26:191-8.

Vellutino, F. 1978. Toward an understanding of dyslexia: Psychological factors in specific reading disability. In *Dyslexia: An Appraisal of Current Knowledge*, eds. A. L. Benton and D. Pearl. New York: Oxford University Press.

Vellutino, F. R. 1979. *Dyslexia: Theory and Research*. Cambridge, MA: The MIT Press.

Vellutino, F. 1983. Dyslexia; Perceptual deficiency of perceptual inefficiency. In *Orthography, Reading, and Dyslexia*, eds. J. P. Kavanagh and R. L. Venezky. Baltimore: University Park Press.

Vellutino, F. 1987. Dyslexia. *Scientific American* 256(3):34–41.

Vellutino, F., and Scanlon, D. M. 1986. Experimental evidence for the effects of instructional bias on word identification. *Exceptional Children* 53:145–56.

Vellutino, F., Steger, J. A., Kaman, M., and DeSetto, L. 1975. Visual form perception in deficient and normal readers as a function of age and orthographic linguistic familiarity. *Cortex* 11:22–30.

Vellutino, F., Steger, J. A., and Kandel, G. 1972. Reading disability: An investigation of the perceptual deficit hypothesis. *Cortex* 8:106–18.

Vellutino, F., Steger, J. A., and Pruzek, R. 1973. Inter- vs. intrasensory deficit in paired associate learning in poor and normal readers. *Canadian Journal of Behavioral Science* 5:111–23.

Venezky, R. L. 1970. *The Structure of English Orthography*. The Hague, Holland: Moulton.

Venezky, R. L. 1976. Prerequisites for learning to read. In *Cognitive Learning in Children: Theories and Strategies*, eds. R. Levin and V. L. Allen. New York: Academic Press.

Venezky, R. L., and Massaro, D. W. 1979. The role of orthographic regularity in word recognition. In *Theory and Practice of Early Reading: Vol. 1*, eds. L. B. Resnick and P. A. Weaver. Hillsdale, NJ: Lawrence Erlbaum Associates.

Vickery, K. S. Reynolds, V. A., and Cochran, S. W. 1987. Multisensory teaching for reading, spelling, and handwriting, Orton-Gillingham based, in a public school setting. *Annals of Dyslexia* 37:189–202.

Vogel, S. A. 1975. *Syntactic Abilities in Normal and Dyslexic Children*. Baltimore: University Park Press.

Vogel, S. A. 1990. Gender differences in intelligence, language, visual-motor abilities, and academic achievement in students with learning disabilities: A review of the literature. *Journal of Learning Disabilities* 23:44–52.

Vygotsky, L. S. 1978. *Mind in Society*, ed. and trans. M. Cole, V. John-Steiner, S. Scribner, and E. Souberman. Cambridge, MA: Harvard University Press.

Wagner, R. K., Torgesen, J. K., Laughon, P., Simmons, K., and Rashotte, C. A. 1993. Development of young readers' phonological processing abilities. *Journal of Educational Psychology* 85:83–103.

Wallach, M. A., and Wallach, L. 1979. Helping disadvantaged children learn to read by teaching them phoneme identification skills. In *Theory and Practice of Early Reading, Vol. 3*, eds. L. A. Resnick and P. A. Weaver. Hillsdale, NJ: Lawrence Erlbaum Associates.

Warrick, N., and Rubin, H. 1992. Phonological awareness: Normally developing and language delayed children. *Journal of Speech Language Pathology and Audiology* 16:7–16.

Warrick, N., Rubin, H., and Rowe-Walsh, S. 1993. Phoneme awareness in language delayed children: Comparative studies and intervention. *Annals of Dyslexia* 43:153–73.

Wasik, B. A., and Slavin, R. E. 1993. Preventing early reading failure with one-to-one tutoring: A review of five programs. *Reading Research Quarterly* 28:179–200.

Wechsler, D. 1989. *Wechsler Preschool and Primary Scale of Intelligence - Revised*. San Antonio, TX: Psychological Corporation.

Wechsler, D. 1991. *Wechsler Intelligence Scale for Children - III*. San Antonio, TX: Psychological Corporation.

Wechsler, D. 1992. *Wechsler Individual Achievement Test*. San Antonio, TX: Psychological Corporation.

Werner, H., and Strauss, A. A. 1940. Causal factors in low performance. *American Journal of Mental Deficiency* 45: 213–18.

Wiederbolt, J. L., and Bryant, B. R. 1992. *Gray Oral Reading Test - 3*. Austin, TX: PRO-ED.

Williams, J. 1993. Comprehension of students with and without learning disabilities: Identification of narrative themes and idiosyncratic text representations. *Journal of Educational Psychology* 85:631–41.

Williams, J. P. 1975. Training children to copy and discriminate letter like forms. *Journal of Educational Psychology* 67:790-95.

Williams, J. P. 1980. Teaching decoding with an emphasis on phoneme analysis and phoneme blending. *Journal of Educational Psychology* 72:1-15.

Williams, J. P. 1985. The case for explicit decoding instruction. In *Reading Education: Foundations for a Literate America*, eds. J. Osborn, P. T. Wilson, and R. C. Anderson. Lexington, MA: D. C. Heath.

Williams, J. P. 1986a. The role of phonemic analysis in reading. In *Psychological and Educational Perspectives of Learning Disabilities*, eds. J. K. Torgesen and B. Y. L. Wong. New York: Academic Press.

Williams, J. P. 1986b. Teaching children to identify the main idea of expository texts. *Exceptional Children* 53:163-68.

Willows, D. M. and Terepocki, M. 1993. The relation of reversal errors to reading disabilities. In *Visual Processes in Reading and Reading Disabilities*, eds. D. M. Willows, R. S. Kruk, and E. Corcos. Hillsdale, NJ: Lawrence Erlbaum Associates.

Willows, D. M., and Jackson, G. April 1992. Differential diagnosis of reading disability subtypes based on the Boder reading spelling test: Issues of reliability and validity. Paper presented at the annual conference of the American Educational Research Association.

Wilson, B. A. 1988a. *Wilson Reading System Program Overview*. Millbury, MA: Wilson Language Training.

Wilson, B. A. 1988b. *Instructor Manual*. Millbury, MA: Wilson Language Training.

Wilson, B. A. 1988c. *Student Reader Seven*. Millbury, MA: Wilson Language Training.

Wilson, B. A. 1995. Wilson reading system: MSLE research report. Unpublished report from Wilson Language Training, 162 West Main Street, Millbury, MA 01527.

Wise, B. W. April 1995. Orthographic and phonological influences in computerized remedial reading. Paper presented at the annual meeting of the American Educational Research Association in San Francisco.

Wise, B. W., Olson, R. K., Anstett, M., Andrews, L., Terjak, M., Schneider, V., and Kostuch, J. 1989. Implementing a long term computerized remedial reading program with synthetic speech feedback: Hardware, software, and real world issues. *Behavior Research Methods, Instruments, and Computers* 21:173-80.

Wolf, B. J. 1985. The effect of Slingerland instruction on the reading and language of second grade children. Ph.D. diss., Seattle Pacific University, Seattle, WA.

Wolf, M. 1986. Rapid alternate stimulus naming in the developmental dyslexias. *Brain and Language* 27:360-79.

Wolf, M. 1991. Naming speed and reading: The contribution of the cognitive sciences. *Reading Research Quarterly* 26:123-41.

Wolf, M., and Goodglass, H. 1986. Dyslexia, disnomia, and lexical retrieval. *Brain and Language* 28:154-68.

Wolff, D. E., Desberg, P., and Marsh, G. 1985. Analogy strategies for improving word recognition in competent learning disabled readers. *The Reading Teacher* 38:412-16.

Wolff, P. H., Michel, G. F., and Ovrut, M. 1990a. Rate variables and automatized naming in developmental dyslexia. *Brain and Language* 39:556-75.

Wolff, P. H., Michel, G. F., and Ovrut, M. 1990b. The timing of syllable repetitions in developmental dyslexia. *Journal of Speech and Hearing Research* 33:281-89.

Wood, F. B. April 1993. Mrs. Orton's now adult dyslexics. Paper presented at the New York Orton Dyslexia Society's annual meeting in New York City.

Wood, F. B., and Felton, R. H. 1994. Separate linguistic and attentional factors in the development of reading. *Topics in Language Disorders* 14:42-57.

Wood, F., Felton, R., Flowers, L., and Naylor, C. 1991. Neurobehavioral definition of dyslexia. In *The Reading Brain: The Biological Basis of Dyslexia*, eds. D. D. Duane and D. B. Gray. Parkton, MD: York Press.

Woodcock, R. 1987. *Woodcock Reading Mastery Tests - Revised*. Circle Pines, MN: American Guidance.

Woodcock, R., and Mather, N. 1989a. *Woodcock-Johnson Tests of Cognitive Ability*. Allen, TX: DLM.

Woodcock, R., and Mather, N. 1989b. *Woodcock-Johnson Tests of Achievement*. Allen, TX: DLM.

Woods, M. L., and Moe, A. J. 1995. *Analytical Reading Inventory*. Columbus, OH: Merrill.

Wright, D. C., and Wright, J. P. 1980. Handwriting: The effectiveness of copying from moving vs. still models. *Journal of Educational Research* 74-95-8.

Yee, A H. 1966. The generalization controversy on spelling instruction. *Elementary English* 43:154-63.

Yopp, H. K. 1988. The validity and reliability of phonemic awareness tests. *Reading Research Quarterly* 23:159-77.

Ysseldyke, J. E., and Algozzine, B. 1983. Where to begin in diagnosing reading problems. *Topics in Learning and Learning Disabilities* 2:60-9.

Zigmond, N. 1966. Intrasensory and intersensory processes in normal and dyslexic children. Ph.D. diss., Northwestern University, Chicago.

Zigmond, N., and Miller, S. E. 1986. Assessment for instructional planning. *Exceptional Children* 52:501-9.

Resource and Teacher Training Guide

The Orton Dyslexia Society
Chester Building, Suite 382
8600 LaSalle Road
Baltimore, Maryland 21204-6020
(410) 296-0232

> This is an extremely useful resource for parents as well as teachers of dyslexic students. The organization has branches in many areas of the United States, and in Canada and Israel. Often the local branches can provide referrals to tutors trained in multisensory techniques or schools specializing in services for children with dyslexia. Some branches also provide training in multisensory techniques or information about local resources for this.

TEACHER TRAINING CENTERS

ALPHABETIC PHONICS

Centers for Youth and Families – Dyslexia Training Center
Stacey L. Mahurin, Director
118 E. 8th Street
Little Rock, AR 72201
(501) 375-0782

Institute in Multisensory Teaching of Basic Language Skills
Judith Birsh, Director
Box 223, Department of Special Education
Teachers College, Columbia University
525 West 120th Street
New York, NY 10027
(212) 678-3080

James Phillips Williams Memorial Foundation
2133 Office Park Dr.
San Angelo TX 76904
(915) 942-9361

Katheryne B. Payne Education Center
Ann Richardson, Director
3240 W. Britton Rd. Suite 104
Oklahoma City, OK 73120
(405) 755-4205

Katheryne B. Payne Education Center
Ginny Little, Director
P.O. Box 1807
Ardmore, OK 73402
(405) 226-2341

Multisensory Structured Language Training of the University of New Mexico
6344 Buenos Aires N.W.
Albuquerque, NM 76120
(505) 345-8531 ext. 378 or (505) 898-7500

Neuhaus Education Center
Lenox Reed, Director
4433 Bissonnet
Bellaire, TX 77401
(713) 664-7676

Scottish Rite Learning Center of West Texas
Jan Morris, Director of Teacher Training
602 Avenue Q
P.O. Box 10135
Lubbock, TX 79401
(806) 765-9150

Southern Methodist University, Learning Therapy Program
SMU Box 750384
Dallas, TX 75275-0384
(214) 768-7323

Southwest Multisensory Training Center
Beverly Dooley, Director
9550 Forrest Ln., Suite 600
Dallas, TX 75243-5933
(214) 349-7272

Texas Scottish Rite Hospital for Children
Connie Burkhalter, Education Coordinator & Coordinator of
   Teacher Training
2222 Welborn St., Rm. 425
Dallas, TX 75219-3993
(214) 559-7800

ALPHABETIC PHONICS ADAPTATIONS

Edmar Educational Services (MTA training)
Margaret Smith & Edith Hogan, Directors
P.O. Box 2
Forney, TX 75126
(214) 552-1500 or (214) 542-2323

Dyslexia Training Program (Training plus videotapes for classroom use)
Martha Sibley, Dyslexia Coordinator
Texas Scottish Rite Hospital for Children
2222 Welborn St.
Dallas, TX 75219-3993
(214) 559-7800

TSRH Literacy Program (Videotapes for adolescents and adults)
Elizabeth Cantrell, Outreach Director
Texas Scottish Rite Hospital for Children
2222 Welborn St.
Dallas, TX 75219-3993
(214) 559-7800

THE ORTON-GILLINGHAM APPROACH

Reading Disabilities Unit of the Language Disorders Unit
A.C.C. – Room 737
Massachusetts General Hospital
Boston, MA 02114
(617) 726-2764

Carroll School
Baker Bridge Road
Lincoln, MA 01773
(617) 259-8342

Wilson Language Training Corporation
Barbara A. Wilson
162 West Main Street
Millbury, MA 01527-1943
(800) 899-8454

DISTAR AND CORRECTIVE READING

Association for Direct Instruction
P.O. Box 10252
Eugene, OR 97440
(503) 485-1293

WRITING TO READ 2000

International Business Machines
Your local IBM office can be identified by calling (800) 237-4824 or you
can call the national EduQuest office with questions about training at:
(800) 772-2227

AUDITORY DISCRIMINATION IN DEPTH

Lindamood-Bell Learning Processes
416 Higuera Street
San Luis Obispo, CA 93401
(805) 489-2823

PROJECT READ (CALFEE)

Robert Calfee
Calfee Project: Project READ
School of Education
Stanford University
Stanford, CA 94305-3096
(415) 723-8698

PROJECT READ (ENFIELD & GREENE)

The Language Circle
P.O. Box 20631
Bloomington, MN 55420
(612) 884-4880

RECIPE FOR READING

Mrs. Connie Russo
323 Concord Street
Dix Hills, NY 11746
(516) 242-8943

SLINGERLAND

The Slingerland Institute
Clara McCulloch, Director
1 Bellevue Center
411 108th Avenue, N.E.
Bellevue, WA 98004
(206) 453-1190

MATERIALS FOR TESTING AND REMEDIATION

Addresses for publishers (see the keys) for the following materials are included at the end of this section.

Alphabetic Phonics	EPS
Blocks for phoneme segmenting (2 cm colored wooden blocks are listed in Delta's math catalog)	Delta
Case Studies in Teaching Beginning Readers: The Howard Street Tutoring Manual (by Darrell Morris, contains his developmental spelling test)	Fieldstream
The Childs Spelling System: The Rules Sound Spelling (teacher guides and references for older students by Sally and Ralph Childs)	EPS
Clear and Lively Writing (a book of ideas for teaching writing by Priscilla Vail)	Walker
Direct Instruction Reading (a book by Carnine, Silbert, and Kameenui about the methods used in the DISTAR and Corrective Reading programs)	Merrill
Dyslexia Training Program DTP print materials DTP tapes	EPS Scottish Rite Hospital
Insta-Learn materials	Step
J & J Language Readers	Sopris

Lindamood materials
    Auditory Discrimination in Depth   PRO-ED
        ADD is the remedial program
    Lindamood Auditory Conceptualization Test   Riverside
        LAC is the test. Both the test and the
        remedial program were originally
        published by DLM.
    Both materials are available from either
        of these publishers

Merrill Linguistic Readers   Merrill

Multisensory Teaching Approach (MTA)   EPS

Preventing Academic Failure   EPS
    Orton-Gillingham program by Phyllis
    Bertin and Eileen Perlman which can
    be used with the Merrill readers.

Primary Phonics   EPS

Recipe for Reading   EPS

Recipe for Spelling   Walker

Test of Analysis of Language Segments (TALS)   PRO-ED
    by Diane Sawyer

Spellmaster   PRO-ED
    curriculum-based spelling tests

Slingerland   EPS
    testing and remedial materials

Story Box Books   Wright
    a series of picture books (both big books
    and little books) with predictable text
    used in Reading Recovery and in many
    grade K-1 classrooms

Test of Auditory Analysis Skills (Rosner, TAAS)   Walker
    in J. Rosner, *Helping children overcome*
    learning difficulties.

Wilson Reading System   Wilson
    Sound Cards, Word Cards, Student Readers,
    Student Workbooks, Supplemental Readers,
    Instructor Manual. etc.

Winston Grammar Program   Hewitt
      parts-of-speech cards, by Paul Irwin

Words: Integrated Decoding and Spelling   EPS
      Instruction Based on Word Origin and
      Word Structure by Marcia Henry

Writing Skills for the Adolescent   EPS
      by Diana King
      teacher's guide and two workbooks
      for grades 4–adult

ADDRESSES FOR PUBLISHERS LISTED ABOVE

Academic Therapy Publishers   Academic
20 Commercial Blvd.
Novato, CA 94949
(415) 883-3314 or (800) 422-7249

Delta Education, Inc.   Delta
P.O. Box 3000
Nashua, NH 03061
(800) 442-5444

Educators Publishing Service   EPS
31 Smith Place
Cambridge, MA 02138-1000
(800) 225-5750

Fieldstream Publications   Fieldstream
Rt. 7 Box 916
Boone, NC 28607

Hewitt Educational Resources   Hewitt
PO Box 9
Washougal, WA 98671
(800) 348-1750

International Business Machines   IBM
EduQuest (Educational materials K-12)
materials and training at:
(800) 772-2227
or your local IBM office can be identified
by calling (800) 237-4824

Lex Press   Lex
P.O. Box 859
Los Gatos, CA 95031

PRO-ED   PRO-ED
8700 Shoal Creek Blvd.
Austin, TX 78757
(512) 451-3246

Riverside Publishing Company   Riverside
8420 West Bryn Mawr Avenue, Suite 1000
Chicago, Illinois 60631
(312) 693-0040

Sopris West, Inc.   Sopris
1140 Boston Avenue
Longmont, CO 80501
(303) 651-2829

Step, Inc.   Step
P.O. Box 887
Mukilteo, WA 98275-0887
(800) 225-7837

Walker and Company   Walker
435 Hudson Street
New York, NY 10014
(212) 727-8300 or (800) 289-2553

Wilson Reading System   Wilson
Wilson Language Training Corporation
162 West Main Street
Millbury, MA 01527-1943
catalog inquiries at:
(508) 865-5699

Wright Group   Wright
19201 120th Avenue, N.E.
Bothell, WA 98011-9512
(800) 523-2371

Glossary of Terms

Affix — a letter or group of letters attached to the beginning or ending of a base word which changes the meaning of that word.

Allomorph — one of two or more forms of the same morpheme (see defintion of morpheme).

C-V-C — a word composed of letters with the consonant-vowel-consonant pattern. These short vowel words are a common starting point for reading phonetically regular words.

Digraph — two successive letters in the same syllable representing a single speech sound.

   a. Consonant digraph — two successive letters representing a single consonant sound, e.g, *sh*.

   b. Vowel digraph — two successive letters representing a single vowel sound e.g., *oa*.

Dipthong — two adjacent vowels in the same syllable whose sounds blend together. Cox lists four English dipthongs: *ou* as in *out*; *ow* as in *cow*, *oi* as in *oil*, and *oy* as in *boy* (1984, p. 15)

Dysgraphia — severe handwriting disorder due to poor eye-hand coordination.

Etymology — the study of the origins and derivations of words.

Gestalt — a pattern or configuration which constitutes, and is conceived as, a unit or whole.

Grapheme — a single letter or letter cluster representing a single speech sound, e.g., *i, igh* (Cox 1984, p. 17)

Inflectional ending — a morpheme added to the end of a word which changes its meaning in terms of grammatical case, number, gender, or tense, e.g., *ing* in *ending, ed* in *ended*

Laterality — the choice of hand, eye, or foot in performing everyday activities.

Lateralization — dominance of one or the other cerebral hemispheres for any form of brain functioning.

Lexicon — a body of word knowledge, either spoken or written.

Morpheme — a meaningful unit of speech. A morpheme may be a whole word e.g., *child*; a base word, e.g., *child* in *childhood*; a suffix, e.g., *hood* in *childhood*; or a prefix, e.g., *un* in *untie*. A single morpheme may have many forms, as for example, the morpheme for plurality: *s* in *dogs, es* in *foxes, a* in *data*. Each of these forms is an allomorph of the morpheme for plurality.

Morphograph — written form of a word part that has meaning, such as the ending *tion*.

Morphological — in linguistic terms, an adjective referring to meaningful units of speech; a suffix, for example, is a morphological (or inflectional) ending.

Multisensory — involving three or more senses, usually visual, auditory, kinesthetic (awareness of muscle movement), or tactile.

Neuron — a nerve cell.

Onset — the initial portion of a word, spoken or written, which, when segmented, leaves the rime, e.g., *c* in *cat* and *str* in *stretch*.

Orthography — the spelling of written language.

Orthographic — pertaining to the spelling of written language.

Phoneme — an individual sound unit in spoken words. The "smallest unit of speech that distinguishes one utterance from another... in the speech of a particular person or particular dialect..." (Webster's Third Edition).

Phonetic — pertaining to "speech sounds and their relation to graphic or written symbols" (Cox 1984, p. 24).

Phonetics — "The study and sytematic classification of sounds made in spoken utterance..." (Webster's Third Edition).

Phonics — 1. "The science of sound" (Webster's Third Edition). 2. "The central use of letter-sound connections in the teaching of reading and spelling" (Cox 1984, p. 25).

Phonogram — "A symbol or symbols used to represent a single speech sound" (Cox 1984, p. 25).

Phonological — pertaining to the speech sounds in words.

Phonology — the science of speech sounds, including the development of speech sounds in one language or comparison of speech sound development in different languages (Webster's Third Edition).

Prefix — a morpheme (letter or combination of letters) attached to the beginning of a base word which changes the meaning of that word, e.g., *tri* in *tricycle*.

Rime — the vowel and final consonant(s) portion of a word, in contrast with the onset or initial consonant(s), e.g., *at* in *cat*, and *itch* in *switch*. The term is sometimes used to indicate printed words alone and sometimes oral rhyme as well.

Scheme — in psychological terms, a theoretical framework of knowledge. Plural form: schemata.

Schwa — an unaccented vowel whose pronunciation approximates the short /u/ sound, as the first and last *a* in *America* or the *o* in *carrot*.

Suffix — a morpheme (letter or combination of letters) attached to the end of a word which changes the meaning of that word, e.g., *s* in *cats*.

Syntax — sentence structure. "That part of grammar which treats the relation of words, according to established usuage" (Cox 1984, p. 31).

Index